ASCP QUICK COMPENDIUM
OF
MOLECULAR PATHOLOGY

Dedication

I dedicate this book to Sarah, Diana,
and the Davids.

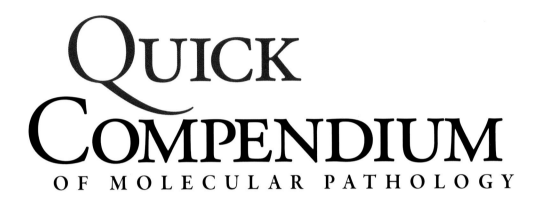

QUICK COMPENDIUM
OF MOLECULAR PATHOLOGY

Daniel D Mais, MD

Medical Director of Hematopathology,
Surgical Pathologist, Department of Pathology
St Joseph's Mercy Hospital and Warde Medical Laboratory
Ann Arbor

Mary Lowery Nordberg, PhD

Director, Molecular Pathology and Cancer Cytogenetics,
Associate Professor of Pathology & Pediatrics,
Feist-Weiller Cancer Center,
Louisiana State University Health Sciences Center
Shreveport

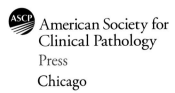 American Society for
Clinical Pathology
Press
Chicago

Publishing Team
Ted Moon and Erik Tanck (design)
Erik Tanck (production)
Joshua Weikersheimer (publishing direction)

Notice
Trade names for equipment and supplies described herein are included as suggestions only. In no way does their inclusion constitute an
endorsement or preference by the American Society for Clinical
Pathology. The ASCP did not test the equipment, supplies, or procedures and therefore urges all readers to read and follow all manufac-
turers' instructions and package insert warnings concerning the proper and safe use of products.

Acknowledgments

My mentor, Dr James L Kelley, taught me to be diagnostician and a doctor. Through his example I saw the way to gain the esteem of clinical colleagues: be prepared, be honest, and, above all, be available. I am grateful to my publisher, Joshua Weikersheimer, who saw the value in this idea and assisted me through to its completion. I am indebted to Dr David F Keren for his teaching and encouragement. I thank Emily for her assistance, friendship, and love.

Preface

A vast quantity of work has contributed to the understanding of disease at the genetic level. A correspondingly expansive body of literature reports this work—we have sought to digest that work into briefly summary statements. The *ASCP Quick Compendium of Molecular Pathology* is not designed to be a definitive textbook of genetics or diagnostic molecular pathology; instead, its purpose is to summarize knowledge relevant to routinely encountered clinical problems.

The book has been organized into sections that reflect the interaction of pathologists with molecular medicine. Several chapters discuss medical diseases with inherited bases about which we are often called upon to guide diagnostic testing. Additional chapters review the molecular basis of and testing for neoplastic diseases. Within each topic, we have included what it is essential to know for both practical and somewhat more esoteric purposes.

Like the other volumes in this *ASCP Quick Compendium* series, our aim has been to provide a distilled and accessible resource for the benefit of pathologists and residents. We hope that this book will serve both as a digestible review and as a useful desktop reference.

— D Mais, MD

Table of

Contents

Chapter 9

Immunologic Disorders, Immunodeficiency, and Autoimmunity

Chapter 13

Inherited Tumor Syndromes

Chapter 14

Solid Tumors

Chapter 15

Neoplastic Hematology

Chapter 1

Molecular Biology and Molecular Assays

The Structure of DNA and Chromosomes

Nucleotides

- Nucleic acids are chains of nucleotides (nucleotide bases). Nucleotides are composed of a nitrogenous base added to a sugar moiety and a phosphate group.

- There are 2 main types of nitrogenous bases: purines (2-ring structures including a hexamer linked to a pentamer) and pyrimidines (single-ring hexamer).

- 5 major nitrogenous bases are found in cells: 2 purines (adenine and guanine) and 3 pyrimidines (thymine, cytosine, and uracil). These are commonly abbreviated as A (adenine), G (guanine), T (thymine), C (cytosine), and U (uracil). The bases found in DNA are A, G, T, and C. In RNA they are A, G, U, and C (thymine is present in DNA but is replaced by uracil in RNA).

- The nitrogenous base, when combined with a sugar moiety, is called a nucleoside. The attached sugar may be ribose (in ribonucleic acid or RNA) or deoxyribose (in deoxyribonucleic acid or DNA). The nucleoside, when added to a phosphate (PO_4) group, is called a nucleotide **T1.1**.

Polynucleotides (Single-Stranded Nucleotide Chains, Single-Stranded DNA or RNA)

- A dinucleotide is 2 nucleotides covalently bonded. This bond forms between the 5'-phosphate of 1 nucleotide and the 3'-hydroxyl of a second, with the formation of a *phosphodiester* bond. A polynucleotide is several nucleotides linked by phosphodiester bonds, with nucleotides being added to the 3' end of the preceding one.

- Note that the formation of these phosphodiester bonds in DNA and RNA exhibits directionality. The primary (linear) structure of polynucleotides proceeds in a 5' to 3' (5'→3') direction. By convention, the primary structure (sequence) of DNA and RNA is written from the 5'→3' direction.

- The 2 ends of a DNA or RNA strand can thus be chemically distinguished as either a free 3' or free 5' end. Importantly, enzymes involved in DNA replication and transcription are capable of distinguishing one end of a nucleic acid from the other. Most such enzymes catalyze the formation of DNA or RNA in only one direction, the 5'→3' direction.

Double-Stranded Nucleotide Chains (Double-Stranded DNA or DNA:RNA Double Strands)

- A nucleotide or polynucleotide is capable of associating noncovalently with a complementary nucleotide or polynucleotide, by the formation of hydrogen bonds. Complementation is as follows: A is complementary to T (or U in the case of RNA), and G is complementary to C. Hydrogen bonding occurs between the constituents of the hexameric rings of the nucleotide bases; thus, protruding outward from the core of the double-stranded DNA molecule are the sugar and phosphate appendages.

- Furthermore, when A associates with T, it does so by the formation of 2 hydrogen bonds. When G associates with C, there are 3 hydrogen bonds. One corollary of this is that double-stranded sequences rich in G and C hold together more stalwartly than (have a higher "melting point" than) sequences rich in A and T. Another is that each 2-ringed purine binds to a

T1.1
Nucleotide Constituents

Base	Nucleoside (base + ribose or deoxyribose)	Nucleotide (base + ribose or deoxyribose + phosphate)
Cytosine (C)	Cytidine	Cytidine monophosphate (CMP)
Uracil (U)	Uridine	Uridine monophosphate (UMP)
Thymine (T)	Thymidine	Thymidine monophosphate (TMP)
Adenine (A)	Adenosine	Adenosine monophosphate (AMP)
Guanine (G)	Guanosine	Guanosine monophosphate (GMP)

1-ringed pyrimidine throughout the length of a DNA double strand, imparting upon the molecule a degree of asymmetry.

- Two adjacent strands of DNA will associate in opposite (antiparallel) directions; that is, 1 strand is oriented 5' to 3' and the other 3' to 5'. The 2 strands will associate strongly (anneal) only if they have highly or entirely complementary sequences in opposite directions.

- As a result of asymmetries in base pairing, longer antiparallel DNA double strands will begin to twist. When viewed 3-dimensionally, long strands of double-stranded DNA appear to have alternating wide and narrow grooves, called the "major" and "minor" grooves. There are several 3-dimensional forms that double-stranded DNA can assume, depending on external conditions. Only 1 of these, the B-form, is common under physiologic conditions. 2 other forms, the Z-form and the A-form, are seen mainly in artificial in vitro conditions. In the B-form, the helix is right-handed, contains 10 base pairs per turn (with each base pair the molecule turns $36°$), with a full turn occurring every 3.4 nm, and contains alternating minor (narrow and deep) and major (wide and deep) grooves.

- Biologically, to replicate or transcribe DNA, the 2 strands must be separated (denatured). In vitro, denaturation is accomplished with heat (thermal denaturation), a sufficient quantity of which can overcome the hydrogen bonds. Again, sequences rich in A-T base pairs will denature at lower temperatures than will sequences rich in G-C base pairs. In thermal denaturation, the point at which 50% of the DNA molecule exists as a single strand is called the "melting" temperature (TM). If allowed to cool, the single-stranded DNA will find complementary DNA and spontaneously associate into double strands (anneal or hybridize).

Nucleic Acid Nomenclature

- A system recommended by the International Union of Pure and Applied Chemistry (IUPAC) for denoting nucleotides and polynucleotides is adhered to with variable tenacity in the remainder of this text and in medical literature. Recommendations for amino acid and polypeptide nomenclature are also listed. Additional guidelines for human gene nomenclature are available from the HUGO Gene Nomenclature Committee (HGNC) International Advisory Committee. All approved human gene symbols can be found in the HGNC database (http://www.gene.ucl.ac.uk/nomenclature/guidelines.html). The IUPAC recommendations are as follows:

  □ DNA and RNA should be used for deoxyribonucleic acid and ribonucleic acid, respectively. The terms "ribonucleoprotein" and "deoxyribonucleoprotein" should not be abbreviated according to the recommendation. Nonetheless, one often sees these species abbreviated RNP and DNP.

  □ Specific functional types of ("fractions" of) RNA and DNA should be denoted as mRNA (messenger RNA, the DNA transcript), tRNA (transfer RNA, the fraction of RNA that transports individual amino acids), rRNA (ribosomal RNA, the RNA structural component of ribosomes), cRNA (complementary RNA, any generic RNA copy), cDNA (complementary DNA, any generic DNA copy), nRNA (nuclear RNA, any RNA within the nucleus), and mtDNA (mitochondrial DNA).

  □ With specific reference to tRNA (transfer RNA), there is a dedicated group of tRNAs for each of the 21 amino acids used in protein synthesis. Each of these can exist in 2 main forms: aminoacylated (amino acid attached) or nonacylated. Aminoacylation refers to the addition of an aminoacyl group to the tRNA molecule, resulting in a tRNA with covalently bound amino acid at the 3' end. Transfer RNAs are designated as follows, using alanine as an example: alanine tRNA or $tRNA^{Ala}$ (for the nonacylated form), alanyl-tRNA or Ala-tRNA, or Ala- $tRNA^{Ala}$ (aminoacylated form).

Chromosomes

- To pack a cell's entire DNA into the nucleus, it must be highly compressed. Chromosomes are the compressed form of DNA, consisting of organized structures of double-stranded DNA and associated proteins (histones).

- Histones (H) are positively charged proteins that are present at regular intervals along the negatively charged DNA helix. They are present as 8-histone complexes, with each complex formed by 2 copies each of H2, H3, H4, and H5. Each histone complex is capable of binding 146 base pairs of DNA; thus, when all DNA is histone-bound, a histone complex may be present roughly every 146 base pairs.

- Whether in mitosis or interphase, the histone complex is capable of wrapping DNA tightly into a supercoiled structure called heterochromatin (appearing in light microscopy as darkly staining portions of the nucleus). Euchromatin (light staining portions of the nucleus) generally is present in variable quantities during interphase and is composed of DNA that is not bound to a histone complex; instead, these segments may only be bound to the monomeric histone protein H1.

- The histone status of a particular segment of DNA exerts some influence on the degree to which it is available for transcription. Furthermore, histone complexes can interfere with attempts to replicate DNA as part of a molecular diagnostic assay; thus, laboratory protocols usually involve a protein digestion step.

- Without histone-induced supercoiling, DNA has a girth of about 2 nm; however, supercoiled histone-associated DNA has a girth of about 1400 nm. When all DNA is supercoiled (eg, in metaphase), the chromosomes are easily visualized with the light microscope.

DNA Replication and Cell Division

The Cell Cycle

- The cell cycle is a process that is guided by a complex set of controls. Broadly speaking, cyclin proteins (cyclins) and cyclin-dependent kinases promote entry of a cell into the cell cycle, whereas several proteins (such as p53) inhibit entry into the cell cycle.

- The cell cycle consists of 4 distinct phases: G1 (gap 1), S (synthesis, in which DNA is replicated), G2 (gap 2), and M (mitosis). Collectively, G1, S, and G2 are called interphase. Entry into the cell cycle is a phrase that refers to a transition from the G1 to the S phase, after which progression through G2 and M is essentially inexorable.

- Cells in G1 have a diploid (2N) quantity of DNA. Cells in late S, G2, and early M have a tetraploid (4N) quantity of DNA.

- Mitosis is the production of 2 genetically identical (assuming all goes well) daughter cells from 1 cell. From the G2 phase of interphase, the cell enters prophase, when the centrioles move to opposite poles of the nucleus, and microtubules begin to assemble, which will ultimately attach the chromosomes (via kinetochores built around the centromeres) to the

centrioles. Prophase is followed by prometaphase, in which the nuclear envelope disappears, and metaphase, in which the chromosomes align along the middle of the nucleus (the metaphase plate). In anaphase the chromosomes are pulled apart, and in telophase the chromatids are located at opposite poles. Lastly, new nuclear envelopes form and the cell divides (cytokinesis).

- Meiosis occurs only in germ cells. It is the process by which 4 nonidentical haploid daughter cells are produced from 1 diploid cell. The overall process consists of meiosis I and meiosis II. DNA replication precedes meiosis, such that the process begins in a cell that has 4N. To better understand this process, it is helpful to recall that at this 4N stage, each chromosome is represented by 4 chromatids, 2 exact copies of the paternal chromosome (paternal homolog) linked together at the centromere and 2 exact copies of the maternal chromosome (maternal homolog) linked together at the centromere. During prophase I, homologous chromosomes become attached to one another via so-called synapses, forming bivalents, each bivalent consisting of 4 chromatids. Furthermore, chiasmata form between the homologs because of the process of crossing-over (genetic recombination) during prophase I. This is followed by prometaphase I and metaphase I, in which the bivalents become aligned at center. In anaphase I, the chromosomes move to opposite poles randomly (a random mixture of paternal and maternal homologs goes to each daughter cell). Furthermore, at the end of this process, each daughter cell is technically haploid (each has 2 chromatid copies of either the maternal or paternal homolog for each chromosome). Meiosis II is very similar to mitosis, resulting in 4 haploid cells.

DNA Replication

- DNA replication commences with the splitting of the double strand into 2 single strands, followed by the creation of a new complementary strand for each. Thus, DNA replication is described as semiconservative (half of the original DNA is preserved in each new double strand).

- Strand splitting is mediated by the enzymes DNA helicase and topoisomerase. It occurs simultaneously at multiple points along the DNA molecule, resulting in several "replication bubbles." At the ends of the bubble, where the split strands converge back into double-stranded DNA, are the "replication forks."

DNA Replication and Cell Division>DNA Replication I Gene Structure, Gene Expression, and Control of Gene Expression>Gene Structure; Transcription

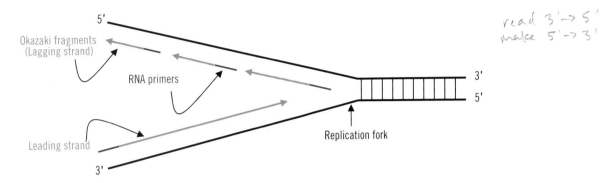

read 3'→5'
make 5'→3'

F1.1 DNA replication

- DNA polymerase binds to the exposed single-stranded DNA and begins to create a complementary sequence for each. Where it sees a C on the template strand, for example, it adds a G to the new strand; where it sees a T it adds an A, and so on. It does so by catalyzing the creation of a phosphodiester bond between the free 3' OH on the growing strand and the 5' phosphate group of an incoming nucleotide. DNA polymerase is capable of adding new bases to a growing strand in only 1 direction: 5'→3'. The template strand is therefore read in the 3'→5' direction.

- Thus, addition of new bases to one of the 2 new strands proceeds towards the replication fork, in the 5'→3' direction, in continuous fashion (the leading strand). On the other new strand replication proceeds away from the replication fork, also in the 5'→3' direction, but in discontinuous fashion (the lagging strand). On this strand, DNA polymerase creates short stretches of DNA (Okazaki fragments) which are later ligated (DNA ligase) to form an intact strand **F1.1**.

- DNA polymerase requires a *primer sequence* to begin replicating. The primer is provided in the form of a short segment of RNA (an RNA primer) laid down by RNA polymerase (which does not require a primer). The RNA primer is later removed and replaced with DNA.

Gene Structure, Gene Expression, and Control of Gene Expression

Gene Structure

- A gene is a segment of DNA that can be *transcribed* into RNA. Most RNA transcripts are subsequently *translated* into protein, but some remains as RNA (noncoding RNA).

- The first portion of a gene, which is typically located the farthest "*upstream*" in the extreme 5' end of the gene, is the promoter sequence.

- Following the promoter is the coding region (the portion of the gene that is actually transcribed into RNA). Most genes contain both *exons* (portions of the coding sequence that are ultimately translated into protein) and *introns* (untranslated sequences). The exon is composed of a specific sequence of nucleotides functionally divided into trinucleotides (codons) that encode a specific amino acid **F1.2**.

- The smallest known human gene, encoding one of the histones, consists of 1 exon (no introns) and around 500 nucleotides. In contrast, the largest known gene, which encodes the protein dystrophin, has 70 exons, 70 introns, and around 2.5 million nucleotides (2500 kilobases).

Transcription *DNA → mRNA*

- Transcription is the production of mRNA from a DNA template.

- The process begins at a sequence of DNA within the promoter region called the *TATA box*. The TATA box is actually a 6-nucleotide TATAAA sequence located 25 nucleotides upstream (minus 25 or -25) from the start of transcription. The TATA box is capable of binding a TATA-binding protein (TBP) which is part of a larger transcription factor complex. The transcription factor complex is capable of binding RNA polymerase.

- Like DNA polymerase, RNA polymerase can elongate a new strand in the 5'→3' direction (thus it reads the template in the opposite or 3'→5' direction). Instead of pairing an A on the template with a T, RNA polymerase pairs A with U.

5

Gene Structure, Gene Expression, and Control of Gene Expression>Transcription; Translation

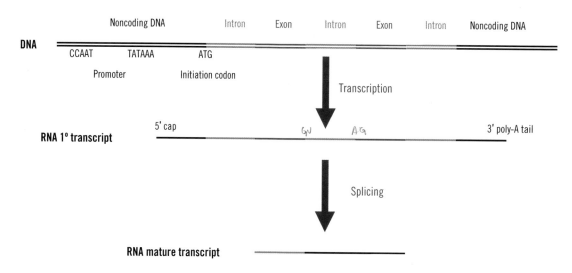

F1.2 Gene structure

- At a certain point, often following the encoding of an AAUAAA sequence, RNA polymerization ceases. A 1° mRNA transcript is thus produced which contains the entire coding sequence, including exons and introns.

- The next step is to reduce the mRNA transcript down to the portions that will be translated into protein—the exons. This is accomplished through a process called *splicing*, in which the intron segments are removed. An RNA-protein complex called the spliceosome is capable of recognizing short RNA sequences (eg, GU and AG) that signal the start and stop of an intron and thus excise it.

- Further modifications to the mRNA transcript follow, including the addition of a 7-methyl guanosine cap to the 5' end (which will function to bind the mRNA to a ribosome) and the addition of a poly-A tail sequence to the 3' end. Finally, the mature mRNA is transported to the cytoplasm for translation. Note that there is a variable quantity of RNA located upstream (5') and downstream (3') from the actual translated portion of the mRNA (ie, that part located between the start and stop codons). These so-called 5' and 3' untranslated regions (5' UTR and 3' UTR) affect the stability (half-life) of the mRNA transcript. In genes that are constitutively expressed, it may be desirable to have more stable transcripts, whereas in genes whose expression a cell would want tight control over, unstable transcripts would be preferable.

Translation mRNA → protein

- Translation is the production of protein from an mRNA template.

- The mRNA strand, by virtue of its 7-methyl guanosine cap, becomes bound to a ribosome. The mRNA strand is passed through the ribosome until a start (initiation) codon is recognized. A codon is a triplet of RNA nucleotides which instructs the ribosome to attach a particular amino acid. Every possible nucleotide triplet has a corresponding amino acid. Because there are more possible triplets than amino acids (only 21 amino acids are used to make protein), several different codons may denote a single amino acid (this is called a degenerate code). For example, any of the following can denote leucine: UUC, UUG, CUU, CUA. A start codon is the triplet AUG, which encodes the amino acid methionine.

- Every amino acid **T1.2** has an amino acid–specific tRNA (transfer RNA). These are small molecules of RNA that have the capacity to bind a specific amino acid as well as a strategically placed trinucleotide sequence (anticodon) that is complementary to the mRNA codon.

- There are Only 3 codons that do not denote an amino acid: UAA, UAG, and UGA. Entry of one of these codons into the ribosome will result in release of the growing polypeptide chain; thus, these are stop (termination) codons.

T1.2
Amino Acid Nomenclature

Amino Acid	Symbol	Abbreviation
Alanine	A	Ala
Cysteine	C	Cys
Aspartate	D	Asp
Glutamate	E	Glu
Phenylalanine	F	Phe
Glycine	G	Gly
Histidine	H	His
Isoleucine	I	Ile
Lysine	K	Lys
Leucine	L	Leu
Methionine	M	Met
Asparagine	N	Asn
Proline	P	Pro
Glutamine	Q	Gln
Arginine	R	Arg
Serine	S	Ser
Threonine	T	Thr
Valine	V	Val
Tryptophan	W	Trp
Tyrosine	Y	Try

- Returning to the start codon, when this trinucleotide is recognized by the ribosome, a methionine-bearing tRNA is brought in. The mRNA strand is then advanced to the next trinucleotide codon and the encoded amino acid–bearing tRNA is brought in next to the methionine **T1.2**. These are then enzymatically connected to one another via peptide bond, and the process repeats until a stop codon is reached.

Control of Gene Expression

- In actuality, only a small portion of the genome encodes proteins, that is, most DNA in the genome is in noncoding (non-gene) segments. Much of this DNA is involved in controlling the expression of genes.

- Selective expression (transcription) of some genes, with simultaneous repression of others, makes it possible to generate various cell types from a single genome. Control of gene expression is exerted through several mechanisms.

- Histones can repressively control gene expression. Most of the DNA in mature cells cannot be transcribed (or is effectively inactivated) because of its tight bundling into nucleoprotein complexes (heterochromatin). Enzymes involved in transcription can more easily gain access to DNA that is unbound from histone complexes—euchromatin.

- Methylation is another repressive genetic control. Most genes are heavily methylated, that is, methyl groups are added to the cytosine residues to produce 5-methyl-cytosine, particularly in the promoter sequence. These regions of the gene contain DNA sequences with a high content of cytosine and guanine (called CpG islands). DNA methylation is catalyzed by DNA methyltransferases. Heavily methylated genes are prevented from transcription, while unmethylated genes can be easily transcribed. The degree of methylation can be assessed by various modalities (see methods section).

- Histones and methylation exert relatively rigid forms of control. They are best suited for genes whose expression is to be switched off for the life of the cell. Dynamic control is desirable for genes that are intermittently expressed. Such control is mediated by promoters, enhancers, silencers, and transcription factors.

  □ Genes are influenced by both cis-acting and trans-acting elements. Cis-acting elements are those that are present on the same DNA strand, usually flanking the coding region of a gene. These include promoters, enhancers, and silencers. Trans-acting elements are encoded elsewhere and usually take the form of DNA-binding proteins (transcription factors). Often, trans-acting proteins recognize and bind to cis-acting elements, thus influencing transcription. Cis-acting elements usually exert control only over the gene they flank, whereas, trans-acting elements may simultaneously influence several genes.

  □ Promoter sequences are found upstream (5') of the gene start codon. RNA polymerases are sensitive to the status of the promoter sequence. Within the promoter sequence

1: Molecular Biology and Molecular Assays

Gene Structure, Gene Expression, and Control of Gene Expression>Control of Gene Expression
Genetic Anomalies: Acquisition>Inherited Defects

usually located at –25 (25 nucleotides upstream from the start of transcription) is a TATAA sequence (the TATA box).

□ Enhancer sequences may be found on either side of a gene, and sometimes are even found in the coding sequence itself. Enhancers bind transcription factors and thereby stimulate transcription of the genes they flank; however, some enhancers are known to influence transcription of entire multigene regions of DNA (locus-activating region).

□ Silencer sequences work in a fashion opposite to that of promoters.

□ Transcription factors are proteins that bind to specific DNA sequences. These proteins contain certain repetitive structural features, also called *motifs*, including so-called zinc fingers.

■ Alternative RNA Splicing

□ A key step in gene expression is mRNA splicing.

□ Some mRNA transcripts can be spliced in various ways, resulting in proteins with variable conformations. Thus, from one gene, several different *isoforms* of a protein can be made, simply by splicing in one or another way.

□ These different isoforms often have different behaviors, being more or less active as enzymes, for example.

Genetic Anomalies: Acquisition

Genetic anomalies come in a multitude of forms, and there are 2 major ways that genetic anomalies are obtained. First, a genetic anomaly may be inherited. Second, a genetic anomaly may be acquired.

Inherited Defects T1.3

■ Inheritance may be Mendelian or non-Mendelian.

■ Mendelian inheritance is generally observed in single-gene disorders that are passed on from parent to offspring. That is, the genetic anomaly is present in the parental DNA and therefore is present in at least some of the gametes (sperm and ova). The child who inherits a defect in this way will express the defect in every cell in his or her body; in such situations, the genetic defect is considered *germline*.

■ Mendelian traits follow a set of principles initially described by Mendel. The law of segregation

(Mendel's first law) holds that alternative versions of genes (alleles) account for variations in inherited traits. For each trait, one allele is inherited from the father and one from the mother. These alleles may be the same (homozygosity) or different (heterozygosity). An allele may be dominant, recessive, or codominant. During gametogenesis, the 2 alleles for each inherited trait segregate. The law of independent assortment (Mendel's second law) holds that individual traits do not affect one another; that is, they are inherited

T1.3
Inheritance of Selected Mendelian Disorders

Autosomal recessive	Phenylketonuria (PKU) and most other inherited metabolic diseases Sickle cell anemia and most other hemoglobin disorders Alpha-1-antitrypsin deficiency Wilson disease Hemochromatosis Cystic fibrosis Infantile polycystic kidney disease Congenital adrenal hyperplasia Spinal muscular atrophy (SMA) Ehlers-Danlos syndrome
X-linked dominant	Hypophosphatemic rickets Incontinentia pigmenti type 1
X-linked recessive	Hemophilia A (factor VIII deficiency) Hemophilia B (factor IX deficiency) Duchenne muscular dystrophy Chronic granulomatous disease Fragile X syndrome Glucose-6-phosphate dehydrogenase deficiency Bruton agammaglobulinemia Lesch-Nyhan syndrome Color blindness Duncan disease (X-linked immunoproliferative disorder) Mencke syndrome.
Autosomal dominant	Huntington disease Peutz-Jegher syndrome Protein C deficiency Osler-Weber-Rendu (hereditary hemorrhagic telangiectasia) Adult polycystic kidney disease Neurofibromatosis 1 & 2 Familial hypercholesterolemia Osteogenesis imperfecta Achondroplasia Familial adenomatous polyposis Myotonic muscular dystrophy Tuberous sclerosis Hereditary spherocytosis Von Willebrand disease Marfan syndrome Ehlers-Danlos syndrome

Genetic Anomalies: Acquisition>Inherited Defects; Acquired Defects; Autosomal Dominant; Autosomal Recessive; X-Linked Recessive

independently. This phenomenon results from genetic recombination (crossing over) in meiosis and is, in fact, not always true. The degree to which 2 traits are independent is proportional to the distance of their genetic loci from one another. Loci found adjacent to one another on a chromosome are less likely to assort independently. For example, the many loci in the HLA (human leukocyte antigen) complex tend to be inherited en bloc.

- Several conditions are inherited in a non-Mendelian pattern. These include multifactorial disorders, disorders affected by genomic imprinting, trinucleotide repeat disorders, mitochondrial disorders, and others.

Acquired Defects

- Acquired defects are those that are not passed from parent to offspring. Generally these represent genetic events that develop after parental gametogenesis: either within the gamete, during embryogenesis, during fetogenesis, or during postnatal life.

- The timing of the defect largely determines how widespread the defect will be felt. For example, mutations acquired at the gamete stage will affect all tissues in the body and behave as *germline* defects. Defects acquired during embryogenesis (*somatic* mutations) may only affect a few cell lines, resulting in mosaicism. Defects acquired later (also considered *somatic* mutations) may affect only 1 cell and its progeny, if any.

- For nearly every known inherited disorder, there are affected patients who do not have affected parents, grandparents, or relatives. Such cases are attributed to new (spontaneous) mutations that arise within gametes or very early in embryogenesis. Such cases are sometimes called *simplex* cases, and such mutations are often transmissible to the next generation (if survival permits). However, genetic diseases having a large proportion of spontaneous cases are generally those that do not permit survival into adulthood.

Autosomal Dominant (AD)

- AD alleles are manifested in those with only 1 copy (manifested in heterozygotes). In fact, for many AD conditions, homozygosity is incompatible with life.

- The degree to which heterozygotes are affected is mitigated by *expressivity* and *penetrance*. Penetrance refers to the proportion of heterozygotes who show manifestations, and expressivity refers to the degree

(severity) of manifestations. Penetrance is expressed as a percentage (if half of all persons with the mutation are affected, then the penetrance is 50%). Furthermore, penetrance is influenced by the age at which the population is surveyed, because many AD diseases are not manifested until late in life. Expressivity has no numerical value, but it is affected by such things as environmental factors and coinherited traits.

- AD disorders are characterized by a family pedigree that shows a *vertical inheritance* pattern, that is, the disorder is passed from generation to generation. Both males and females are affected, and phenotypically normal individuals do not pass the disorder to their offspring. Either parent can transmit to a child of either sex.

- A child with 1 affected parent has a 50% chance of being affected.

- Unlike many autosomal recessive (AR) conditions, AD ones usually permit survival into adulthood (otherwise the allele would cease to exist in the population). Furthermore, unlike AR conditions, AD diseases rarely result from the impaired activity of an enzyme (because 50% activity is adequate for most enzymes). Instead, AD conditions are usually the result of mutations affecting either structural proteins, membrane receptor proteins, or regulatory proteins.

Autosomal Recessive (AR)

- An allele that is manifested only in those with 2 copies (homozygotes).

- AR disorders display what is called *horizontal transmission*, that is, they affect several members in a generation but not the parents (and not the following generation). Both males and females are affected.

- A child of 2 carrier parents has a 25% chance of being affected.

- Consanguinity is commonly involved.

- Recessive disorders, which are mostly enzyme deficiencies, tend to impair the affected individual's ability to reproduce, by causing either death in childhood or infertility.

- In contrast to AD disorders, penetrance and expressivity tend not to vary significantly.

X-Linked Recessive (XLR)

- Alleles that are expressed recessively and whose loci are found on the X chromosome.

Genetic Anomalies: Acquisition>X-Linked Recessive; Structural and Numerical Chromosomal Disorders; Microdeletion Syndromes; Multifactorial Inheritance

- Males are essentially homozygous for all alleles on the X chromosome; thus, an allele that is disease-causing will be manifested (whereas females are heterozygous, except in very rare instances). The heterozygous female is usually asymptomatic; however, subtle abnormalities can sometimes be detected (eg, mild creatine kinase elevations in Duchenne carriers or mild hemolysis in glucose-6-phosphate dehydrogenase [G6PD] carriers). Because of the random nature of X inactivation in females, however, very rare examples have been reported of women with lyonization that is too heavily weighted toward the abnormal allele. Furthermore, women with Turner syndrome may be affected if their sole X chromosome bears an abnormal allele.

- XLR disorders are characterized by a pedigree that has skipped generations, with males affected solely or affected more often than females.

- Daughters of affected males are obligate carriers, and male offspring of affected males are completely spared. Male offspring of carrier moms have a 50% chance of being affected.

- X-linked dominant inheritance is quite rare, as is Y-linked inheritance (because it nearly always causes infertility).

Structural and Numerical Chromosomal Disorders (Chapter 2)

- Chromosomal disorders, such as Down syndrome (trisomy 21), are seldom inherited. Usually, these are the result of sporadic events, but uncommonly a parent harbors a transmissible rearrangement, such as a balanced translocation.

- A chromosomal anomaly should be suspected in a child with mental retardation (especially when accompanied by dysmorphic features), with 2 or more major birth defects, 3 or more minor defects, or 1 major and 2 minor defects.

- A transmissible anomaly should be considered in the differential diagnosis of multiple pregnancy losses or infertility.

Microdeletion (Contiguous Gene) Syndromes (Chapter 2)

- These are disorders caused by the deletion of a portion of a chromosome, sufficiently large to simultaneously affect several genes, but too small to be visualized with conventional cytogenetic preparations. DiGeorge

syndrome T1.4 is the prototypical microdeletion syndrome.

- Microdeletions are usually sporadic events and are not commonly inherited. The clinical features may closely resemble a monogenetic disorder.

Multifactorial Inheritance

- Multifactorial disorders are those that appear to have a real genetic basis (cluster within families, increased risk among siblings of affected persons, high concordance among identical twins) but also appear to be influenced by multiple factors (more than 1 genetic influence, environmental influences, gender influences, etc).

- The rate of recurrence among first-degree relatives generally runs between 2% to 7% for most multifactorial disorders (if parents have had 1 affected child, the risk of another affected child will be around 2% to 7%), and the concordance risk among identical twins runs between 20% and 40%.

T1.4
Selected Non-Mendelian Inherited Disorders

Multifactorial	Cleft lip/palate Diabetes mellitus Hypertrophic pyloric stenosis Congenital heart disease Neural tube defect
Mitochondrial	Kearns-Sayre syndrome Pearson syndrome Progressive external ophthalmoplegia Myoclonic epilepsy with ragged red fibers (MERRF)
Genomic imprinting	Prader-Willi syndrome Angelman syndrome Beckwith-Wiedemann syndrome
Trinucleotide repeat	Fragile X Friedreich ataxia Myotonic muscular dystrophy Spinobulbar muscular atrophy (Kennedy disease) Huntington disease Dentatorubral-pallidoluysian atrophy Spinocerebellar ataxia
Chromosomal instability	Ataxia telangiectasia Bloom syndrome Fanconi anemia Xeroderma pigmentosum Nijmegen syndrome

1: Molecular Biology and Molecular Assays

Genetic Anomalies: Acquisition>Mitochondrial Inheritance; Genomic Imprinting; Trinucleotide Repeat Disorders |
Genetic Anomalies: Types>Mutations

Mitochondrial (Maternal) Inheritance (Chapter 10)

- Mitochondrial inheritance is the pattern in which mutations in mitochondrial DNA (mtDNA) are inherited.

- The clinical manifestations are dominated by expressions of impaired oxidative phosphorylation; thus, the neuromuscular system is largely affected.

- The expressivity is highly variable.

Genomic Imprinting

- The hallmark of disorders affected by genomic imprinting is that the gender of the transmitting parent affects expression. Prader-Willi and Angelman syndromes are prototypes for this pattern of inheritance (chapter 2).

- Genomic imprinting is not in itself a pathologic process. The term refers to a phenomenon that affects certain genetic loci in which the alleles inherited from 1 parent are inactivated in the gamete; thus, there is germline inactivation of either the maternal or paternal alleles.

- Maternal imprinting refers to inactivation of the maternal allele, and paternal imprinting refers to inactivation of the paternal allele.

- Imprinting is generally mediated by hypermethylation.

- Genomic imprinting is an operant mechanism in normal individuals. However, if maternal alleles are normally inactivated at a particular locus and the paternal allele is aberrant, then the result will essentially be homozygosity for the mutant allele. This is the case, for example, in Prader-Willi syndrome.

Trinucleotide Repeat Disorders

- Scattered throughout the normal genome, usually within noncoding regions, are trinucleotide repeats. Trinucleotide repeats are stretches of, for example, GAG or CGG repeats. Generally, these stretches are at the same locus and roughly the same number from person to person. Trinucleotide repeat disorders are caused by expansion of a stretch of trinucleotides.

- As long as the number of trinucleotide repeats at a given locus remains below a certain threshold (the number varies), the locus will generally remain stable from 1 generation to the next. Beyond a certain threshold, the locus becomes unstable, that is, it is likely to progressively enlarge from generation to generation. In this range, the allele is considered "premutation." After further expansion, the allele can become a full mutation, implying that it can adversely affect gene expression.

- The distinctive clinical feature in all trinucleotide repeat disorders is *anticipation*—the tendency of the clinical disorder to worsen or present at an earlier age with each successive generation.

- Interestingly, the tendency of a trinucleotide repeat locus to expand depends to some degree on the parent of origin. In Huntington disease, for example, it has been shown that paternal inheritance is associated with locus expansion, whereas in fragile X, the opposite is true.

- Trinucleotide repeat disorders have also been called "unstable DNA disorders," because they display such lability from generation to generation. This term may cause confusion with the "chromosomal instability/chromosomal breakage" syndromes. These terms refer to a wholly unrelated group of diseases caused by mutations in DNA repair enzymes, leading to observable chromosomal breakage in cytogenetic preparations. Trinucleotide repeat (unstable DNA) disorders, by contrast, usually show no cytogenetic abnormalities, although when quite markedly expanded, the trinucleotide repeat may be visible.

Genetic Anomalies: Types

Mutations

- A mutation is a harmful alteration in the nucleotide sequence of a gene. This should be contrasted with a polymorphism, which is a genetic alteration that (1) is harmless and (2) is present in more than 1% of the population.

- 1 way to classify mutations is based on their effect on the function of the encoded protein. From this perspective, mutations are broadly divided into loss-of-function and gain-of-function types. By far, loss-of-function mutations are more common, implying a mutation resulting in an absent or dysfunctional protein. Less common are the gain-of-function mutations. In this type of mutation, the result is a protein with enhanced function.

1: Molecular Biology and Molecular Assays

Genetic Anomalies: Types>Mutations; Structural or Numerical Chromosomal Anomalies |
Molecular Diagnostic Methods>Cytogenetics

- A common way of classifying mutations is based on their effect upon the transcript. A *missense* mutation results from a nucleotide substitution that alters a codon such that a different amino acid is encoded in the ultimate protein. A *silent* or *conservative* mutation is a nucleotide substitution that alters a codon without changing the encoded amino acid. A nonsense mutation may be a substitution, deletion, or insertion that results in a premature stop codon. mRNA *splice site* mutations corrupt a true mRNA splice site or create a novel one.

- Yet another grouping is based on the nature of the genetic change at the DNA level. A *point* mutation is a single base substitution in the DNA sequence. *Deletions* and *insertions* are the removal or addition of 1 to several nucleotides. If these are in multiples of 3, then while they may cause the gain or loss of several amino acids, they do not alter the reading frame; if not in multiples of 3, they result in a *frameshift* mutation.

Structural or Numerical Chromosomal Anomalies

- These are rarely inherited. Instead, germline cases are usually attributed to dysfunctional meiosis in the process of gametogenesis. Somatic anomalies may arise at any point after fertilization; like somatic mutations, very early changes (in embryogenesis) give rise to mosaicism, while late changes may give rise to neoplasms.

- Chromosomal anomalies can be detected by cytogenetics, fluorescence in situ hybridization (FISH), or (when associated with an abnormal fusion gene) polymerase chain reaction (PCR). Anomalies must be quite large—several megabases (Mb)—or distinct to be visible by cytogenetics. Smaller or more subtle anomalies may require FISH, which can detect anomalies several kilobases (Kb) in size. For example, older studies that used cytogenetics for chronic lymphocytic leukemia (CLL), reported anomalies in a few cases. With more recent FISH studies, however, it appears that CLL has chromosomal anomalies in more than 80% of cases.

- Microdeletions are deletions that affect a large amount of DNA (usually a sequence of several genes) but that are undetectable by routine cytogenetics (see chapter 2).

Molecular Diagnostic Methods

Cytogenetics

- Classic cytogenetics is the manipulation of cells so that their metaphase chromosomes can be visualized.

- Cells are generally obtained from a clinical sample, such as peripheral blood, bone marrow, or tumor, which must be fresh and viable.

- The cells are grown in culture, either resuspended from the specimen and attached directly to the surface of a coverslip (the in-situ method) or in a flask.

- The cells are arrested in metaphase by the addition of an inhibitor of microtubule elongation (colchicine). Prometaphase studies can provide significantly enhanced resolution and may be indicated when subtle chromosomal anomalies are suspected.

- The cells are subjected to a hypotonic solution (to separate the chromosomes), fixed, treated to enhance banding, stained, and then mounted on a slide. Staining methods exploit A-T– and G-C–rich areas to provide staining contrast. The most commonly used staining method uses a Giemsa stain (G banding). Banding patterns are highly reproducible, and the banding pattern of each chromosome is unique.

- With experience, a cytogeneticist can distinguish like-sized normal chromosomes from one another and visually detect subtle chromosomal abnormalities. The normal karyotype has 46 chromosomes (22 pairs of autosomes and 2 sex chromosomes). In a metaphase spread, the chromosomes exist as paired chromatids connected at the centromere. The chromosomes are arranged by the cytogeneticist in order of decreasing length, with the sex chromosomes last **F1.3**.

- When chromosomally abnormal cells are found, the first question is whether the abnormality affects all cells or a subset. If only a subset of cells is involved, particularly if only a single cell is abnormal, then an anomaly that arose in culture (a common artifact) must be distinguished from true mosaicism. This distinction may be easier to make if more cells are studied (in true mosaicism, one expects to find the same abnormality in more than 1 cell).

Molecular Diagnostic Methods>Cytogenetics

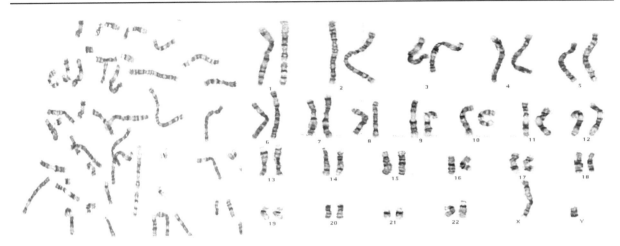

F1.3 Karyotype

- Karyotypes are usually reported using a standard shorthand in the following order: number of chromosomes, sex chromosomes, abnormalities. For example, a normal male karyotype is written 46,XY. A typical case of Down syndrome in a male will be reported as: 47,XY,+21. Other notes on standard shorthand:

  □ The short arm of a chromosome is called p.

  □ The long arm of a chromosome is called q.

  □ Distinct regions of an arm of a chromosome are numbered beginning at the centromere and moving outward; these are then subdivided according to bands within the regions. Thus the location of the cystic fibrosis (*CFTR*) gene, which is on the long arm of chromosome 7, in sub-band 2 of band 1 of region 3, is denoted 7q31.2.

- The normal chromosomes are divided into several chromosome types:

  □ Metacentrics—1, 3,16, 19, 20—have the centromere near the center.

  □ Acrocentrics—13, 14, 15, 21, 22—have the centromere at one end. Their short arm consists of a small knob (satellite) connected to the centromere by a thin stalk.

  □ Submetacentrics—the rest—have centromeres eccentrically located.

- Applications of cytogenetic studies are numerous (list follows). Some laboratories supplement (or replace) classic cytogenetics with FISH (molecular cytogenetics) for greater sensitivity, and there is some overlap in the clinical indications for these 2 studies.

  □ Diagnosis of suspected chromosomal anomalies.

  □ Evaluation of parents for a balanced chromosomal translocation (as the cause for recurrent miscarriages or a child with a chromosomal anomaly).

  □ Diagnosis of fragile X syndrome. While other modalities can be applied to this diagnosis, the so-called fragile site, which is created by a massively expanded trinucleotide repeat, can often be visualized (particularly with prometaphase studies). (Note: Fragile X syndrome is now more commonly diagnosed using molecular genetic approaches.) Molecular genetic determination (by PCR and Southern blot) are considered to be standard of care for the diagnosis of Fragile X. Cytogenetic analysis is useful to rule out any other underlying chromosomal anomaly that may be a cause of developmental delay.

  □ Diagnosis of chromosomal breakage syndromes (eg, Fanconi anemia, Ataxia-telangiectosia, Bloom syndrome). Metaphases in these syndromes often display chromatid breaks, cruciate forms, etc. Sometimes the cell cultures must be performed under special conditions (ie, cultures containing diepoxybutane (DEB) or mitomycin C (MMC)) which provide adequate in vitro stress on the chromosomes to demonstrate fragility/breakage. Chromosome breakage analysis is considered to be diagnostic for many of these conditions as each demonstrates unique structural aberrations under these conditions. For example, Fanconi anemia will characteristically show quadriradial formations and an increased level of chromosome breakage on exposure to DEB. Bloom syndrome shows an increased level of sister chromatid exchanges (SCEs) in cultures performed in the presence of bromodeoxyuridine (BrDU).

□ Evaluation of products of conception (chorionic villi). Around 50% of spontaneous miscarriages are associated with a chromosomally anomalous abortus. Cytogenetic study may provide important information about the cause of fetal loss and provide a foundation for predicting a recurrence risk in future pregnancies.

□ Tumors. Chromosomal anomalies can provide both diagnostic and prognostic information in tumor pathology.

Fluorescence In Situ Hybridization

■ FISH is sometimes called molecular cytogenetics. Because cells in any phase of the cell cycle may be evaluated (metaphase cells not required), this technique has also been referred to as "interphase cytogenetics." FISH can be performed on direct clinical samples—fresh tissue, frozen tissue, cytologic preparations, or formalin-fixed paraffin-embedded tissue—and viable cells are not required. It has certain advantages over other molecular techniques, chief among which is that it permits direct microscopy.

■ FISH uses fluorescence-tagged DNA oligonucleotide probes designed to be complementary to DNA regions of interest. The process has much in common with immunohistochemistry, with steps for paraffin-embedded tissues typically including (1) sectioning and deparaffinization, (2) microwave or heat-induced target retrieval, (3) protein digestion and DNA denaturation, (4) hybridization, and (5) microscopic examination. Because the hybridization step usually requires an overnight incubation, a FISH assay typically requires 2 days; however, results on fresh tissue can be obtained within 2 hours if needed.

■ 3 types of probes are used commonly: locus-specific or gene-specific probes that adhere to a specific target DNA sequence, centromeric probes (identify a particular chromosome by its centromere), and painting probes (identify an entire chromosome). Locus-specific or gene-specific probes are most commonly used, and these must usually be in excess of 30 Kb to provide a visible signal. Centromeric probes,

often called centromere-enumerating probes (CEPs) are well suited for (1) detecting gains or losses or entire chromosomes (trisomies, monosomies, etc) and (2) serving as a control (or denominator) when looking for gene amplification. However, locus-specific or painting probes can also be used for this purpose.

■ Compared with PCR, FISH can more readily identify whether a specific DNA sequence has been duplicated or deleted, particularly in the context of cellular/nuclear architecture which is retained in the process. PCR, by contrast, has traditionally been poor at detecting deletions or duplications; however, quantitative PCR techniques are now demonstrating increased usefulness in these areas. With regard to translocations (rearrangements), the comparison between FISH and PCR is trickier. In general, PCR is an excellent means of detecting translocations that result in fusion genes with highly reproducible breakpoints. However, some fusion genes (notoriously the *BCL1/IGH* fusion gene of mantle cell lymphoma) are highly variable with respect to breakpoints and are better detected with FISH. In these cases, a primer capable of detecting some rearrangements will not detect others; in fact, some rearrangements that can be seen easily with cytogenetics can be missed entirely by PCR. This limitation has been mitigated somewhat through the use of multiple simultaneous primers (multiplex PCR), but in some entities (such as mantle cell lymphoma) multiplex PCR remains far less sensitive than FISH. Thus, FISH is, in some respects, less sensitive than PCR: the alteration in question must be large enough to be detected by FISH (about 30 Kb, the typical size of a FISH probe), and FISH cannot detect small (point) mutations. However, PCR is less sensitive than FISH in other respects: it performs poorly in the detection of rearrangements that form in highly variable ways, and it does poorly in mixed populations of cells.

■ Compared to cytogenetics, FISH is more sensitive to small chromosomal alterations. The limit of detection in conventional cytogenetic studies is an alteration several megabases (Mb) in size; whereas normally formatted FISH assays can detect anomalies of several kilobases (Kb).

■ FISH and loss-of-heterogeneity (LOH) studies have similar sensitivity, but in fact, the 2 studies provide different information. FISH can determine the number of copies of a gene present, but LOH studies can determine how many alleles are present for a gene.

- For detecting translocations by FISH, combination probes are used, which hybridize to the opposite sides of the translocation breakpoints. 2 main strategies are employed: break-apart (segregation) probes and fusion probes. With break-apart probes, the germline form of the gene produces a single signal of one color; a translocation separates the 2 probes, generating 2 signals of different colors. With fusion probe, the opposite is true.

- For detecting aneuploidy, probes for a constant portion of a chromosome (eg, the centromere) can be used. For example, a probe for chromosome 12 can be used to screen for trisomy 12 in chronic lymphocytic leukemia (CLL).

- Like immunohistochemistry, several artifacts can affect FISH interpretation.

  □ Truncation artifact refers simply to the sectioning through of a nucleus such that not all of its chromosomal material is present in the section being evaluated. This can lead to a falsely negative signal or, in the case of a targeted deletion, a false-positive signal. Smears and other cytologic specimens do not have a problem with truncation.

  □ Aneuploidy and polyploidy, if present in the neoplastic cells, can lead to apparent gene duplications. For this reason, duplication analysis is often performed using a centromeric probe as an internal control.

  □ Autofluorescence is similar to endogenous enzymatic activity in immunohistochemistry, and like immunohistochemistry, has morphologically different features than a true-positive signal. In immunohistochemistry, a blocking step is critical, while in FISH, color filters are used to block these signals. Wash conditions before and after hybridization may help eliminate inherent autofluorescence.

- Applications of FISH include many of the applications of classic cytogenetics with the following caveat: FISH can only find what is sought after, and it can (and probably will) miss other anomalies. Thus, if a centromeric probe is used to look for trisomy 12, one can fail to notice that there is loss of 11q, t(9;22) or other anomaly.

  □ **Diagnosis of suspected structural and numerical chromosomal anomalies**. Conventional cytogenetic studies are capable of most abnormalities relevant to prenatal diagnosis and evaluation of products of conception, and they offer the advantage that one does not need to know prospectively what one is looking for. Panels of probes have been developed for use in FISH, for example with probes for chromosomes 13, 18, 21, X, and Y. Such panels are capable of detecting the most common expected disorders. In other settings, the usefulness of classic cytogenetics goes only so far as the anomaly is large (megabase-level resolution). In particular, microdeletion syndromes (see chapter 2) are generally only detectable by FISH. Furthermore, cells must be mitotically active to complete a successful cytogenetic study.

  □ **Tumors.** Panels of probes can be useful to screen for common anomalies in, for example, multiple myeloma. Furthermore, it is a relatively simple thing to look for a tumor-defining anomaly if suspected [eg, t(X;18) in synovial sarcoma]. Lastly, oncogene amplification and deletion of tumor suppressor genes can be detected by FISH. Such chromosomal anomalies can provide both diagnostic and prognostic information in tumor pathology.

  □ **Characterization of a marker chromosome.** Marker chromosomes are extra chromosomes of unknown origin. Using probes for components of known chromosomes, FISH is an effective way to determine the origin of a marker chromosome.

Derivatives of FISH

- Spectral karyotyping imaging (SKI or SKY, also called multicolor fish or MFISH) is an extension of FISH in which 23 sets of different chromosome-specific painting probes of 23 different "colors" (fluorescent spectra) are used as a form of cytogenetic study. Instead of a sequence-specific probe, several chromosome-specific probes are applied that bind to the chromosome at numerous places. SKI actually evolved from whole chromosome paint techniques, in which a cocktail of probes to several genes known to be present on a given chromosome are applied. Thus a "painted" chromosome is produced. More than simply visualize a chromosome, this technique has proven valuable in untangling complex chromosomal rearrangements. However, there are not enough distinct fluorescent "colors" to paint the entire karyotype. Spectral karyotyping uses 5 fluorochromes, extremely sensitive detectors, and software with which all 46 chromosomes can be simultaneously visualized and distinguished from one another, despite having colors that are indistinguishable to the naked eye. It then digitally creates a picture with colors that the human eye can distinguish.

- Comparative genomic hybridization (CGH) is another technique derived from FISH that is used to identify copy number changes in the genome. In CGH, probes of 2 different colors are applied to normal control DNA and tumor DNA (eg, a red probe for the normal control and a green probe for the tumor). Both labeled samples are mixed in a 1:1 ratio (in the presence of repetitive DNA [COT1 DNA]) and are incubated with normal metaphase chromosomes, such that tumor and control DNA compete for hybridization with the normal metaphase chromosomes. The metaphase chromosomes are then examined for fluorescence. Thus, if relatively more green (tumor) signal is hybridized to the chromosomes, this indicates a gain in copy number for the gene of interest; however, if the signal is relatively more green (control), it indicates a loss of copy number. Anomalous hybridization is indicative of alterations in gene copy number in the tumor DNA.

- Tissue microarray (TMA) is an extension of FISH in which multiple tiny tissue fragments are examined simultaneously on a single slide. Typically, hundreds of sections of a lesion of interest, normal tissue, and control tissue are present for evaluation. In the research setting, the FISH probes are often selected based on preceding gene expression profiling (GEP) studies. Array CGH (aCGH) is the marriage of FISH and TMA in the context of additions and deletions of genomic sequences. Clinical laboratories now incorporate aCGH to detect genomic imbalances in patients with developmental delay (grossly normal at the chromosomal level).

- Chromogenic in situ hybridization (CISH) has some advantages over FISH, especially the peristance over time of the chromogenic signal (fluorescent signals fade rapidly). Thus far, major factors limiting CISH are the unavailability of multiple colors and the reduced specificity of the chromogenic probes compared with fluorescent probes.

Polymerase Chain Reaction

- PCR is used to amplify a specific DNA sequence. Amplification may target a sequence known to be present, to further study it, or it may amplify a sequence merely to see if it is present. If the target sequence is present, there will be millions of identical copies of it at the end of a PCR procedure. Thus, if the PCR product is subjected to electrophoresis, the copies will form a single prominent band. Furthermore, the location of this band can be compared to a standard to ensure that it is in the appropriate location.

- PCR amplification begins with primers—sequences complementary to those that flank the genomic DNA target—on which DNA polymerase can begin the work of creating a complementary sequence.

- The sample DNA, primers, and excess nucleotides (A, T, G, and C) are incubated together in the presence of a heat-stable DNA polymerase obtained from the *Thermus aquaticus* bacterium (Taq polymerase) and carried through numerous hot then cold (denaturation, replication, then annealing) cycles so that amplification can take place.

- The reaction products are then available in large quantity for additional study. Most often, they are subjected to electrophoresis on agarose gels and visualized under UV light to determine whether a product has been obtained (confirming the presence, in the original sample, of the target sequence). Alternatively, the reaction products may be sequenced or hybridized with allele-specific oligonucleotide (ASO) or reverse dot blot hybridization.

Derivatives of PCR

- Nested PCR is a highly sensitive qualitative assay, in which an initial amplification product (amplicon) is subjected to a second round of PCR using a new set of primers intrinsic to the first. The major disadvantage of nested PCR is the high rate of contamination that can occur.

- Real-time PCR can produce either qualitative or quantitative results. Also called homogeneous PCR, Q-PCR, or kinetic PCR, real-time PCR refers to methods in which reaction product is detected simultaneously with amplification. These methods require special thermal cyclers with optics capable of monitoring small amounts of fluorescence. The PCR primers are labeled with fluorescent dye, so that the PCR product can be detected and/or quantified.

Molecular Diagnostic Methods>Derivatives of PCR

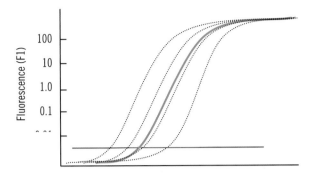

F1.4 Real-time PCR. Dotted lines represent standards (controls) of known quantity. The solid gray line represents signal from the patient sample. The concentration of DNA template is proportional to the crossing point (solid red line) at which signal exceeds background 'noise' and enters the log-linear phase

The quantity of PCR product (amplicon) is directly proportional to the number of target DNA sequences in the sample. This method makes possible the serial measurement of tumor burden (eg, in chronic myelogenous leukemia) or viral load (eg, in hepatitis C virus [HCV] or human immunodeficiency virus [HIV]). Competitive PCR (cPCR) is a broad term that refers to PCR techniques that are quantitative by way of comparison with a known standard. While the quantity of PCR product is theoretically proportional to the starting quantity, there are too many confounding variables for this assessment to be made directly. The basic concept underlying cPCR is the simultaneous amplification, within the same reaction chamber, of 2 targets having similar size. The starting amount of 1 of the templates is known and, after amplification, products from both templates are compared **F1.4**.

- Reverse-transcriptase PCR (RT-PCR) is used when RNA is the target of study. RNA is first converted to complementary DNA (cDNA) using reverse transcriptase. The cDNA can then be subjected to standard PCR. Since RNA is not as stable as DNA, fresh samples are generally required for RT-PCR analysis. Archival formalin-fixed paraffin-embedded material cannot usually be used; however, advances in technology have shown promising results for RNA recovery from paraffin-embedded tissue. Combined RT-PCR and Q-PCR is used for assessment of HIV and HCV viral load.

- Multiplex PCR makes use of 2 or more primers in the same reaction mix. Such a reaction is capable of simultaneously detecting a number of different sequences. This approach must be used, for example, to detect fusion proteins with multiple breakpoints or when looking for multiple mutations within 1 gene (eg, *CFTR* mutations in cystic fibrosis).

- Allele-specific oligonucleotides (ASO) are synthetic oligonucleotides, 15 to 18 bases in length, that are designed to be complementary to and capable of hybridizing with a sample of DNA only if a particular sequence is present. ASOs can be used after amplification to generate dot blots, and is often used in laboratories that offer diagnosis of genetic disease testing (eg, for cystic fibrosis or hereditary hemochromatosis), where relatively high throughput is desired. In such settings, linkage analysis (with Southern blot and restriction fragment length polymorphism [RFLPs]) is often an alternative. PCR is considerably more efficient than linkage analysis because the process is largely automated. However, PCR requires knowledge of the gene sequence so that appropriate primers can be developed, and it helps if there is a single common mutation (or a small number of most common mutations). For example, in hereditary hemochromatosis, most (60%-90%) affected individuals are homozygous for the C282Y mutation, and the remaining cases are the result of compound heterozygosity for C282Y and the H63D mutation. 3 ASO probes may be used in this setting, each about 20 bases in length: 1 for the C282Y allele, 1 for the H63D allele, and 1 for the normal allele. Using a dot blot procedure, these ASO probes are added to a filter paper. The amplified patient DNA is then added to the filter paper **F1.5**.

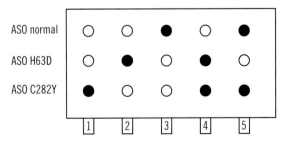

F1.5 Hereditary hemochromatosis dot blot. Patient 1 is homozygous for the C282Y allele. Patient 2 is homozygous for the H63D allele. Patient 3 is homozygous for the normal allele. Patient 4 is a compound heterozygote. Patient 5 is a heterozygote.

Direct Sequence Analysis (DNA Sequencing)

- The traditional way to sequence a segment of DNA is the Sanger (chain termination) method, which is essentially PCR with a clever twist. The ddNTP (2',3'-dideoxynucleotide triphospate) is the key to this reaction; ddNTPs are molecules that differ from deoxynucleotides by having hydrogen attached to the 3' carbon instead of an OH group. This inert hydrogen results in the termination of DNA replication.

- A Sanger reaction is PCR carried out as follows: the target or template strand is added to DNA primer (with a radio-labeled 5' end), DNA polymerase, excess of normal dNTPs (dATP, dCTP, dGTP, and dTTP) and 1 ddNTP (eg, ddATP).

- The reaction is permitted to proceed to completion. What will happen during this process is that complementary DNAs (cDNAs) of several different lengths will be produced. Each time a potential copy happens to incorporate a ddATP instead of a dATP, the elongation of that copy will cease; thus, if enough cDNAs are made, the result is a mixture of cDNAs of varying lengths, each length representing the location of an adenosine residue.

- The reaction is carried out 4 times: one each with ddATP, ddCTP, ddGTP, and ddTTP. At the end of these reactions, the reaction products are added to 4 separate lanes of a polyacrylamide gel and subjected to electrophoresis. The location of the fluorescent bands relative to controls of known length provides the length of every given band. Thus, one can deduce all the positions at which an A, C, G, or T is present in the cDNA. As an oversimplified example, for a theoretical 20 nucleotide segment of DNA, if the lane for the A reaction results in bands migrating to positions of 4, 12, 15, and 18 compared with control segments, it implies that A is present at nucleotides 4, 12, 15, and 18.

Southern Blot Analysis (SBA)

- Southern blotting is a procedure named in honor of its inventor, Edward M. Southern. In it, DNA that has been subjected to electrophoresis in a gel is blotted onto a membrane so that it can be further manipulated and studied.

- The procedure usually involves the following (simplified) steps: (1) DNA is digested with restriction enzymes (2) the digest is subjected to electrophoresis on a gel, (3) the DNA is denatured (eg, with NaOH) to separate double-stranded DNA into single-stranded DNA (double-stranded DNA does not transfer well), (4) DNA is transferred, by blotting, to the membrane (nitrocellulose or nylon, typically), (5) the membrane is subjected to UV light (helps bind the DNA to the membrane), (6) the membrane is probed (hybridized) with labeled (radiolabeled, chemiluminescent, etc) ssDNA sequences, and (7) the membrane is visualized, either with light or as an autoradiograph, depending on the chosen label, to look for the band in question **F1.6**. The transfer step usually involves placing the membrane down flat on the gel and overlaying it with a large quantity of absorbent paper; thus, it is driven by capillary action and can require several hours. This can be expedited by application of a vacuum.

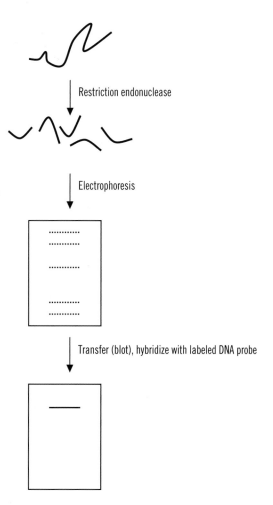

F1.6 Southern blot

- Polymorphisms are DNA sequence variants that are common in the population and generally have no clinical effects. Polymorphisms may be in coding or noncoding sequences.

- Restriction enzymes (restriction endonucleases) are enzymes that cut DNA wherever they recognized a specific sequence—the particular sequence differing from 1 endonuclease to another—called the "restriction site." Generally these are short, palindromic sequences (both strands have identical sequences running in opposite directions).

- If a polymorphism occurs in a restriction site, it will alter the way a segment of DNA is cut; for example, a segment of DNA that is normally cut into 3 segments may be altered such that it is cut into either 2 (longer) or 4 (shorter) segments. Such polymorphisms (that alter restriction sites) are called *restriction fragment length polymorphisms (RFLPs)*.

- In a typical RFLP analysis, 3 restriction enzymes are applied to recovered DNA. The digested fragments are subjected to separation by electrophoresis, blotted, and probes are applied that are complementary to the sequence of interest and capable of exposing X-ray film.

- SBA with RFLP analysis has been useful when the responsible gene is not known or the specific mutation is not known. SBA has been particularly useful in documenting clonality in lymphoid neoplasms. The process of immunoglobulin (Ig) gene and T-cell receptor (TCR) gene rearrangement plays directly into the hands of SBA by providing digestion fragments of distinctly different lengths than the background.

- In the diagnosis of inherited disease, SBA is particularly useful for diseases in which a particular mutation has not been identified or in which there is a large number of possible mutations. In these cases, several family members may need to be tested with the construction of a pedigree. DNA usually obtained from the white blood cells in peripheral blood is digested with restriction enzymes, the resulting fragments separated by electrophoresis, and the gel blotted onto a membrane. Standard controls are processed in parallel for size comparisons. A labeled single-stranded DNA probe is then applied to the Southern blot. Using this procedure, for example, patients can be tested for BRCA1 and BRCA2 mutations, and a test for fragile X (see chapter 2) can differentiate full mutations, premutations, and normal alleles.

Variable Number Tandem Repeats (VNTR)

- Scattered throughout the genome are loci composed of a DNA sequence repeated many times, one after another (tandem repeats), which have largely forensic applications. These loci are usually found in noncoding DNA, and they have no known function. The repeated sequence itself may be 10 to 100 bases in length, but the sequence may be repeated from 5 to 50 times per tandem repeat locus.

- While such loci are usually several hundred bases in length, the precise length varies among individuals; hence they have been called variable number tandem repeats (VNTRs). If several VNTR loci are examined simultaneously, the probability of any 2 people with the exact same pattern is exceedingly small. This process is called DNA fingerprinting.

- For forensic purposes, VNTRs are considered more practical than RFLP analysis. Nonetheless, from a methodologic standpoint, SBA with restriction endonucleases are used to examine VNTRs in a region of DNA that has been amplified by PCR.

- There are 2 main types of VNTR: minisatellites (usually 11-16 bases repeated thousands of times) and microsatellites (1-6 bases repeated 20-50 times). Microsatellites (also called short tandem repeats or STR) can be useful in the molecular pathologic study of tumors (see chapter 14).

Mutation Scanning

- In several genetic conditions, cases can be diagnosed by studying the underlying gene to detect a single mutation (eg, activated protein C resistance), pair of mutations (eg, hereditary hemochromatosis), or limited number of mutations. However, many genetic conditions can be caused by a large number of different mutations within a single gene (eg, cystic fibrosis). In some such cases, there may be a unique mutation for every identified kindred. In such cases, there are 2 major options for genetic diagnosis in a particular patient: direct gene sequencing and mutation scanning. Direct gene sequencing is an option when the gene in question is relatively small and simple or when the vast majority of mutations are confined to 1 or 2 exons; however, mutation scanning may be preferable when mutations are numerous and scattered throughout a large gene.

- Denaturing high-pressure liquid chromatography (DHPLC) and denaturing gradient gel electrophoresis (DGGE)

  □ In this method, PCR is used to simultaneously amplify normal (wild-type) and patient (possible mutant) genes. The PCR products (amplicons) are mixed and heated (so that they undergo denaturation) then cooled (so that they anneal). The result is a mixed population of homoduplexes (normal:normal, patient:patient) plus heteroduplexes (normal:patient). If the patient does indeed have a mutation, then the heteroduplexes will contain some mismatched bases.

  □ If the mixture is subjected to HPLC, 2 separate elution peaks indicate a mutant, while a single elution peak indicates that all of the DNA is identical (no mutation detected).

  □ DGGE is similar to DHPLC.

- Conformation-sensitive gel electrophoresis

  □ This is a mutation scanning modality, somewhat analogous to the foregoing, that looks for mismatched pairing in the patient's DNA.

  □ Appropriate primers are used to amplify the gene region of interest by PCR. The amplified DNA is then treated to induce denaturation and reannealing, then subjected to electrophoresis. The procedure is run in parallel with a normal control.

  □ Several outcomes are possible: (1) in the patient with a normal gene, electrophoresis will result in a single band (normal DNA sequence hybridized to normal DNA sequence, a homoduplex of normal:normal) that is in the same location as the control band, (2) in the patient who is heterozygous for a mutation, electrophoresis will show 4 bands (1 normal:normal homoduplex, 1 abnormal:abnormal homoduplex, and 2 abnormal:normal heteroduplexes), or (3) in the homozygous mutation status, a single band will be found in a different location than the control.

- Single-stranded conformational polymorphism (SSCP)

  □ This is a type of mutation scanning that is based on the differing electrophoretic behaviors of mutated DNA strands, because of a mutation-induced change in the folded conformation.

- Melting point analysis

- In this context, melting point refers to the temperature at which a double-stranded DNA molecule dissociates into 2 strands.

- Melting point analysis has been applied, for example, to detection of *JAK2* mutations in myeloproliferative diseases. The most common JAK2 mutation is the V617F mutation resulting from a G→T substitution.

- In a typical melting curve analysis, a synthetic fluorescence-tagged oligonucleotide probe is added to DNA from the patient, which has been amplified by PCR. When heated to the melting point, the fluorescent probe will elute. If the patient's gene achieves perfect complementation with the probe, the melting point will be high. If a mutation is present that creates less-than-perfect complementation, the melting point is lowered.

- The method is sensitive enough to detect single-nucleotide changes.

DNA Microarrays (Gene Expression Profiling)

- Gene expression profiling (GEP) is a way to look at a particular sample (eg, from a tumor) to simultaneously assess the expression of multiple genes. The tools used to assess gene expression are the DNA (cDNA) microarray and the DNA (oligonucleotide) chip.

- Because this method seeks to determine which genes are being expressed, it must look at what mRNA is present in the sample. A cDNA microarray has a substrate (eg, a glass slide) to which are bound a wide range of cDNA sequences, each designed to be complementary to an mRNA of interest. The immobilized cDNA sequences serve as probes to which mRNA from the sample may hybridize, if present (if the gene is expressed). The mRNA extracted from the sample is first labeled with a fluorescent dye, such that fluorescence at each immobilized cDNA probe is indicative of gene expression. The slide is usually "read" by an automated microarray reader and produces a colored grid.

- At this time, these technologies are primarily a research tool; however, from these studies several genes emerge as highly reproducible for diagnostic or prognostic purposes. Based on such findings, smaller (more practical) chips/slides can be commercially produced. Alternatively, knowledge of these genes can lead to the development of FISH probes for rapid assessment.

Proteomics

- Proteomics is highly analogous to GEP. Instead of using mRNA to signify gene expression, proteomics targets proteins as indicators of gene expression. The protein may be extracted from lesional tissue or from the serum of patients with a known tumor. The tool most widely used in this study is 2-dimensional gel electrophoresis; recently, 2-dimensional electrophoresis has been coupled with mass spectrometry to further characterize electrophoretic isolates.

- Like GEP, proteomic studies are capable of providing a "fingerprint" for each tumor type. Thus, even without knowing the identity of a particular electrophoretic peak (or peaks), 2 tumors can be compared on the basis of their presence or absence.

- Furthermore, if a recurrent peak is found in the serum samples of patients with a particular tumor (that is not found in other sera) it can be further characterized in hopes of discovering a tumor marker.

Loss of Heterozygosity (LOH)

- When a cell has different alleles at a particular locus (mutant recessively expressed allele on 1 chromosome and normal dominant allele on the other), this state of heterozygosity protects the cell from expression of the mutant allele. If, however, the normal allele is altered or lost, it is termed LOH (hemizygosity), which permits dominant expression of the mutant allele.

- This is a common mechanism in tumorigenesis. For example, in the case of LOH when 1 tumor-suppressor gene is mutated, a deletion or second mutation in the normal homolog can lead to tumor initiation. LOH can underlie tumors in both sporadic tumors and hereditary settings; in sporadic tumors, both alleles are normal at conception, while in hereditary tumors, 1 mutant allele is present at conception.

- An LOH study is a method used to detect LOH.

Methylation Assays

- The nucleotide cytosine is capable of undergoing methylation. Significant methylation leads to inactivation of a region of DNA. For example, this mechanism underlies X inactivation in females. On a smaller scale, this is used to suppress gene expression in what has been called "epigenetic genome modification." For example, hypermethylation of mismatch repair genes appears to cause many sporadic cases of microsatellite instability associated colon tumors.

- Certain assays are available for assessing the methylation status of a region of DNA. In 1 such method, DNA is treated with sodium bisulfite, which is capable of converting unmethylated cytosine residues into uracil. The DNA is then subjected to methylation-specific PCR, restriction endonucleases, or other assays capable of distinguishing C from U.

Applications

The methods discussed above can be used in a variety of ways. Often, more than 1 method can be used for the same clinical purpose (eg, *BCR/ABL* in CML may be detected, with various advantages and disadvantages, by conventional cytogenetics, FISH, or PCR). In diagnostic tumor pathology (see chapter 14), molecular methods may be used (1) to support or exclude a diagnosis (eg, when unsure about the diagnosis of synovial sarcoma, mantle cell lymphoma, etc), (2) to provide prognostic information (eg, prognostic FISH panel in multiple myeloma, FISH for Her2 in breast cancer), (3) or as an inherent part of diagnosis and management (*BCR/ABL* in CML). In infectious diseases (see chapter 12), molecular methods may be applied to (1) primary diagnosis (eg, viruses, difficult-to-culture bacteria, mycobacteria), (2) monitoring therapy (HIV, HCV), or (3) detection of antimicrobial resistance. Pharmacogenomics (see chapter 16) is the study of genomic influences on the effect of medication (efficacy, toxicity). It appears that pretreatment genotypic studies may soon become the standard of care in the use of some agents (eg, coumadin). With regard to inherited disease the diagnosis depends on the demonstration of a definitive anomaly at the DNA or protein (enzyme) level. Diagnosis may be pursued in utero (*prenatal diagnosis*), or during postnatal life when symptoms arise (*clinical diagnosis*). In addition, there is a group of disorders in which presymptomatic diagnosis is routinely sought (*neonatal screening*). Lastly, prospective parents may desire to know whether they harbor a recessive allele that can be passed on to offspring (*carrier testing*). These diseases are the subject of multiple chapters in this book, and what follows is a general discussion of the approach to diagnosis. In the discussion of the individual disease entities, any relevant exceptions or peculiarities have been highlighted. Lastly, molecular testing has been applied to HLA typing, primarily in transplantation medicine.

Clinical Diagnosis

- In the realm of inherited disease, this is the most common scenario in which the general pathologist becomes involved. With regard to other forms of inherited disease testing (carrier testing, prenatal diagnosis, neonatal screening), those involved generally do not require our guidance. However, when a single gene disorder is suspected (based either on clinical presentation or a compelling family history) clinicians often desire guidance.

- In many cases, even when the genetic basis for a disease has been fully elucidated, genetic testing is not available. Most often, this is because the test is financially nonviable, perhaps because requests for testing are rare. Testing for a disease that is known to have a genetic basis may not be possible if the responsible gene has not been found. Sometimes the gene has been localized to a particular chromosome segment (the locus is known), but the gene has not been isolated. When a disease-associated locus has been identified, testing can sometimes be developed on the basis of linkage analysis (SBA with RFLP) using several family members for testing. Once a gene is identified, assuming there is a limited number of causative mutations, other modalities may be developed. The gene must first be sequenced so that primers can be synthesized, permitting the application of PCR-based diagnostic modalities. Some conditions, such as cystic fibrosis, have several possible disease-causing mutations. This makes PCR-based testing difficult, and results must be interpreted with caution (a negative test result for the several most-common mutations does not exclude disease). Lastly, even after a test has been developed, it takes time to acquire sensitivity, specificity, and precision data. Thus, genetic testing, while theoretically possible in a large number of conditions, may not be clinically available.

- Furthermore, tests are rapidly changing and it is difficult to keep abreast of their availability. *GeneTests.org* is 1 of the best and most complete resources currently available. This site is continually updated and has, in addition to thorough reviews of many conditions, links to laboratories that offer testing for each condition (either for clinical or research purposes). It is publicly funded (by the National Institutes of Health) and therefore relatively free of commercial bias. Another valuable resource is the site maintained by the Association for Molecular Pathology (amp.org) which has directories for infectious disease, hematopathology, and solid tumor test strategies.

- Some generalizations can be made about testing strategy:

  □ For diseases that are regularly caused by a single known mutation (eg, sickle cell anemia), so-called direct mutation analysis may be applied. Direct mutation analysis refers to such methods as Southern blot analysis with allele-specific probes or PCR-ASO (dot-blot).

  □ In diseases caused by several different mutations in a gene (eg, β-thalassemia and cystic fibrosis), the direct approach may be impractical. However, in some diseases, 2 to 3 different mutations will capture the vast majority of cases, and in these instances direct methods may be used as a first-line test; followed by other methods if needed. For diseases lacking a predominant mutation subset, the situation is more complex. Alternatives include direct sequence analysis, linkage analysis (Southern blot with RFLP of a pedigree), and phenotypic assays (eg, sweat chloride in cystic fibrosis). Such methods are considered forms of indirect mutation analysis.

  □ In diseases caused by gene deletions, failure to amplify the gene by PCR or failure to hybridize the gene (by ASO or dot-blot) is consistent with the presence of the disease (the absence of the gene). This principal is applied to the molecular diagnosis of α-thalassemia, for example, which is often caused by large gene deletions (it is not applicable to most cases of β-thalassemia, however, which is usually caused by a point mutation).

  □ For diseases caused by unknown mutations in a known gene or locus, linkage analysis is usually applicable, provided an "informative marker" can be identified. Linkage analysis can also be used to identify carrier status. The usefulness of a marker (and the specificity of the assay) is limited by meiotic crossing over. When a marker is closely linked to the disease-associated locus, the specificity is better, but it is never 100%. Despite these caveats, linkage analysis provides a diagnosis in many cases in which a specific mutation has not been identified or those with too many possible mutations in a known gene.

Neonatal Screening

- Phenylketonuria (PKU) is an example of an inherited disease that is excellently suited for neonatal screening: easily diagnosed by simple tests, easily treated with dietary restriction, and a profound impact of such treatment. The Guthrie test (bacterial inhibition assay) is a test in which a blood specimen on filter paper is placed on agar plates with a strain of bacteria that requires phenylalanine for growth. The presence of growth is indicated by a halo surrounding the filter paper. If positive, quantitative blood phenylalanine can be measured and/or phenylalanine hydroxylase activity measured.

- Newborn screening programs are usually administered by the state. All states currently require newborn screening for metabolic disorders but the details differ. Currently, all states include screening for PKU and congenital hypothyroidism. Nearly all states require testing for galactosemia and sickle cell disease. Many mandate testing for biotinidase deficiency, homocystinuria, maple syrup urine disease, cystic fibrosis, and/or congenital adrenal hyperplasia. Testing is typically performed by elution of dried blood spots from heel sticks placed on filter paper (Guthrie) cards.

Prenatal Diagnosis

- Samples
  - □ Amniocentesis is usually performed in the second trimester but may be performed as early as 13 to 14 weeks. The procedure is relatively safe but appears to carry a risk of fetal loss that is about 1% over baseline. Chorionic villus sampling (CVS) and amniocentesis can provide essentially the same information—chromosomal status, enzyme levels, and mutation status—but measurement of α-fetoprotein (AFP) levels requires amniocentesis.
  - □ CVS allows prenatal diagnosis in the first trimester. The risk of fetal death is roughly the same as or slightly greater than that of amniocentesis.
  - □ Fetal blood sampling can be performed by percutaneous umbilical blood sampling (PUBS), also called cordocentesis. Fetal blood can be used in hematologic diagnosis as well to evaluate hemolytic disease of the newborn (HDN) or clotting factor deficiencies. PUBS can be performed from about 18 weeks onward. The risk of fetal loss is somewhat high, possibly as high as 3%. For cytogenetic studies, it is necessary to ensure that samples of fetal and not maternal blood are collected.
  - □ Cystic hygromas are often quite large and associated with oligohydramnios; thus, it may occasionally be easier to obtain cystic hygromal fluid than amniotic fluid. Cystic hygromas are most commonly associated with 45X (Turner syndrome), but they are also associated with trisomy 21, trisomy 18, and several mendelian disorders.
  - □ Like cystic hygromas, bladders can become quite large in utero. This is often the result of a congenital genitourinary anomaly (posterior urethral valve) and is, like cystic hygroma, usually associated with oligohydramnios. This makes the urine a more approachable specimen for cytogenetic studies. The danger in this circumstance is the so-called oligohydramnio sequence, a group of anatomic lesions that result from oligohydramnios, most importantly including pulmonary hypoplasia and death. If there is intervention, in the simple form of a vesicoamniotic shunt, these consequences are avoidable. This may not be undertaken without evidence of normal cytogenetics, and urine can provide acceptable cytogenetic studies in more than 95% of cases.
  - □ A fetal skin biopsy may be performed for the prenatal diagnosis of primary skin or systemic disorders. Some have advocated the use of skin biopsies to clarify questions of mosaicism.

- Diagnosis of cytogenetic disorders
  - □ This can be performed using any of the above-described samples The most common indication for prenatal cytogenetic studies is advanced maternal age. The incidence of trisomy 21, trisomy 13, trisomy 18, 47,XXX, and 47,XXY all increase with maternal age. Generally, prenatal diagnosis is offered to all women who will be older than 35 years at the time of delivery (although the most recent recommendation of the American College of Obstetricians and Gynecologists (ACOG) is for use of the integrated screening test instead of maternal age; see chapter 2).
  - □ The risk of a 35-year-old woman bearing a Down syndrome fetus at the time of amniocentesis is 1 in 270; note that the risk is actually somewhat lower for delivering a Down syndrome baby, because these pregnancies have a higher-than-normal fetal mortality rate. The risk for all pregnant women is

about 1 in 800. For women younger than 35 years, the results of prenatal maternal serum screening tests (triple screen or quad screen) are used to guide detection efforts. Women who have given birth to a child with a cytogenetic disorder are at increased risk of having a second affected child—eg, the recurrence risk for trisomy 21 is about 1%. In some cases, 1 of the parents is found to harbor a balanced translocation, imparting a very high risk of affected offspring.

□ Chromosome abnormalities account for approximately half of all spontaneous pregnancy losses, and recurrent spontaneous abortion is 1 possible indication for prenatal cytogenetic studies (or studies on an abortus).

□ Although classic cytogenetic studies may be performed, FISH panels are commonly available for the most likely anomalies, such as aneuploidies of 21, 13, 18, X, and Y.

□ Interpretation of cytogenetic studies performed on CVS or amniotic fluid specimens is associated with some difficulties. First, unless an XY karyotype is obtained, one can never be entirely certain that a normal karyotype is fetal and not maternal in origin. In actual practice, this occurs only rarely, and the risk can be minimized (by examining the CVS specimen for villi under a dissecting scope and by discarding the first several milliliters of amniotic fluid). Another problem is that of chromosomal anomalies that arise spontaneously in culture, mimicking true mosaicism. This is a common artifact that should be suspected whenever an anomaly is found only in 1 cell or clone (pseudo-mosaicism).

■ Diagnosis of Mendelian disorders can usually be performed from 1 of these samples. Sometimes enzymatic assays are used to make these diagnoses (eg, metabolic disorders), sometimes hematologic parameters are used (hemoglobinopathies, clotting factor deficiencies), and at other times a metabolic by-product can be used (eg, 17α-hydroxyprogesterone in the 21-hydroxylase deficiency form of congenital adrenal hyperplasia). Increasingly, direct DNA methods are being applied, especially if the enzyme defect is not manifested in amniotic fluid (eg, phenylketonuria).

T1.5

Autosomal Recessive Diseases with High Incidence Among Ashkenazi Jews

Tay-Sachs disease
Cystic fibrosis
Gaucher disease
Niemann-Pick disease
Canavan disease
Fanconi anemia
Bloom syndrome
Familial dysautonomia

Carrier Testing

■ Carrier testing is intended to identify couples who are at risk of having offspring with a genetic disorder. Carrier testing is usually guided by history (prior offspring, family history, ethnicity).

■ Ashkenazi Jewish couples, for example, are at risk for a set of AR disorders **T1.5**.

■ Couples of Mediterranean and Southeast Asian descent may be offered testing for thalassemia and other hemoglobinopathies.

■ Informed consent must be obtained before testing, and testing results must be conveyed in association with genetic counseling.

HLA Typing

■ HLA type compatibility is essential in transplantation medicine. Both the likelihood of graft failure and the incidence of graft-vs-host disease increase with HLA incompatibility.

■ HLA typing is sometimes important in the diagnostic arena. A growing number of diseases, especially autoimmune diseases (chapter 9), are associated with specific HLA types (alleles). For example, over 90% of patients with ankylosing spondylitis are positive for HLA-B*27. (A note on nomenclature: when speaking of the antigen, it is often written simply as HLA-B27; when speaking of the genotype, the locus is listed first [HLA-B], followed by an asterisk and the allele designation [*27].) Only about 10% of the normal population is positive for HLA-B27. The overall risk of developing ankylosing spondylitis in HLA-B27–positive persons is only about 3%, so the value of HLA-B27 testing is largely its negative predictive value (ie, being HLA-B27–negative makes ankylosing spondylitis unlikely). Like ankylosing spondylitis, narcolepsy is strongly tied to the HLA genotype. Nearly all patients with narcolepsy are positive for the DQB1*0602 allele (the overall incidence of this allele in the general population is about 25%).

- The genes for the human lymphocyte antigens (HLA) are located in a cluster on chromosome 6p, also called the major histocompatibility complex (MHC). Each gene locus within the HLA cluster is highly polymorphous (there exist multiple alleles within the population). For the 6 major loci involved in histocompatibility—HLA-A, HLA-B, HLA-C (class I loci), and HLA-DR, HLA-DQ, HLA-DP (class II loci)—there is a combined total of more than 1000 alleles.

- Traditionally, HLA typing has been based on immunochemical methods or in vitro reactivity assays (similar to red cell crossmatching). Briefly, Southern blot with RFLP was used. Presently, however, PCR is the preferred method for molecular HLA typing. Methods currently in use include ASO probes (dot blot), sequence-specific primer amplification, RFLP of amplified products, and double-strand sequence conformation polymorphism.

Definitions and Nomenclature

Allele

- For any given locus, usually more than 1 possible DNA coding sequence (allele) is present in the population. Such a locus may be a coding sequence (gene) or a noncoding sequence. Usually 1 sequence is associated with a normal phenotype—the wild-type (normal) allele. Other coding sequences may result in a normal phenotype; these alleles, if present in more than 1% of the population, are called polymorphisms. Variant coding sequences that are associated with an abnormality are called mutant alleles.

- Any 1 of a number of coding sequences that are compatible with life can be considered an allele for a given genetic locus.

Allele (gene) frequencies

- For every gene locus there is at least 1 allele. Most gene loci have 2 major alleles. Some gene loci, such as

the hemoglobin beta chain gene, have several alleles, and others, such as some of the HLA loci, have a great many alleles.

- The frequency of all the alleles for a gene can be determined by working backward from the observed phenotypes using the Hardy-Weinberg equation. In this equation p is the frequency of homozygotes for the first allele, pq is the frequency of heterozygotes, and q is the frequency for homozygotes for the second allele. The sum of all the gene frequencies at a locus must equal 1.

$$p^2 + 2pq + q^2 = 1$$

- Pedigrees are commonly used to illustrate a genetic disease within a family. By looking at a pedigree, you can tell how the disease is inherited and make predictions about whether offspring will be affected **F1.7**.

Aneuploidy

- This is the gain or loss of individual entire chromosomes, such that the total number is not an even multiple of 23; eg, a cell with 47,XX,+21 is aneuploid.

- A monosomy is the loss of a complete chromosome. A monosomy leads to aneuploidy.

- A trisomy is the gain of a complete chromosome. A trisomy leads to aneuploidy.

- In contrast, polyploidy refers to excess complements of 23 chromosomes so that the total number is divisible by 23; eg, a cell with 69,XXY is polyploid (triploid).

Anticipation

- The tendency of a disease to manifest more severely or at an earlier age with successive generations.

- Anticipation is a common feature of trinucleotide repeat disorders.

Autosomal

- Chromosomes 1 through 22, numbered in order of decreasing length. The sex chromosomes are called X and Y.

Definitions and Nomenclature

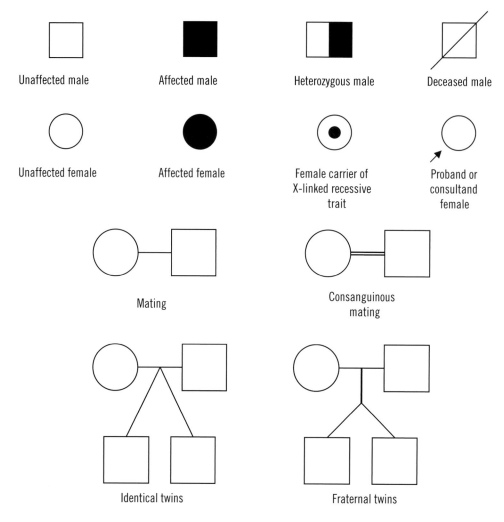

F1.7 Pedigrees

Chromosomal breakage (trinucleotide repeat, chromosomal instability) syndromes

- Most of these disorders are caused by the expansion of a repeated sequence of 3 nucleotides (trinucleotide repeat) in the coding or noncoding sequence of a given gene. These trinucleotide repeat regions are present in the normal gene, polymorphic in length throughout the population, but within a range that is short enough to be stable. When expanded beyond a certain length, they become unstable. Others are due to defective repair of spontaneous chromosomal breakage.

- The diagnosis was traditionally based on demonstration of chromosome breakage (fragility) in culture. A unique feature of trinucleotide repeat expansions is that they tend to expand more with each successive generation; thus, they phenotypically either display greater severity or present at a younger age in offspring (anticipation).

Congenital

- Present from birth. Congenital anomalies are not necessarily inherited.

Definitions and Nomenclature

Contiguous gene syndrome (see chapter 2)

- Syndromes due to deletion of several contiguous genes on a chromosome.

- These deletions are often called "microdeletions," because they are usually too small to be seen on conventional cytogenetic study. Often, FISH is required to identify the abnormality.

Deletion

- The loss of a portion of DNA, ranging in size from a single nucleotide to a portion of a chromosome to an entire chromosome (the latter resulting in monosomy and aneuploidy).

- The term "deletion" implies that the genetic material has not been transferred to another chromosome.

- For example, loss of the long arm of chromosome 7 at band 28 of the long arm is written as 46,XX,del(7)(q28).

- Deletions result from 2 breaks occurring on a single arm, leading to loss of material.

- Derivative

- A derivative (der) is an abnormal chromosome formed from portions of 2 or more chromosomes.

DNA index

- The DNA content of the cell expressed as a multiple of normal (eg, a cell with an unperturbed diploid genome has a DNA index of 1.0). The DNA index is usually determined by flow cytometry.

Dominant negative mutation

- A dominant negative mutation results in a defective gene product that has negative effects on the products of other genes.

- Examples include mutations in platelet glycoproteins. Normally, these are expressed as complexes, eg, the GP Ib/V/IX complex. So a mutation in any 1 member of the complex can affect the expression of the other (nonmutated) members. Another example is the mutation in a collagen chain. Again, because collagen exists as polymers, loss of any member of a polymer will prevent polymerization, thus affecting expression of the other collagen chains.

Duplication

- A duplication (dup) is the presence of an extra segment of DNA (from the same chromosome), usually resulting in redundant copies of a gene or portion of a gene.

First-degree relative

- First-degree relatives include parents, siblings, and offspring. These are individuals with whom one shares essentially half the genetic information.

- In contrast, a second-degree relative shares about a fourth of the genetic information. Examples of second-degree relatives are uncles, aunts, grandparents, grandchildren, nephews, nieces, half-brothers, and half-sisters.

Founder effect

- The predominance of a particular mutation with a population whose gene pool is restricted, because the population is relatively isolated and has descended from just a few individuals.

Genotype

- The genetic constitution of a person or cell.

- Sometimes used to refer to a single gene; that is, the alleles present at a genetic locus.

- Genotyping refers to the assessment of the genotypic status.

- Genotype-phenotype correlation refers to the degree to which an allele alters the clinical phenotype. Genotype-phenotype correlation is considered strong when the phenotype can be reliably predicted from knowledge of the genotype, or vice versa.

Germline

- An allele or anomaly that is present in the DNA of all cells of the body.

- Implies that the allele was present in 1 or both gametes (sperm or egg).

- Insertions

- An insertion (ins) is the incorporation into a chromosome of a portion from the same or a different chromosome.

Definitions and Nomenclature

Inversion

- An inversion (inv) results from 2 breaks within a single chromosome. Instead of loss of the intervening DNA (which would form a deletion), there is reattachment with a reversal (inversion) of the reading frame.

- Inversions may be paracentric (spares centromere) or pericentric (involves centromere), eg, inv(9)(q21q31) is paracentric.

Isochromosome

- An isochromosome (i) is the presence of only short or long arm material on either side of the centromere; eg, a chromosome 12 with only short arm material is i(12p).

Mendelian disorders

- Mendelian disorders are those that result from alterations (mutations) in a single gene and therefore are transmitted in simple (Mendelian) patterns.

Microdeletion/microduplication disorders (contiguous gene syndromes)

- A group of disorders that share a common molecular basis: the loss or gain of a portion of chromosome that is small by cytogenetic standards but large enough to affect multiple genes.

- They can usually be diagnosed by high-resolution cytogenetic studies or FISH. Prader-Willi and Angelman syndromes are diagnosed by parent-of-origin (methylation) studies.

Monosomy

- The loss of a complete chromosome. A monosomy leads to aneuploidy.

Polymorphism

- A genetic alteration that (1) results in no disease and (2) is present in more than 1% of the population.

Polyploidy

- Excess complements of 23 chromosomes so that the total number is divisible by 23, eg, a cell with 69,XXY is polyploid (triploid). A cell or clone may be haploid (1n, 23 chromosomes), diploid (2n, 46 chromosomes), aneuploid (not an even multiple of 23), triploid (3n), or tetraploid (4n). (See also DNA index.)

Ring chromosome

- A ring chromosome (r) results from a break in both arms of a chromosome that are rejoined to form a ring, often with loss (deletion) of some material, eg, r(7)(p12;q34).

- The clinical phenotype can range from near-normal to severe phenotypic anomalies and mental retardation.

Somatic

- Present in only some cells in the body, ie, a genetic alteration that arises after formation of the germline DNA.

Subtelomeric rearrangements

- These are relatively common anomalies that are increasingly thought to be a cause of mental retardation. Subtelomeric rearrangements are found in as many as 10% of children with unexplained moderate to severe mental retardation. Usually these cases are free of overt morphologic abnormalities.

- Regions near the ends of chromosomes (subtelomeric regions) are the frequent site of small deletions and duplications. FISH using telomeric probes can be used to detect these.

Translocation

- Translocations are the physical rearrangement of 2 chromosomes by which material is transferred from 1 to the other. A translocation occurs when there is a break in 2 chromosomes and the material is traded between the chromosomes. Translocations may be inherited from a parent or arise de novo.

- A translocation may be Robertsonian or reciprocal (balanced). A Robertsonian translocation arises when the breaks occur at centromeric regions of 2 acrocentric chromosomes which, when joined, result in the loss of minimal material on the short end of each centromere (the "satellite" material). The loss of this short arm material of acrocentric chromosomes is thought to have no deleterious effect. The new chromosome is composed of the long arms of the 2 fused chromosomes, hence the resulting cell has only 45 chromosomes. Carriers of a Robertsonian translocation are usually phenotypically normal, but their offspring are likely to have effective monosomy or trisomy, resulting in miscarriages and phenotypic abnormalities. A balanced translocation arises whenever there is no net loss of DNA following a translocation. Like the carriers of Robertsonian translocations, carriers of balanced translocations are usually themselves normal, but their offspring are at risk for miscarriages and phenotypic abnormalities.

- Translocations are denoted, for example, as 46, XX, t(9;22)(q34;q11), such that the first location (q34) pertains to the break point on chromosome 9, and the second location(q11) refers to the break point on 22.

Trisomy

- The gain of a complete chromosome. A trisomy leads to aneuploidy.

Uniparental disomy (UPD)

- Both copies of a chromosome, part of a chromosome, or gene come from just 1 parent.
- This arises because of nondisjunction during meiosis such that 1 gamete gets both homologs and the other gamete gets neither.
- The offspring is effectively homozygous for either paternal or maternal alleles.

References

American College of Obstetrics and Gynecology (ACOG) practice bulletin. Screening for fetal chromosomal abnormalities. *Obstet Gynecol* 2007; 109: 217-227.

American College of Obstetrics and Gynecology (ACOG) committee opinion. Prenatal and preconceptional carrier screening for genetic diseases in individuals of Eastern European Jewish descent. *Obstet Gynecol* 2004; 104: 425-428.

Aylward EH, Sparks BF, Field KM, et al. Onset and rate of striatal atrophy in preclinical Huntington disease. *Neurology* 2004; 63: 66-72.

Bagg A, Braziel RM, Arber DA, et al. Immunoglobulin heavy chain gene analysis in lymphomas: a multi-center study demonstrating the heterogeneity of performance of polymerase chain reaction assays. *J Mol Diagn* 2002; 4: 81-89.

Barness LA. An approach to the diagnosis of metabolic diseases. *Fetal Pediatr Pathol* 2004; 23: 3-10.

Beggs AH. Dystrophinopathy, the expanding phenotype: dystrophin abnormalities in X-linked dilated cardiomyopathy. *Circulation* 1997; 95: 2344-2347.

Bennett RL, Steinhaus KA, Uhrich SB, et al. Recommendations for standardized human pedigree nomenclature: Pedigree Standardization Task Force of the National Society of Genetic Counselors. *Am J Hum Genet* 1995; 56: 745-752.

Bernard PS, Wittwer CT. Real-time PCR technology for cancer diagnostics. *Clin Chem* 2002; 48:1178-1185.

Canu A, Abbas A, Malbruny B, et al. Denaturing high-performance liquid chromatography detection of ribosomal mutations conferring macrolide resistance in gram-positive cocci. *Antimicrob Agents Chemother* 2004; 48: 297-304.

Cao A, Saba L, Galanello R, et al. Molecular diagnosis and carrier screening for beta thalassemia. *JAMA* 1997; 278: 1273-1277.

Debelenko LV, Brambilla E, Agarwal SK, et al. Identification of MEN1 gene mutations in sporadic carcinoid tumors of the lung. *Hum Mol Genet* 1997; 6(13): 2285-2290.

References

Diaz-Cano SJ, Blanes A, Wolfe HJ. PCR techniques for clonality assays. *Diagn Mol Pathol* 2001; 10: 24-33.

DiMauro S, Schon EA. Mitochondrial DNA mutations in human disease. *Am J Med Genet* 2001; 106: 18-26.

Donnenfeld AE, Lamb AN. Cytogenetics and molecular cytogenetics in prenatal diagnosis. *Clin Lab Med* 2003; 23: 457-480.

Einerson RR, Kurtin PJ, Dayharsh GA, et al. FISH is superior to PCR in detecting t(14;18)(q32;q21)-IgH/bcl-2 in follicular lymphoma using paraffin-embedded tissue samples. *Am J Clin Pathol* 2005; 124: 421-429.

Emmert-Buck MR, Lubensky IA, Dong Q, et al. Localization of the multiple endocrine neoplasia type I (MEN1) gene based on tumor deletion mapping. *Cancer Res* 1997; 57: 1855-1858.

Emmert-Buck MR, Vocke CD, Pozzatti RO, et al. Allelic loss on chromosome 8p12-21 in microdissected prostatic intraepithelial neoplasia. *Cancer Res* 1995; 55: 2959-2962.

Falls JG, Pulford DJ, Wylie AA, Jirtle RL. Genomic imprinting: implications for human disease. *Am J Pathol* 1999; 154: 635-646.

Gerlach JA. Human lymphocyte antigen molecular typing. *Arch Pathol Lab Med* 2002; 126: 281-284.

Gozzetti A, Crupi R, Tozzuoli D. The use of fluorescence in situ hybridization (FISH) in chronic lymphocytic leukemia (CLL). *Hematology* 2004; 9: 11-15.

Grady WM. Genetic testing for high-risk colon cancer patients. *Gastroenterology* 2003; 124: 1574-1594.

Hanna WM, Kwok K. Chromogenic in-situ hybridization: a viable alternative to fluorescence in-situ hybridization in the HER2 testing algorithm. *Mod Pathol* 2006; 19: 481-487.

Harper PS, Clarke A. Should we test children for "adult" genetic diseases? *Lancet* 1990; 335: 1205-1206.

Herrington CS. In situ hybridization. *J Clin Pathol: Mol Pathol* 1998; 51: 8-13.

Irons M. Use of subtelomeric fluorescence in situ hybridization in cytogenetic diagnosis. *Curr Opin Pediatr* 2003; 15: 594-597.

Jeuken JW, Sprenger SH, Wesseling P. Comparative genomic hybridization: practical guidelines. *Diagn Mol Pathol* 2002; 11: 193-203.

Joyce JA, Schofield PN. Genomic imprinting and cancer. *J Clin Pathol: Mol Pathol* 1998; 51: 185-190.

Keller G, Hartmann A, Mueller J, Höfler H. Denaturing high pressure liquid chromatography (DHPLC) for the analysis of somatic p53 mutations. *Lab Invest* 2001; 81: 1735-1737.

Kricka LJ. Nucleic acid detection technologies: labels, strategies, and formats. *Clin Chem* 1999; 45: 453-458.

Kuerer HM, Goldknopf IL, Fritsche H, et al. Identification of distinct protein expression patterns in bilateral matched pair breast ductal fluid specimens from women with unilateral invasive breast carcinoma: high-throughput biomarker discovery. *Cancer* 2002; 95: 2276-2282.

Lai P, Salazar PA, Hudis CA, et al. HER-2 testing in breast cancer using immunohistochemical analysis and fluorescence in situ hybridization: a single-institution experience of 2279 cases and comparison of dual-color and single-color scoring. *Am J Clin Pathol* 2004; 121: 631-636.

Lazar A, Abruzzo LV, Pollock RE, et al. Molecular diagnosis of sarcomas: chromosomal translocations in sarcomas. *Arch Pathol Lab Med* 2006; 130: 1199-1207.

Liotta L, Kohn EC, Petricoin EF. Clinical proteomics: personalized molecular medicine. *JAMA* 2001; 286: 2211-2214.

Lynch HT, de la Chapelle A. Hereditary colorectal cancer. *N Engl J Med* 2003; 348: 919-932.

Medeiros LJ, Carr J. Overview of the role of molecular methods in the diagnosis of malignant lymphomas. *Arch Pathol Lab Med* 1999; 123: 1189-1207.

Min T. FISH techniques. *Methods Mol Biol* 2003; 220: 193-212.

References

Min T, Swansbury J. Cytogenetic studies using FISH: background. *Methods Mol Biol* 2003; 220: 173-179.

Moss GP. *IUPAC-IUB Commission on Biochemical Nomenclature (CBN). Abbreviations and Symbols for Nucleic Acids, Polynucleotides and their Constituents Recommendations.* Available at: http://www.chem.qmul.ac.uk/iupac/misc/naabb.html. Accessed September 6, 2007.

Netto GJ, Saad RD. Diagnostic molecular pathology: an increasingly indispensable tool for the practicing pathologist. *Arch Pathol Lab Med* 2006; 130: 1339-1348.

Pusztai L, Ayers M, Stec J, Hortobagyi GN. Clinical application of cDNA microarrays in oncology. *Oncologist* 2003; 8: 252-258.

Tai A, Mak W, Ng P, et al. High-throughput loss-of-heterozygosity study of chromosome 3p in lung cancer using single-nucleotide polymorphism markers. *Cancer Res* 2006; 66: 4133-4138.

Tantravahi U, Wheeler P. Molecular genetic testing for prenatal diagnosis. *Clin Lab Med* 2003; 23: 481-502.

Taylor AM, Byrd PJ. Molecular pathology of ataxia telangiectasia. *J Clin Pathol* 2005; 58: 1009-1015.

Teixeira MR. Combined classical and molecular cytogenetic analysis of cancer. *Eur J Cancer* 2002; 38: 1580-1584.

Vallance H, Ford J. Carrier testing for autosomal-recessive disorders. *Crit Rev Clin Lab Sci* 2003; 40: 473-497.

Van der Heiden IP, van der Werf M, Lindemans J, van Schaik RHN. Sequencing: not always the "gold standard". *Clin Chem* 2004; 50: 248-249.

Waters JJ, Barlow AL, Gould CP. FISH. *J Clin Pathol: Mol Pathol* 1998; 51: 62-70.

Weiss MM, Hermsen M, Meijer GA, et al. Comparative genomic hybridization. *J Clin Pathol: Mol Pathol* 1999; 52: 243-251.

Williams TM. Human leukocyte antigen gene polymorphism and the histocompatibility laboratory. *J Mol Diag* 2001; 3: 98-104.

Chapter 2

Chromosomal and Microdeletion Disorders

Numerical Disorders T2.2

Spontaneous Abortus

- Cytogenetic studies identify chromosomal anomalies in about 50% of cases of spontaneous abortus or spontaneous miscarriage specimens, whereas only about 0.5% of live born infants have them T2.1.

- The most common abnormalities to be found in a spontaneous abortus are monosomy X (45, X), triploidy (eg, 69, XXY), and trisomy 16 (eg, 47, XX + 16). Among live births, trisomy 21 is the most common finding.

Down Syndrome (Trisomy 21)

- The karyotype in more than 95% of individuals with Down syndrome has trisomy 21, about 4% have unbalanced translocations (which is important because it indicates that 1 of the parents harbors a translocation that can be passed to additional offspring), and most of the remaining 1% are mosaics.

- The extra chromosome 21 in most cases is maternally derived, resulting from meiotic nondisjunction in a karyotypically normal female. Both parents of such children have a normal karyotype and are normal in all respects. In 4% to 5% of cases, the extra chromosome 21 material derives from a Robertsonian translocation in 1 of the parents, usually the mother. Most often, the translocation is between 21 and another acrocentric chromosome (eg, 22 or 14). The parent in this case is usually phenotypically normal, but cytogenetic study will reveal the abnormal karyotype. In such cases, there is a theoretical 1 in 3 chance of an affected child; in fact, the incidence is much lower, probably because of the decreased viability of such fetuses.

- About 1% of patients with Down syndrome are mosaics; that is, they have some cells with a normal karyotype and others with trisomy 21. This results from *mitotic* nondisjunction at some point in embryogenesis and has no relation to maternal age. The manifestations depend on the particular distribution of affected cell lines. Symptoms in such cases are variable and milder, depending on the proportion of abnormal cells.

- Down syndrome affects about 1 in 800 newborns. The incidence increases with maternal age: in mothers younger than 20 years of age, the incidence is about 1 in 2000, while in mothers older than 45 years, the incidence is 1 in 25. Because most births occur to young women, however, more than 80% of infants with Down syndrome are born to mothers younger than 35 years.

- In the neonate, the cardinal features are hypotonia, hyperflexibility, excess skin on the back of the neck, flat facial profile, slanted (oblique) palpebral fissures, epicanthal folds, abnormal auricles, cardiac anomalies (especially of the endocardial cushion—ostium primum atrial septal defect, atrioventricular valve malformations, ventricular septal defect), and a single transverse palmar (simian) crease. A significant minority of affected infants have an intestinal atresia and/or Hirschsprung disease. Over time, additional features may manifest, including mental retardation, hearing loss, autoimmune thyroid disease, immunodeficiency, atlantoaxial instability, and leukemia (especially transient myeloproliferative disorder; see chapter 15). Virtually everyone with trisomy 21 who survives past 40 years will develop the neuropathologic findings of Alzheimer disease.

T2.1
Cytogenetics: Spontaneous Abortions vs Live Births

	Spontaneous Abortions	Live Births
Incidence of anomalies	50% (1st trimester)	1 in 200
Most common anomaly	Trisomy 16 (1st trimester) Monosomy X (all trimesters)	Trisomy 21
Additional notes	95% numerical 5% structural Trisomy 16 most common autosomal trisomy 20% are 45, X 15% are triploid (molar)	60% numerical 40% structural abnormalities 1 in 5000 have 45, X

Numerical Disorders>Down Syndrome

- Prenatal screening for Down syndrome (and other aneuploidies)

  □ Currently, the most effective screening is provided by a combination of 3 categories of tests: (1) maternal age, (2) serum biochemical markers, and (3) ultrasonography. Sensitivity and specificity are maximized through the combined use of all 3 modalities, which has been called the *integrated screen*. However, this approach is limited by the availability of proficient (and certified) ultrasonographers. Thus, the most widely used approach remains a combination of serum biochemical markers (*quadruple screen*) and maternal age. Amniocentesis and chorionic villus sampling are considered confirmatory tests. Note that these modalities are also useful for certain anatomic defects (neural tube defects) and other trisomies. In fact, currently available screening modalities detect trisomy 18 with much greater sensitivity than Down syndrome.

  □ *Qualitative ultrasound findings* indicative of aneuploidy include gross anatomic defects, such as cardiac defects, cystic hygroma, hydrops, hydronephrosis, and intestinal atresia (gastric double-bubble sign). More subtle anatomic findings include hyperechoic bowel, an intracardiac echogenic focus (echogenicity of a papillary muscle), and nasal bone hypoplasia. Major or several anatomic defects are significantly more common in trisomy 18 or 13 than in trisomy 21. Overall, the incidence of gross anatomic defects in Down syndrome is about 15%.

  □ *Quantitative ultrasound measurements (biometry)* include femur length, humerus length, and nuchal fold thickness. Femoral and humeral shortening are indicative of Down syndrome, with a sensitivity of about 20% to 60%. Increased nuchal skin fold thickness is the most sensitive sonographic marker, found in about 40% to 50% of Down syndrome fetuses; however, this measurement requires great skill and adherence to strict standards.

  □ *Second trimester biochemical tests* include maternal serum α-fetoprotein (MSAFP), human chorionic gonadotropin (hCG), unconjugated estriol (uE), and inhibin A. Average MSAFP and uE are decreased in Down syndrome pregnancies, while hCG is elevated. For over a decade, these 4 markers (the *quadruple, or "quad," screen*) in combination with maternal age have been the standard screening panel for Down

syndrome. Inhibin A is elevated in Down syndrome pregnancies and, importantly, quite stable throughout the second trimester. Thus, inhibin A can mitigate the impact of slight errors in the estimation of gestational age. The risk calculated from these parameters has been compared with that of an average 35-year-old woman (1:270) to determine whether the screening result was positive (risk >1:270) or negative. With maternal age and the triple screen (the previously used HCG, uE, and MSAFP), a roughly 70% sensitivity was possible, with a 5% false-positive rate. With the quad screen, a roughly 80% sensitivity is possible, with a 5% false-positive rate.

  □ *First trimester biochemical tests* include the free β chain of hCG and pregnancy-associated plasma protein-A (PAPP-A). Addition of first trimester PAPP-A to the second trimester quad screen can increase sensitivity further.

  □ Through the use of all available modalities—first trimester biochemical tests, nuchal-fold ultrasonography, second trimester biochemical tests, and maternal age—a sensitivity of 90% is achievable with a 5% false-positive rate.

  □ In January 2007, the American College of Obstetricians and Gynecologists (ACOG) issued revised recommendations for Down syndrome screening. The salient points were as follows:

  - Screening and diagnostic testing should be available to all pregnant women who present for prenatal care before 20 weeks' gestation, *regardless of maternal age.*

  - First-trimester screening, including nuchal translucency measurement and biochemical markers (PAPP-A), results in sensitivity comparable to the second-trimester quadruple screen (and superior to both nuchal translucency alone and the second-trimester triple screen), with the same false-positive rates. Women found to have increased risk for aneuploidy based on first-trimester screening should be offered confirmatory chorionic villus sampling (1st trimester) or amniocentesis (2nd trimester). Women who receive only first trimester screening for aneuploidy should be offered second trimester neural tube defect screening (MSAFP).

  - Integrated first- and second-trimester screening is more sensitive than either first-trimester (nuchal fold plus PAPP-A) or second-trimester (quad screen) alone.

Edward Syndrome (Trisomy 18)

- Few survive beyond 1 year of age.

- Incidence of approximately 1/3000 live births and increases with maternal age.

- Typical features in the neonate include clenched fists (with second digit overlapping third and fifth digit overlapping fourth), intrauterine growth retardation, inguinal and/or umbilical hernias, cardiac defects, prominent occiput, low-set ears, micrognathia, and rocker-bottom feet. Beyond this stage, profound mental retardation becomes evident.

- 50% die within the first week of life, and less than 10% survive first year.

Patau Syndrome (Trisomy 13)

- Few survive beyond 1 year of age.

- The incidence is approximately 1/5000 live births and increases with maternal age.

- At birth, evident features include holoprosencephaly, polydactyly, microcephaly, sloping forehead, cleft lip and/or palate, retinal anomalies, microphthalmia, abnormal ears, single umbilical artery, omphalocele, cardiac defects, and genitourinary malformations. Over time, seizures, profound mental retardation, and deafness may become apparent.

- 50% die within first month, and less than 30% survive the first year.

Turner Syndrome (Monosomy X; 45, X)

- 45, X is the most common chromosomal finding in spontaneous abortions; however, most of those born alive with 45, X survive into adulthood. It is estimated that 99% of 45, X conceptions abort spontaneously. This apparent paradox is answered in part by the fact that only about half of those born alive with Turner syndrome have complete loss of 1 X chromosome; instead, the remainder of these patients have 45, X mosaicism.

- In conventional cytogenetic preparations, 3 main karyotypes are found in Turner syndrome. In 55% to 60%, the entire X chromosome is missing (45, X). About 30% have mosaicism. The remaining have structural anomalies resulting in partial monosomy X: deletion of the small arm of the X chromosome (resulting in an isochromosome of the long arm), deletion of portions of the short arm, and deletion of portions of both arms (resulting in the formation of a ring chromosome). With more sensitive techniques (eg, fluorescence in situ hybridization [FISH]), even more mosaics can be found, accounting for up to 75% of cases. If studied in detail, all surviving patients with Turner syndrome may in fact be mosaics or complex translocations and that all true 45, X conceptuses are nonviable.

- Up to 10% of those with Turner syndrome have some Y chromosome material in their genome. Such individuals may have some degree of masculinization and are at risk for the development of gonadoblastoma.

T2.2
Numerical Disorders

Syndrome	Incidence	Manifestations
Down syndrome (trisomy 21))	1 in 800 live births	Hypotonia, flat face, upwardly slanted palpebral fissures, epicanthal folds, Brushfield spots, mental retardation, cardiac malformations (of the endocardial cushion), simian crease, hypoplasia of middle phalanx of 5th digit, intestinal atresia, high arched palate
Edward syndrome (trisomy 18)	1 in 3,000 live births	Small for gestational age, microcephaly with prominent occiput, mental retardation, clenched fists, 2nd digit overlapping 3rd, 5th digit overlapping 4th, short sternum, hernias, rocker-bottom feet cardiac malformations, renal malformations
Patau syndrome (trisomy 13)	1 in 5,000 live births	Sloping forehead, single umbilical artery, cleft lip/palate, polydactyly, ocular hypotelorism, low-set ears, microcephaly, holoprosencephaly, microphthalmia, cardiac malformations, visceral anomalies

- The incidence of Turner syndrome is about 1 in 2000 live female births (1 in 4000 births). Many present as neonates with lymphedema, predominantly on the dorsum of the hands, feet, and neck (cystic hygroma). Other findings include a webbed neck, broad chest, widely spaced inverted nipples, short stature, and a low hairline on the back of the neck. Coarctation of the aorta and bicuspid aortic valve are common cardiac anomalies. Hypertension frequently occurs even in the absence of coarctation. Intelligence is usually normal to just subnormal, and lifespan is essentially normal. Autoimmune thyroid disease is very common, as is diabetes mellitus and obesity.

- Ovaries that are normal in utero are progressively depleted of ova and end up as fibrous streaks of tissue. Recall that in the normal female fetus, the ovaries contain many million oocytes. These begin to disappear so that the normal pubescent female has about half a million. These dwindle further during reproductive life, leaving several thousand by menopause. In Turner syndrome, this death of oocytes is accelerated such that they are depleted by infancy.

- Only about 10% of cases are detected at birth, usually because of an abnormal karyotype performed for advanced maternal age or findings on neonatal examination (cystic hygroma or acral edema). Another 10% to 25% of cases are found during childhood when short stature is investigated. The remaining cases are discovered as a result of amenorrhea or infertility. At the age of puberty, the genitalia remain unchanged, amenorrhea develops, and secondary sex characteristics do not develop. Turner syndrome is among the most common causes of primary amenorrhea.

- Noonan syndrome was once referred to as "male Turner syndrome," because of their morphologic similarities. In particular, short stature, abnormal-appearing chest, a webbed neck, and high incidence of lymphatic malformations give rise to a superficial resemblance to Turner syndrome. However, Noonan syndrome affects females and males equally and is molecularly distinct, and the associated congenital heart disease is right-sided, including most commonly pulmonic stenosis. Prolonged coagulation times are frequently observed because of a wide range of defects (von Willebrand disease phenotypes, factor V deficiency, factor VIII deficiency, etc). Mental retardation affects a significant minority. A characteristic facial dysmorphism includes low-set ears, blue-green irides,

and hypertelorism. The incidence of Noonan syndrome is estimated to be about 1 in 1000, making it among the more common inherited syndromes. It is inherited in an autosomal dominant manner, but many cases are sporadic (de novo mutations). Noonan syndrome is caused by mutations in either the *PTPN11* gene (12q) or the *KRAS* gene (12p). Interestingly, the *PTPN11* gene has also been implicated in some examples of LEOPARD syndrome and juvenile myelomonocytic leukemia.

Klinefelter Syndrome (47, XXY)

- While present in 1 in 1000 live male births, Klinefelter syndrome is diagnosed at birth in only about 10% of affected boys. Most cases are detected during childhood, but it is found during adulthood in 25% of cases.

- Affected males tend to be tall, with disproportionately long arms and legs (relative to torso). Some develop gynecomastia, and the testes are small. Most have a mild mental retardation. There is an increased risk of breast cancer and predominantly *extragonadal* germ cell tumors. The incidence of autoimmune disease and osteoporosis is also higher than in other males.

- Klinefelter syndrome is among the most common causes of male hypogonadism, and many cases come to clinical attention through evaluation for infertility. Almost all men with a 47, XXY karyotype will be infertile, and Klinefelter syndrome accounts for 5% infertile men with oligo- or azoospermia. The testicular biopsy shows hyalinized atrophic, nonspermatogenic seminiferous tubules.

- In about 80% of affected males, the karyotype shows 47, XXY. Like other trisomies, (21, 18, 13), this results most commonly from meiotic nondisjunction. However, the proportion that results from paternal meiotic nondisjunction is high (about 50%-60%). About 15% of patients have some kind of mosaicism.

Deletions and Microdeletions (Contiguous Gene Syndromes) T2.4

Wolf-Hirschhorn Syndrome (4p–)

- Result from deletion of the short arm of chromosome 4 (4p-).

- Affected individuals are described as having a "Greek helmet" facies (ocular hypertelorism, prominent glabella, and frontal bossing). They also have microcephaly, dolichocephaly, a hypoplastic eye socket, bilateral epicanthic folds, cleft lip and palate, a beaked nose, hypospadias, cardiac malformations, and mental retardation.

Cri-du-Chat Syndrome (5p–)

- Results from deletion of the short arm of chromosome 5 (5p–).

- A characteristic cry gives the syndrome its name. Other features include hypotonia, small stature, microcephaly, moonlike face, hypertelorism, bilateral epicanthic folds, a high arched palate, wide and flat nasal bridge, and mental retardation.

Angelman Syndrome and Prader-Willi Syndrome (15q–)

- 2 syndromes with vastly different clinical manifestations that result from the same deletion of 15q11.2. Prader-Willi syndrome is characterized by mental retardation, short stature, hypotonia, obesity, small hands and feet, and hypogonadism. It is usually the result of a deletion of band 15q12; importantly, the deletion must be in the paternally derived chromosome 15. In contrast, Angelman syndrome is caused by a deletion in the same band affecting the maternally derived chromosome 15. Patients with Angelman syndrome are also mentally retarded, but manifest an ataxic gait, seizures, and inappropriate laughter (happy puppets).

- Imprinting forms the basis for most of these phenotypic differences and refers to the preferential inactivation of an allele based on the parent of origin. Hypermethylation is the means by which the cell inactivates either the maternal or paternal 15q11.2. If 1 allele is inactivated and the other is missing, then the cell has no 15q11.2 to transcribe.

- About 15% of instances of Prader-Willi syndrome result from uniparental disomy, which occurs when part or all of a chromosome comes from just 1 parent. This arises because of nondisjunction during meiosis such that 1 gamete gets both homologs and the other gamete gets neither. Most (about 70%) cases of Prader-Willi are the result of a microdeletion in the paternally derived chromosome 15, at 15q11-13 **T2.3**. About 25% are caused by uniparental maternal disomy of chromosome 15 (both copies of chromosome 15 are from the mother). Of the remaining cases, some have an abnormality in the imprinting (methylation) process, resulting in underexpression of the paternal chromosome. A methylation assay is available, which uses a methylation-sensitive probe for detecting abnormal methylation within the

T2.3
Prader-Willi vs Angelman Syndrome

Molecular Basis	Prader-Willi	Angelman
Lost 15q11	Paternal	Maternal
Class I (deletion)	65%-75%	65%-75%
Class II (uniparental disomy)	20%-30%	5%
Class III (imprinting defect)	5%	5%
Class IV (gene mutation)	0.1%	10%
Class V (balanced translocation)	0.1%	10-15%
Clinical features	Hypotonia, short stature, hypogonadism, hyperphagia, obesity, moderate mental retardation	Microcephaly, seizures, ataxia, inappropriate laughter, severe mental retardation

Prader-Willi syndrome critical region (15q11-13). This should be sensitive to all of the aforementioned underlying molecular abnormalities, about 97% of cases. In addition, a FISH-based assay is available for identifying the deletion on chromosome 15q11-q13, and this should be sensitive to about 70% of cases.

■ Most (about 70%) cases of Angelman syndrome are caused by a microdeletion in the maternally derived chromosome 15 at 15q11-13. About 5% are caused by uniparental paternal disomy of chromosome 15 (both copies of chromosome 15 are from the father). About 5% of cases have an abnormality in the imprinting (methylation) process, resulting in underexpression of the maternal chromosome. Another 5% of patients with Angelman syndrome have a point mutation in the *UBE3A* gene, located in the critical 15q11-13 region. Using the methylation assay, the presence of only a paternal methylation pattern is diagnostic, and this would be sensitive to about 80% of cases. Those who

test negative by methylation studies may be considered for direct sequencing of the *UBE3A* gene, but this will only detect about one fourth of the remaining cases. *UBE3A* encodes the E6-AP ubiquitin ligase protein, expressed within brain tissue. In about 70% of cases, FISH is sensitive enough to detect microdeletions in 15q11-q13.

Smith-Magenis Syndrome (17p–)

■ Many of the features of Smith-Magenis syndrome are subtle in infancy and early childhood, and the diagnosis is often made in later childhood. Infants tend to be hypotonic and lethargic, with minor morphologic anomalies, such as brachydactyly, subtle craniofacial features, laryngeal abnormalities causing a hoarse voice, and an inverted circadian sleep schedule (because of inverted circadian melatonin secretion). As they grow, morphologic anomalies, such as prominent

T2.4
Selected Microdeletion Syndromes

Syndrome	Microdeletion	Manifestations
DiGeorge, Catch 22, velo-cardio-facial (see chapter 9)	22q11.2	Thymic aplasia/hypoplasia (immunodeficiency), parathyroid aplasia/hypoplasia (hypocalcemia, tetany), abnormal facial features, mental retardation, conotruncal cardiac anomalies
WAGR (see chapter 13)	11p13	Wilms tumor, aniridia, genital hypoplasia (in males), gonadoblastoma, mental retardation
Alagille (see chapter 8)	20p12	Bile duct paucity, heart defects (pulmonary artery stenosis), ocular defects (posterior embryotoxin), butterfly vertebrae, long nose with broad midnose
Kallman	Xp22.3	Anosmia, hypogonadism
Prader-Willi	15q11.2 (paternal)	Hyperphagia, obesity, hypogonadism, mild mental retardation
Angelman	15q11.2 (maternal)	Hyperactivity, inappropriate laughter, aphasia, ataxia, mental retardation, seizures
Smith-Magenis	17p11.2	moderate mental retardation, prominent forehead, prognathism, maladaptive and self-mutilating behavior, disturbed sleep
Williams	7q11.23	elfin face, abnormal dentation, stellate pattern in iris, growth deficiency, heart malformations, infantile hypercalcemia, mental retardation, very friendly personality
Wolf	4p deletion	Intrauterine growth retardation, heart malformations, microcephaly, cleft lip and palate, broad nasal root, severe mental retardation
Miller-Dieker	17p13	microcephaly, lissencephaly, mental retardiation, heart malformations, renal malformations, seizures, prominent forehead, vertical furrowing of brow
CHARGE sequence	22q11.2	colomba, heart malformations, choanal atresia, genital hypoplasia, deafness, mental retardation

2: Chromosomal and Microdeletion Disorders

Deletions and Microdeletions>Smith-Magenis Syndrome; Y Chromosome Microdeletion Syndrome |
Trinucleotide Repeat Disorders>Fragile X Syndrome

forehead, progressive prognathism, and short stature become more apparent. They begin to manifest mental retardation, visual problems, hearing loss, and behavioral problems, and their sleep difficulties persist.

■ The diagnosis is confirmed by cytogenetic studies or FISH, displaying a deletion in 17p11.2. A very small number of cases lack an anomaly detectable by FISH, and these cases have mutations in the *RAI-1* (retinoic acid induced-1) gene, located in the 17p11.2 band.

Y Chromosome Microdeletion (YCMD) Syndrome

■ This syndrome is caused by microscopic deletions in the Y chromosome, specifically within Yq11. Within this band is the azoospermia factor (AZF) region.

■ Y microdeletion is the most frequent (10%) genetic cause of spermatogenic failure, and most present with azoospermia.

Trinucleotide Repeat Disorders T2.6

Fragile X Syndrome (FRAXA)

■ Fragile X **T2.5** is the most common inherited form of mental retardation, and the second most common cause of mental retardation overall (second to Down syndrome). The incidence is about 1 in 2000 male births (1 in 4000 births), and fragile X accounts for about 5% of all instances of mental retardation, spanning all races and ethnicities.

■ In addition to mental retardation, affected individuals also commonly manifest autistic behavior and attention deficit hyperactivity disorder. Physical findings include large head size, prominent ears, prominent jaw, and macroorchidism that arises during or after puberty (the most consistent physical finding). Often the stature is tall. In female carriers, the phenotype may be normal, or there may be mild mental retardation.

■ Before the genetic basis for this disorder was understood, when fragile X was considered just another X-linked recessive disorder, some aspects of its inheritance were confusing. In particular, while predominantly affecting males, a significant number of females were also affected. Second, there was a tremendous range in clinical severity. Third, and most perplexing, the number of family members affected increased with successive generations. This latter

T2.5
Clinical Features of Fragile X

Physical features	Large ears
	Prominent forehead
	Macrocephaly
	Tall stature
	High-arched palate
	Macroorchidism (after puberty)
	Hyperextensible fingers
Neurologic features	Mental retardation/developmental delay
	Hyperactivity/attention deficit disorder/autism
	Seizures

feature became the Sherman paradox and is now known to be merely an example of anticipation.

■ The underlying defect is found in the distal long arm of the X chromosome, at Xq27.3. A series of CGG trinucleotide repeats normally is present in this location, called the FRAXA locus, which is very near the promoter sequence of the *FMR1* (familial mental retardation-1) gene. Normal individuals have approximately 29 CGG repeats at the FRAXA locus, and alleles with up to 200 CGG repeats are compatible with normal *FMR1* gene expression. When the number of trinucleotide repeats exceeds 200, for unclear reasons the *FMR1* promoter region becomes methylated, thus inactivating the gene.

■ When less than 50 repeats are present, the FRAXA site can remain stable for many generations, rarely undergoing expansion. Once there are more than 50 repeats, the locus becomes *unstable,* that is, subsequent increases in size are very likely. FRAXA sites with 52 to 200 repeats are considered premutations. Note, however, that carriers of premutations are phenotypically normal. Sites with more than 200 repeats are considered a full mutation, because these are associated with *FMR1* inactivation and phenotypic abnormalities.

■ FMRP, the product of *FMR1*, is a protein with widespread expression. It is found in greatest concentration in the brain and testis, but its exact function is unknown. Rare cases of fragile X syndrome are the result of mutations within the *FMR1* coding sequence.

Trinucleotide Repeat Disorders>Fragile X Syndrome

- The fragile site is visible in cytogenetic culture only under special culture conditions, eg, folate or thymidine deprivation culture. In such conditions, a discontinuity of staining or a constriction in the long arm of the X chromosome develops, such that the X chromosome appears "broken"; this reproducible site has been called the "fragile site." In all, over 80 such fragile sites have been found in the human genome, many of which are folate sensitive; the significance of most of these is unknown. The originally discovered fragile site is called FRAXA. Since then, additional fragile sites associated with the fragile X syndrome have been discovered, and these are called FRAXB, FRAXC, FRAX D, and FRAXE.

- The molecular diagnosis of fragile X syndrome may be made by Southern blot, which can demonstrate an expanded segment of DNA from the Xq27.3 region or methylation analysis of the *FMR1 gene*. An additional method, possibly applicable to widespread screening, was recently described, based on the principle that the fragile site expansion prevents effective polymerase chain reaction (PCR) amplification. DNA is isolated from a Guthrie card blood spot, and subjected to PCR. Those subjects with no amplified product can then undergo a confirmatory test via 1 of the more traditional methods (eg, Southern blot).

T2.6
Trinucleotide Repeat Disorders

Syndrome	Fragile Site	Trinucleotide	Location	Affected Gene or Protein
Fragile X	FRAXA (FMRI)	CGG	Xq27.3	*FMR-1* (FMRP protein)
Friedreich ataxia	X25	GAA	9q13-21.1	*FRDA* (Frataxin)
Myotonic muscular dystrophy (see chapter 11)	DMPK	CTG	19q13	Myotonic dystrophy protein kinase (DMPK)
Spinobulbar muscular atrophy (Kennedy disease)	AR	CAG	Xq13-21	Androgen receptor (AR)
Huntington disease (see chapter 11)	HD	CAG	4p16.3	Huntingtin
Dentatorubral-pallidoluysian atrophy (Haw River syndrome)	DRPLA	CAG	12p13.31	Atrophin-1
Spinocerebellar ataxia type 1	SCA1	CAG	6p23	Ataxin-1
Spinocerebellar ataxia type 2	SCA2	CAG	12q24.1	Ataxin-2
Spinocerebellar ataxia type 3 (Machado-Joseph disease)	SCA3 (MJD1)	CAG	14q32.1	Ataxin-3
Spinocerebellar ataxia type 6	SCA6	CAG	19p13	α1A voltage-dependent calcium channel subunit
Spinocerebellar ataxia type 7	SCA7	CAG	3p12-13	Ataxin-7

2: Chromosomal and Microdeletion Disorders

Trinucleotide Repeat Disorders>Friedreich Ataxia I Short Stature, Idiopathic Short Stature, and Dwarfism: Summary and Approach>Achondroplasia

Friedreich Ataxia

- An autosomal recessive disorder in which affected individuals suffer deterioration of the spinal dorsal root ganglia, posterior columns, corticospinal tracts, and spinocerebellar tracts. This manifests initially with gait ataxia, usually no later than age 20 years, with eventual limb ataxia and dysarthria. Afterward, there is loss of deep tendon reflexes, impaired proprioception, and decreased pain and temperature sensation. A minority display optic atrophy or sensorineural hearing loss. About 60% develop a hypertrophic cardiomyopathy.

- Caused by a GAA trinucleotide expansion in the *FRDA* gene (9q13). Those with fully manifested Friedreich ataxia display homozygosity for pathologic trinucleotide GAA expansion with more than 500 repeats. Normal alleles are those up to 65 repeats, with those between 66 and 500 considered premutations.

- The expansion size correlates with age at onset and disease severity. There is a direct correlation between the length of the trinucleotide expansion and the thickness of the interventricular septum.

- The uniqueness of Friedreich ataxia is that, unlike other trinucleotide repeat disorders, anticipation is not observed. This is because 2 copies of an abnormal allele must be inherited for the disease to occur; thus, the disease is not directly transmitted from 1 generation to the next.

Short Stature, Idiopathic Short Stature, and Dwarfism: Summary and Approach

Chromosomal disorders represent one of the many causes of short stature **T2.7**. Other categories to consider include chronic disease, monogenetic disorders, and endocrine diseases. Most cases are simply familial (genetic) or constitutional, but these are considered diagnoses of exclusion. The characteristic features of *familial short stature* are a normal growth velocity, predicted adult height (based on published tables) that is appropriate when compared with the heights of parents, and bone age that is appropriate for chronologic age. *Constitutional short stature* (growth delay) is characterized by a normal growth velocity, predicted adult height that is appropriate when compared with that of parents, but a bone age that is inconsistent with chronological age. Typically, those with constitutional short stature also achieve puberty at a later age and reach their final height at a later-than-average age (over 18 years). Weight gain that is out

T2.7
Causes of Short Stature

Monogenetic disorders of bone growth	Achondroplasia Chondrodysplasia Osteogenesis imperfecta
Chromosomal disorders	Down syndrome Turner syndrome
Chronic disease (genetic and acquired)	Malabsorption (Crohn, celiac sprue) Asthma Cystic fibrosis Congenital heart disease Chronic renal failure
Endocrine	Hypothyroidism Growth hormone deficiency (may be genetic) Panhypopituitarism (pituitary dwarfism) Cushing syndrome (including iatrogenic) Precocious puberty

of proportion to height gain is the hallmark of endocrine causes of growth failure.

- Although the definition of idiopathic short stature is controversial, it is necessary to exclude the aforementioned known causes. Furthermore, most definitions specifically exclude those with significant intrauterine growth retardation or significantly low birth weight (excluding most forms of congenital dwarfism). The laboratory evaluation should initially include serum growth hormone, serum insulinlike growth factors, thyroid stimulating hormone, cytogenetics, and erythrocyte sedimentation rate. Tests to evaluate nutritional status (prealbumin) and tests to exclude cystic fibrosis should be considered. Radiographic imaging may be necessary to exclude chondrodysplasia and other primary defects of the growth plate.

- Idiopathic short stature may be defined as (1) height 2 standard deviations or more below the mean, (2) essentially normal weight and body proportion, and (3) known causes excluded (normal growth hormone levels, normal growth hormone response to provocative testing, and appropriate bone age).

Achondroplasia

- Achondroplasia is the most common form of dwarfism, despite an overall incidence of only about 1 in 15,000 to 1 in 40,000.

2: Chromosomal and Microdeletion Disorders

Short Stature, Idiopathic Short Stature, and Dwarfism: Summary and Approach>Achondroplasia; Hypochondroplasia; Thanatophoric Dysplasia | References

- Inheritance is autosomal dominant, but about 80% of cases are sporadic (simplex) and caused by new (spontaneous) mutations. Couples in which only 1 parent has achondroplasia have a 50% chance of having an affected child, whereas couples in which both parents have achondroplasia have a 75% chance (homozygosity is lethal).

- Achondroplasia is characterized by short stature associated with disproportionately short arms and legs, a large head with frontal bossing, and characteristic facial features. The thorax is unusually narrow, and there is risk of death in infancy from upper airway obstruction or spinal stenosis; despite this, the overall lifespan is essentially normal.

- Nearly all cases are caused by mutations in the *FGFR3* gene (4p16.3) for which testing is clinically available. Furthermore, virtually all cases are caused by 1 of 2 mutations in *FGFR3*, permitting targeted mutation analysis. More than 95% of cases are the result of the G1138A mutation (resulting in G380R in the amino acid sequence), and most remaining cases are caused by the G1138C mutation.

Hypochondroplasia

- Hypochondroplasia is characterized by short stature with disproportionately short arms and legs; broad, shortened hands and feet; and macrocephaly. Thus the overall features tend to resemble achondroplasia but are usually milder. In contrast to achondroplasia, the diagnosis is difficult to make in infancy.

- Hypochondroplasia is also the result of *FGFR3* mutations; however, these differ from the ones seen in achondroplasia. Instead, the C1620A and C1620G mutations, both of which result in the same lysine-for-asparagine substitution, cause most cases of hypochondroplasia.

Thanatophoric Dysplasia

- Thanatophoric (meaning "tending toward death") dysplasia is a condition that is usually lethal in the neonate.

- Characteristic features include bent (telephone receiver) femurs and a cloverleaf skull deformity. Neonates with this condition die of respiratory insufficiency shortly after birth.

- Like the preceding conditions, the *FGFR3* gene is responsible for thanatophoric dysplasia.

References

Avgidou K, Papageorghiou A, Bindra R, et al. Prospective first-trimester screening for trisomy 21 in 30,564 pregnancies. *Am J Ob Gynecol* 2005; 192: 1761-1767.

American College of Obstetrics and Gynecology (ACOG) Practice Bulletin. Screening for fetal chromosomal abnormalities. *Obstet Gynecol* 2007; 109: 217-227.

Bahado-Singh RO, Choi S-J, Cheng CC. First- and midtrimester Down syndrome screening and detection. *Clin Perinatol* 2004; 31: 677-694.

Broughton BC, Berneburg M, Fawcett H, et al. Two individuals with features of both xeroderma pigmentosum and trichothiodystrophy highlight the complexity of the clinical outcomes of mutations in the XPD gene. *Hum Mol Genet* 2001; 10: 2539-2547.

Chasen ST, Sharma G, Kalish RB, et al. First-trimester screening for aneuploidy with fetal nuchal translucency in a United States population. *Ultrasound Obstet Gynecol* 2003; 22: 149-151.

Egan JFX, Benn PA, Zelop CM, et al. Down syndrome births in the United States from 1989 to 2001. *Am J Ob Gynecol* 2004; 191: 1044-1048.

Ellis NA, Ciocci S, Proytcheva M, et al. The Ashkenazic Jewish Bloom syndrome mutation blmAsh is present in non-Jewish Americans of Spanish ancestry. *Am J Hum Genet* 1998; 63: 1685-1693.

Ellis NA, German J. Molecular genetics of Bloom's syndrome. *Hum Mol Genet.* 1996; 5: 1457-1463.

Foucault F, Vaury C, Barakat A, et al. Characterization of a new BLM mutation associated with a topoisomerase II-alpha defect in a patient with Bloom's syndrome. *Hum Mol Genet.* 1997; 6: 1427-1434.

Francomano CA. Achondroplasia. Available at GeneTests. org. Accessed January 9, 2006.

Gennery AR, Slatter MA, Bhattacharya A, et al. The clinical and biological overlap between Nijmegen Breakage Syndrome and Fanconi anemia. *Clin Immunol* 2004; 113: 214-219.

References

Gropman A, Duncan W. Neurologic and developmental features of the Smith-Magenis syndrome (del 17p11.2). *Pediatr Neurol* 2006; 34: 337-350.

Gruber SB, Ellis NA, Scott KK, et al. BLM heterozygosity and the risk of colorectal cancer. *Science* 2002; 297: 2013.

Gubitosi-Klug RA, Cuttler L. Idiopathic short stature. *Endocrinol Metab Clin N Am* 2005; 34: 565-580.

Haddow JE, Palomaki GE, Knight GJ, et al. Screening of maternal serum for fetal Down's syndrome in the first trimester. *N Engl J Med* 1998; 338: 955-961.

Kabbani H, Raghuveer TS. Craniosynostosis. *Am Fam Physician* 2004; 69: 2863-2870.

Khalifa MM, Struthers JL. Klinefelter syndrome is a common cause for mental retardation of unknown etiology among prepubertal males. *Clin Genet* 2002; 61: 49-53.

Kratz CP, Niemeyer CM, Castleberry RP, et al. The mutational spectrum of PTPN11 in juvenile myelomonocytic leukemia and Noonan syndrome/myeloproliferative disease. *Blood* 2005; 106: 2183-2185.

Lanfranco F, Kamischke A, Zitzmann M, et al. Klinefelter's syndrome. *Lancet* 2004; 364: 273-283.

Lee MM. Idiopathic short stature. *N Engl J Med* 2006; 354: 2576-2582.

Poppe B, Van Limbergen H, Van Roy N, et al. Chromosomal aberrations in Bloom syndrome patients with myeloid malignancies. *Cancer Genet Cytogenet* 2001; 128: 39-42.

Pryor JL, Kent-First M, Muallem A, et al. Microdeletions in the Y chromosome of infertile men. *N Engl J Med* 1997; 336: 534-540.

Ranke MB, Saenger P. Turner's syndrome. *Lancet* 2001; 358: 309.

Rapin I, Lindenbaum Y, Dickson DW, et al. Cockayne syndrome and xeroderma pigmentosum. *Neurology* 2000; 55: 1442-1449.

Sagi L, Zuckerman-Levin N, Gawlik A, et al. Clinical Significance of the parental origin of the X chromosome in Turner syndrome. *J Clin Endocrinol Metab* 2007; 92: 846-852.

Smyth CM, Bremner WJ. Klinefelter syndrome. *Arch Intern Med* 1998; 158: 1309.

Snijders RJM, Noble P, Sebire N, et al. UK multicenter project on assessment of risk of trisomy 21 by maternal age and fetal nuchal translucency thickness at 10-14 weeks of gestation. Lancet 1998; 352: 343-346.

Spencer K, Macri JN, Aitken DA, Connor JM. Free beta hCG as first trimester marker for fetal trisomy. *Lancet* 1992; 339: 1480.

Sybert VP, McCauley E. Turner's syndrome. *N Engl J Med* 2004; 351: 1227-38.

Tzeng C, Lin S, Chen Y, et al. An effective strategy of using molecular testing to screen mentally retarded individuals for fragile X syndrome. *Diag Mol Pathol* 2001; 10: 34-40.

Van Kerckhove CW, Ceuppens JL, Vanderschueren-Lodeweyckx M, et al. Bloom's syndrome: clinical features and immunologic abnormalities of four patients. *Am J Dis Child* 1988; 142: 1089-1093.

Wapner R, Thom E, Simpson JL, et al. First-trimester screening for trisomies 21 and 18. *N Engl J Med* 2003; 349: 1405-1413.

Zenker M, Buheitel G, Rauch R, et al. Genotype-phenotype correlations in Noonan syndrome. *J Pediatr* 2004; 144: 368-374.

Chapter 3

Disorders of Coagulation and Thrombosis

Hemophilia Caused by Inherited Platelet Defects

Bernard-Soulier Syndrome (BSS)

- BSS is a cause of excessive platelet-type bleeding **T3.1** in which platelet aggregation studies resemble those of von Willebrand disease (platelets aggregate with all agonists except ristocetin) and the peripheral blood smear resembles immune thrombocytopenic purpura (thrombocytopenia with large and giant platelets **T3.2**.

- BSS platelets have a paucity and/or dysfunction of the GPIb/V/IX complex **T3.3**. GPIb is the von Willebrand factor (vWF) receptor, and the interaction of these 2 molecules is needed for platelet adhesion to denuded subendothelial tissue. In the laboratory, this defect results in decreased ristocetin-induced platelet aggregation. Failure to aggregate even in the presence of normal plasma distinguishes BSS from von Willebrand disease (vWD).

- BSS is inherited as an autosomal recessive trait. 2 genes—$Ib\alpha$ and $Ib\beta$—encode the GPIb receptor. 2 additional genes—V and IX—encode the remaining components of the GPIb/V/IX complex. The $Ib\alpha$ and $Ib\beta$ genes are found on chromosomes 17 and 22, respectively, $Ib\alpha$ having a single exon, and $Ib\beta$ having 2. While most cases of BSS are caused by mutations in the $Ib\alpha$ gene, the $Ib\beta$ gene may be affected in the DiGeorge (22q) microdeletion. Note that because the receptor is expressed as a complex, mutations in IX or V may also result in reduced expression of GPIb and a BSS phenotype.

T3.2
Conditions Associated with Giant Platelets

Bernard-Soulier syndrome
May-Hegglin anomaly (giant platelets with Döhle bodies)
Fechtner syndrome (giant platelets with hearing loss, cataracts, and nephritis)
Sebastian syndrome (giant platelets with leukocyte inclusions)
Immune thrombocytopenic purpura

- Mediterranean macrothrombocytopenia, a relatively common cause of mild thrombocytopenia in Southern Europe, is caused by a mutation in $Ib\alpha$ (chromosome 17) which results in decreased expression of the GPIb/IX/V complex (the vWF receptor). This syndrome is essentially the same as the BSS carrier state.

- Platelet-type (pseudo) vWD is caused by a gain-of-function mutation that enhances the avidity of GPIb for vWF. The high affinity leads to low plasma levels of vWF, mimicking VWD.

Platelet Dense Granule Disorders (Hermansky-Pudlak, Chédiak-Higashi, Wiskott-Aldrich Syndromes)

- Together, the dense granule disorders and the alpha granule disorders are considered "storage pool disorders" **T3.4**. Platelet dense granules are similar in many respects to neurosecretory granules. They are membrane-bound organelles with an electron-dense center that store small molecules such as serotonin, adenosine 5′-diphosphate (ADP), and adenosone triphosphate (ATP).

T3.1
Platelet- vs Coagulation-Type Bleeding Disorders

Variable	Platelet-type bleeding	Coagulation-type bleeding
Onset	Spontaneous Following trauma, immediate	Spontaneous Following trauma, delayed
Location	Skin, mucous membranes (epistaxis, gingival hemorrhage, menorrhagia)	Deep soft tissue, joints (hemarthroses)
Cutaneous findings	Petechiae, purpura	Hematomas

T3.3
Platelet Receptors

Receptor	Ligand	Notes
GP Ib/V/IX complex	vWF	CD42 Bernard-Soulier syndrome Platelet-type von Willebrand disease
GP IIb/IIIa complex	Fibrinogen	PL^A = GP IIIa Bak = GP IIb CD41 = GP IIb/IIIa CD61 = GP IIIa Glanzmann thrombasthenia
GP Ia/IIa complex	Collagen	Br^a/ Br
GP Ic/IIa complex	Fibronectin	

GP = glycoprotein.

- In the dense granule disorders, only first-wave aggregation occurs in platelet aggregation studies. Dense granule secretion, as quantified by ATP secretion using chemiluminescence, is markedly diminished. The absence of dense granules can be confirmed on electron microscopy.

  □ Hermansky-Pudlak syndrome and Chédiak-Higashi syndrome manifest *oculocutaneous albinism*, because the underlying defects appear to affect the dense granules (melanosomes) of melanocytes as well. Epistaxis occurs frequently, particularly in childhood. Platelet counts are usually normal, but the bleeding time is often prolonged.

  □ In Hermansky-Pudlak syndrome, the macrophages contain ceroidlike inclusions. Hermansky-Pudlak syndrome is particularly common in Puerto Rico. Several genes have been associated with the syndrome, including *HPS1, HPS3, HPS4, HPS5, HPS6, ADTP3A,* and *DTNBP1. HPS1,* found at 10q23, is implicated in nearly all cases in people of Puerto Rican ancestry; in fact, a single mutation—a 16 base-pair duplication in exon 15—is found in nearly all Puerto Rican cases. Among those cases of non-Puerto Rican descent, mutations are more variable or yet uncharacterized, and testing is not clinically available. Pulmonary fibrosis and granulomatous colitis complicated by bleeding have been reported in a significant minority of affected persons. Biopsies in affected tissues show ceroidlike material within macrophages (eg, within alveolar macrophages).

  □ In Chédiak-Higashi syndrome, granulocytes and platelets (and melanocytes) contain giant granules rather than ceroid bodies. A lymphoproliferative disorder ultimately arises in the vast majority of those with this syndrome. The responsible gene has been mapped to chromosome 13.

  □ Wiskott-Aldrich syndrome (WAS) is an X-linked recessive disorder that presents with the *triad of thrombocytopenia, eczema, and immunodeficiency.* A partial form of the disease manifests only with thrombocytopenia (X-linked thrombocytopenia). The platelets are small and demonstrate decreased aggregation with ADP, epinephrine, and collagen. Rather than a real deficiency of dense granules, WAS appears to be due to a problem relocating granules to the cell surface - due to cytoskeletal anomalies. The *WASP* gene (see chapter 9) is responsible for the WAS.

Platelet α Granule Disorders (Gray Platelet Syndrome, White Platelet Syndrome, and Quebec Platelet Syndrome)

- The α granules store larger molecules than those found in the dense granules, including vWF, platelet-derived growth factor, platelet factor 4, and fibrinogen, and give platelets their characteristic granular appearance.

- Gray platelet syndrome is a recessively inherited mild bleeding disorder. Aggregation is blunted with all agents except ADP. The lack of platelet alpha granules imparts a uniform pale-grey tinctorial quality in Wright-stained blood films. Platelets fail to express CD62 following stimulation with high-dose thrombin, and enzyme-linked immunosorbent assay shows abnormally low PF4. Thrombocytopenia is common.

- White platelet syndrome is named not for the microscopic appearance of the platelets but rather for the Minnesota family in whom this syndrome was described. It is characterized by a mild bleeding disorder with thrombocytopenia, mildly enlarged platelets, and impaired responses to all agonists. Ultrastructurally, the platelets have persistent Golgi complexes and poorly formed alpha granules.

- Quebec platelet disorder is a mild bleeding disorder with autosomal dominant inheritance. Unlike gray platelet syndrome, the alpha granules form normally but fail to fully mature and appear to lack factor V; thus the tinctorial quality of platelets is unaltered. Platelet aggregation in response to epinephrine is abnormal.

Glanzmann Thrombasthenia

- First described in Switzerland by Glanzmann in 1918, Glanzmann thrombasthenia is an autosomal recessive deficiency of GPIIb/IIIa complexes. It is the function of GPIIb to bind fibrinogen, thus cross-linking platelets within a thrombus. Because this complex is responsible for the PLA1 antigen, affected platelets are PLA1-negative. GPIIb represents the extracellular portion of a transmembrane integrin protein known as αIIb, and GPIIIa is the extracellular portion of a transmembrane protein known as β3.

- The peripheral smear shows a normal number of small, dispersed platelets.

- In aggregometry studies, there is a normal initial slope of ristocetin-induced aggregation (normal plasma vWF and normal GPIb/V/IX complex) but a blunted second wave of ristocetin-induced aggregation (because of decreased IIb/IIIa).

- Clot retraction is poor or absent.

T3.4
Platelet Storage Pool Disorders

Disease	Defect	Notes
Gray platelet syndrome	Absent α granules	Autosomal recessive Splenomegaly Pulmonary fibrosis
Quebec platelet syndrome	Immature α granules that lack factor V	Autosomal dominant
White platelet syndrome	Immature α granules	Autosomal dominant Mild bleeding Enlarged platelets
Hermansky-Pudlak syndrome	Absent dense granules	Autosomal recessive Oculocutaneous albinism Pulmonary fibrosis Neutropenia Recurrent infections
Chediak-Higashi syndrome	Absent dense granules Large lysosomes	Autosomal recessive Oculocutaneous albinism Recurrent infections Accelerated phase

Hemophilia Caused by Inherited Platelet Defects>Glanzmann Thrombasthenia; Inherited Thrombocytopenia; Familial Thrombotic Thrombocytopenia Purpura

- The *αIIb* gene is large, consisting of 30 exons. The *β3* gene has 15 exons. Both are found at 17q. A large number of mutations in both genes can produce the Glanzmann phenotype. As such, molecular diagnosis is complicated, and flow cytometry for cell-surface expression of GPIIb/IIIA is the preferred diagnostic modality.

Inherited Thrombocytopenia

- This designation refers to a quantitative abnormality of functionally normal platelets. It should be suspected when thrombocytopenia presents in the first year of life or when episodes are chronic or recurrent. Note that milder disorders may be noted only much later, either at the time of menarche, trauma, or surgery, or on a routine complete blood count.

- A poor response to steroids but good response to transfused platelets is consistent with an inherited syndrome (in contrast to immune thrombocytopenic purpura).

- Many of the inherited syndromes have recognizable changes in platelet morphology, and examination of the peripheral blood smear may disclose giant platelets (megathrombocytes), very small platelets (microthrombocytes), abnormal platelet granules, and Döhle bodies.

- May-Hegglin anomaly presents as the triad of giant platelets, thrombocytopenia, and Döhlelike leukocyte inclusions. Several similar disorders are known to be closely related to May-Hegglin (Fechtner, Sebastian, and Epstein syndromes), some with an Alportlike nephritis and sensorineural hearing loss. All are autosomal dominant giant platelet disorders, and all are linked to anomalies on chromosome 22q12-13, where the *MYH9* gene, encoding a nonmuscle type of myosin heavy-chain, is found. Aggregates of this heavy chain appear to comprise the Döhlelike bodies found in neutrophils. Mutations of *MYH9* have also been identified in an autosomal dominant form of sensorineural hearing loss without hematologic anomalies.

- Congenital amegakaryocytic thrombocytopenia (CAMT) is an autosomal recessive disorder that should be considered in a neonate with severe thrombocytopenia and the absence of megakaryocytes in the marrow. Patients with CAMT develop progressive thrombocytopenia and eventual pancytopenia by the second decade of life. Thus, they may be mistaken for other marrow failure syndromes (Fanconi anemia, dyskeratosis congenita, etc). Mutations of the thrombopoietin receptor (*MPL*) gene are the cause of CAMT.

- The thrombocytopenia with absent radii (TAR) syndrome comprises defective development of the bilateral radii and severe thrombocytopenia. Thrombocytopenia is most profound at birth, and becomes *less* severe during the first year of life. The molecular origin of TAR remains unknown.

Familial Thrombotic Thrombocytopenia Purpura (TTP)

- The classic pentad of TTP includes thrombocytopenia, microangiopathic hemolytic anemia, neurologic findings, renal impairment, and fever. TTP is usually an acquired, idiopathic condition that affects young adults and, if survived, is an isolated event. Some cases of acquired idiopathic TTP have recurrent bouts. Familial (chronic relapsing) TTP (Schulman-Upshaw syndrome) is rare in comparison, but it is characterized by juvenile onset and frequent recurrence.

- Endothelial cells release vWF as large multimers. These normally undergo proteolysis to form smaller multimers, dimers, and monomers. Proteolysis of vWF multimers is catalyzed by the vWF-cleaving protease known as ADAMTS-13.

- In both acquired and inherited TTP, predominantly large vWF multimers are found in the circulation. This is now known to be the result of a deficiency of ADAMTS-13 caused, in acquired cases, by an antibody against it and in inherited cases by a mutation in its gene.

- Mutations in the *ADAMTS13* gene are responsible for nearly all inherited cases.

Hemophilia Caused by Coagulation Defects

von Willebrand Disease

- While vWD affects the function of both clotting factors and platelets, the primary defect lies in vWF. vWD is the *most common inherited bleeding diathesis* (*hemophilia A is considered the most common cause of severe hemophilia*), with incidence varying from 1 in 100 in Italy to 1 in 100,000 in Great Britain.

- vWF has 2 main functions: it assists in platelet aggregation by binding platelet GPIb, and it binds factor VIII in plasma, protecting it from degradation. The clinical manifestations of vWD reflect this dual role, with a combination of platelet-type and coagulation-type bleeding.

- The *VWD* gene is located on chromosome 12 and is transcribed primarily in endothelial cells and megakaryocytes. It is stored in Weibel-Palade bodies of endothelium and α granules of megakaryocytes. vWF is initially synthesized as the very large pro-vWF which is then cleaved into the vWF propeptide (vWF II) and finally into mature vWF. Mature vWF consists of monomers linked by disulfide bonds into large multimers. vWF is released by these cells as a large multimer and broken down in serum, by the ADAMTS-13 protease, into variably sized multimers, most commonly dimers. The multimeric distribution of vWF can be evaluated by electrophoresis. In the normal individual, this will disclose a ladderlike pattern of multimers with the darkest bands toward 1 end (the smaller multimers) and the lightest bands toward the other (the large multimers).

- Levels of vWF are lowest in blood type O individuals; however, there is no greater incidence of vWD in any particular blood type. In 1 study, the mean vWF in each blood type was as follows: O, 75%; A, 105%; B, 117%; and AB, 123%. The ABO blood type is thus an example of a genetic modifier in vWD. For a given genotype, affected individuals with the O blood type will be relatively more severely affected, and those with A, B, or AB will be less severely affected.

- There are several types of vWD **T3.5** and a type of pseudo-vWD. Type I vWD is a quantitative defect, type III is a severe quantitative defect, and the type II variants are qualitative (functional) defects.

  □ Type I, an autosomal dominant condition, is the most common type of vWD, responsible for more than 70% of cases. It is clinically mild. The prothrombin time (PT) and platelet count are typically normal, the partial thromboplastin time (PTT) and bleeding time prolonged, and factor VIII, vWF antigen, and vWF activity levels decreased. Multimers are normally distributed but globally dim in comparison with normal adults. However, these parameters vary, and in fact the diagnosis of type I vWD can be challenging, sometimes requiring repeated testing over extended periods. Despite being responsible for 70% to 80% of vWD cases, remarkably little progress has been made in characterizing the underlying molecular defect. This may reflect the possibility that loci outside the *VWF* gene—perhaps those involved in biosynthesis or transport—are responsible. A Canadian

T3.5
Von Willebrand Disease Types

Type	Factor VIII	vWF antigen	Ristocetin-induced platelet aggregation	Multimeric analysis
I	↓	↓- NI	↓	Normally distributed but slightly decreased
IIa	NI - ↓	NI -↓	↓↓	Decreased high molecular weight
IIb	NI - ↓	NI - ↓	↑	Decreased high molecular weight
III	↓↓	↓↓	↓↓	Globally decreased

study found a single dominant mutation, Tyr1584Cys, in about 15% of type 1 families.

□ Type IIa (10%-15% of vWD cases) is a moderately severe bleeding disorder that results largely from missense mutations in the *VWF* gene. Multimer analysis shows absence of high-molecular-weight multimers. The PT, fibrinogen, and thrombin time (TT) are normal, while the PTT may be slightly prolonged. The factor VIII and vWF antigen are normal to decreased. The ristocetin cofactor is decreased (<50%). Thus, there may be *discordance* between the markedly decreased ristocetin cofactor assay and normal to mildly decreased factor VIII and vWF:Ag. Type IIa is the most common of the type II variants and is caused by 1 of several missense mutations in exon 28 that is involved with multimer formation or multimer stability. This impaired multimerization results in the electrophoretic finding of decreased high-molecular-weight multimers.

□ Type IIb, like IIa, shows decreased high-molecular-weight multimers; however, IIb is unique in 2 important respects: ristocetin-induced platelet aggregation is *enhanced*, and profound thrombocytopenia and bleeding are seen on exposure to 1-deamino-8-d-arginine vasopressin (DDAVP); which is therefore contraindicated. Type IIb results from spontaneous binding of vWF to platelets. Most cases are caused by a gain-of-function point mutation in the GP1b-binding domain. Type IIb vWD must be distinguished from platelet-type vWD, which is the result of mutations in the gene that encodes the platelet GP1b receptor. In both cases, the enhanced binding is selective for high-molecular-weight multimers and results in clearance of both platelets and high-molecular-weight multimers from the blood. Thus, thrombocytopenia and decreased high-molecular-weight multimers are characteristic laboratory features in both disorders. In most other laboratory assays, it mimics type IIa.

□ Type IIM is extremely rare and caused by loss-of-function mutations in the GP1b-binding domain. The basic defect prevents binding of vWF to GPIb. Multimer analysis appears entirely normal. Normal multimeric distribution distinguishes this from IIA and IIB.

□ Type II N (Normandy) is caused by a mutation in the domain that binds factor VIII, encoded in exons 18 to 20. This results in low levels of circulating factor VIII, mimicking hemophilia A. vWF quantity and function are otherwise unaffected. The resulting clinical disease resembles mild hemophilia A with the exception of an autosomal pattern of inheritance, ie, females are affected as commonly as males. 3 mutations (T791M, R816W, and R854Q) appear to account for most 2N cases. Multimer analysis is normal, radioimmunoprecipitation assay findings are normal, and vWF antigen is normal.

□ Type III is a severe disorder with virtually no vWF. Factor VIII is low, vWF antigen and activity level are low, and multimers are quite faint across the size spectrum. It results from frameshift mutations, nonsense mutations, and deletions in the *VWF* gene. Type III must be considered in kindreds in whom apparent hemophilia follows an autosomal recessive rather than X-linked inheritance.

□ Pseudo- or platelet-type vWD mimics some of the laboratory findings of type IIb. It is caused by an abnormality in platelet GPIb, leading to *increased* avidity for vWF. It can be distinguished by the observation that in pseudo-vWD, the platelets aggregate if exposed to cryoprecipitate, while in IIb they do not.

□ Type Vicenza vWD is believed to be the result of increased clearance of vWF from the blood. This variant is characterized by discrepant plasma (low) and platelet (normal) vWF and unusually large vWF multimers.

Hemophilia A (Factor VIII Deficiency)

■ Hemophilia A **T3.6** is the most common form of inherited *severe* hemophilia, with an incidence of about 1 in 5000 live male births. Inheritance is X-linked recessive, implying that affected persons are male, and all mothers and daughters are obligate carriers. A female carrier has a 50% chance of passing the disease to a male offspring. A family history of hemophilia is present only about 60% to 70% of the time, however, because 30% of cases are the result of a new spontaneous mutation.

Hemophilia Caused by Coagulation Defects>Hemophilia A

- The degree of hemophilia is considered severe when spontaneous bleeding occurs, and this develops when factor VIII is less than 1 U/dL (<1%). In moderate hemophilia, in the range of 1 to 5 U/dL, bleeding with minor trauma is noted. With factor VIII levels higher than 5 U/dL, the patient is noted to have excessive bleeding after surgery or other significant trauma. The factor VIII activity level must be less than 30% to prolong the PTT. The bleeding severity and factor VIII level are relatively constant in an individual patient and within a family, but there is variation among kindreds.

- Diagnosis of hemophilia A in the coagulation laboratory

- □ The diagnosis of hemophilia A is usually straightforward and can be made in the coagulation laboratory. In screening tests, the platelet count, PT, and thrombin time are normal, while the PTT is prolonged. Note that often the PTT is prolonged in the cord blood of normal infants because of an intrauterine vitamin K deficiency and a relative deficiency in contact factors (XI, XII). However, assays for factor VIII activity level can be reliably performed in utero, from cord blood, and from neonatal and adult blood. In affected persons, the factor VIII level is less than 30%.

T3.6
Inherited Factor Deficiency

Deficiency	Prevalence	Chromosome	Inheritance
I (fibrinogen)	1 in 1 million	4	AR
II (prothrombin)	1 in 2 million	11	AR
V	1 in 1 million	1	AR
VII	1 in 500,000	13	AR
VIII	1 in 10,000	X	XLR
IX	1 in 50,000	X	XLR
X	1 in 1 million	13	AR
XI	1 in 1 million (higher in Ashkenazi Jews)	4	AR
XIII	1 in 1 million	6 (XIIIA) 1 (XIIIB)	AR
Combined (V & VIII, others)	1 in 1 million	18q and others	AR

AR = autosomal recessive; XLR = X-linked recessive.

- □ Female carriers usually have factor VIII activity level of at least 50%, and often their factor VIII activity level falls within the normal range. They have a normal PTT, and no history of abnormal bleeding (rare exceptions exist). *The ratio of factor VIII to vWF, however, is usually about 1:2 (normal ratio is 1:1).* Note that both factor VIII and vWF are positive acute phase reactants and may both be elevated during pregnancy. Clinically apparent hemophilia has arisen rarely in females, for which there are *3 possible mechanisms: very asymmetric lyonization, homozygosity (offspring of an affected male and carrier female), and hemizygosity (Turner syndrome).*

- □ There are several caveats. First, factor VIII is a labile factor, making expeditious measurement (or freezing for later measurement) important. Second, the effect of high hematocrit or inappropriately low-volume blood draws into citrated tubes, on function clotting assays should be borne in mind. Lastly, once factor VIII deficiency is documented, the primary differential diagnostic consideration is vWD. Especially difficult to exclude is vWD type N (Normandy).

- ■ Diagnosis of hemophilia A in the molecular laboratory

- □ The factor VIII gene is found at Xq28, not far from the factor IX gene, but far enough that it is independent of linkage. The gene is transcribed in, and most factor VIII is produced in, hepatic endothelial cells. On entering the circulation, most factor VIII is bound rapidly to circulating vWF, an association that prolongs its half-life.

- □ The factor VIII gene is 1 of the largest in the genome, 186 kilobases long with 26 exons, and with many different disease-causing mutations. Most instances of mild to moderate hemophilia A are caused by point mutations, and most of these are missense mutations (about 70%). The remaining cases of mild to moderate hemophilia A result from nonsense mutations, splicing error mutations, frameshift mutations, small deletions, large deletions, small insertions, and inversions. However, *in severe hemophilia A,* a small inversion accounts for about 45% of cases. This *common partial inversion* in the factor VIII gene can be found with Southern blot analysis, a useful assay for prenatal diagnosis and carrier detection. The remaining cases are the result of missense, nonsense, and frameshift mutations. However,

a negative test result fails to exclude about half of all cases of severe hemophilia A and most of the cases of mild to moderate hemophilia A.

- □ The development of anti-factor VIII antibodies has been a major problem in hemophilia. Certain mutations correlate with an increased likelihood of developing factor VIII antibodies. In particular, mutations, such as inversions, gross deletions, and nonsense mutations, that lead to production of no factor VIII or truncated factor VIII—confer a higher risk of antibody development. Mutations associated with even minimal production of factor VIII have a lower risk of antibody formation, but so far, inexplicable difference in risk among these individuals exist.

- □ The primary role for molecular testing in hemophilia A is in carrier detection and prenatal diagnosis. Detecting carriers through coagulation testing is fraught with difficulty. Both the PTT and the factor VIII acitivity are normal in most carrier females. A more useful assay is the ratio of factor VIII antigen to vWF antigen, which should normally be about 1. Carrier females often, but not always, have ratios less than 0.7. However, pregnancy and any use of exogenous estrogen can artificially raise this ratio.

- □ The first step in making the molecular diagnosis is to identify the causative mutation in an affected family member (a proband). If an affected family member is unavailable, testing can be performed on an obligate female carrier. For families with a history of severe hemophilia, the testing should be first performed for the intron 22 inversion which can be detected by Southern blot analysis. This will be positive and thus provide a marker in about 45% of such families. In the remaining families with severe hemophilia and the vast majority of families with mild to moderate hemophilia who do not have an intron 22 inversion, additional molecular testing is required. This can include direct sequence analysis and/or analysis for the intron 1 inversion (present in about 5% of families with severe hemophilia). Lastly, consideration should be given to testing for vWD, type 2N.

- □ If a specific mutation is identified, carrier or prenatal testing can be carried out by inversion 22 testing (if this defect is present), direct DNA analysis, or restriction fragment length polymorphism (RFLP)-based linkage analysis.

When attempting carrier detection or prenatal diagnosis in the face of an unidentified factor VIII mutation, RFLP linkage analysis can be applied if family members of the affected relative from 2 generations are available and willing to give blood samples.

Hemophilia B (Factor IX Deficiency, Christmas Disease)

- Because factors VIII and IX work together as part of the tenase complex and both are encoded on the X chromosome, the clinical and laboratory features of hemophilia A and B are essentially identical. The incidence of hemophilia B is about 1 in 25,000 male births.

- Diagnosis of hemophilia B in the coagulation laboratory

  □ As with hemophilia A, there are some things to note. First, most commercially available PTT reagents are insensitive to mild factor IX deficiency, with the result that up to 30% of affected persons may show a normal PTT. Second, while not nearly as labile as factor VIII, factor IX is vitamin K-dependent, and vitamin K deficiency (as well as liver disease and coumadin ingestion) should be excluded. Third, unlike factor VIII, factor IX levels are low in neonates; actually, levels of factor IX increase progressively with age, even into old age.

  □ While up to 10% of carrier females manifest a bleeding diathesis, the majority have a normal PTT and factor IX level.

- Diagnosis of hemophilia B in the molecular laboratory

  □ The factor IX gene is much smaller than the factor VIII gene, having 33 kb and 8 exons. It is found at Xq27, close to factor VIII, but far enough away to assort independently. Factor IX is synthesized in hepatocytes and released as the inactive form (IX). It is converted to the active form (IXa) by factor VII, combines with its cofactor (factor VIII), and activates X to Xa.

  □ The considerations for detecting carrier females and for prenatal diagnosis are similar to those for hemophilia A. The factor IX gene, being considerably smaller than the factor VIII gene, is more amenable to direct sequence analysis. Using this method, a specific mutation in the factor IX gene can be detected in more than 99% of affected individuals. Like hemophilia A,

molecular testing in hemophilia B is primarily applied to carrier detection and prenatal testing.

  □ Mild to moderate hemophilia B is most commonly caused by missense point mutations in the factor IX gene. Severe hemophilia B is usually associated with a nonsense mutation, microdeletion, gross deletion, or frameshift mutation.

  □ As is the case with hemophilia A, mutations resulting in essentially no production of antigenic factor IX (nonsense mutations and gross deletions) are associated with the greatest likelihood of developing anti-factor IX antibodies.

- Factor IX Leiden is a particular type of hemophilia B characterized by spontaneous remission after puberty. A severe bleeding disorder is present during childhood, with factor IX level less than 1%. With either puberty or the exogenous administration of androgens, factor IX levels rise to more than 30% and the bleeding disorder abates. Normal individuals experience a modest increase in factor IX activity level at puberty as well. Interestingly, the genetic defect in factor IX Leiden appears to be located in the promoter region.

Factor VII Deficiency

- Factor VII deficiency is the most common of the autosomal recessive coagulation factor deficiencies. With the exception of factors XII and XIII, the autosomal recessive factor deficiencies (II, V, VII, X, XI) have several features in common. Heterozygotes have factor levels of approximately 50%, while homozygotes have activity levels in the range of 1% to 5%. Heterozygotes are usually asymptomatic. Homozygotes tend to have somewhat milder disease than the X-linked recessive disorders, hemophilia A and B. The autosomal recessive deficiencies in general are rare, with prevalence only in regions that practice consanguineous marriage. Factor VII deficiency has an incidence of about 1 in 500,000.

- Factor VII is a vitamin K-dependent factor synthesized in the liver. Circulating factor VII is activated by tissue factor to VIIa, which can catalyze the formation of additional VIIa and activate factors X and IX. Thus, it is capable of driving both the extrinsic and intrinsic pathways.

- Factor VII deficiency is essentially the only cause of an isolated prolongation of the PT. The PTT, TT, and bleeding times are usually normal. A factor VII assay will confirm the diagnosis.

- A unique feature of factor VII deficiency is the poor association between factor levels and bleeding severity. In general, a complete absence of factor VII is incompatible with life, and while a severe bleeding phenotype is mainly seen in those with factor VII activity levels lower than 1% to 2%, many individuals with levels in this range have only mild disease or no disease.

- The factor VII gene is located on chromosome 13q, adjacent to the factor X gene. A wide variety of mutations have been reported with varying clinical phenotypes. Clinical severity appears only weakly associated with genotype, suggesting other counterbalancing influences. Molecular assays for factor VII gene mutations require direct DNA sequence analysis and are not widely available.

Factor V Deficiency

- Inherited isolated hereditary factor V deficiency is a very rare autosomal recessive condition that is often associated with a consanguineous pedigree.

- The factor V gene is located at 1q21-25. It has a high degree of homology with the factor VIII gene, and like the factor VIII gene it is quite large with a wide variety of described mutations. Most appear to cluster in exon 13, which encodes the domain removed from factor V during activation by thrombin. Of course, the most common factor V gene mutation overall, discussed later, is that leading to factor V Leiden.

- Factor V is synthesized in the liver (plasma factor V) and in megakaryocytes (platelet factor V, stored in α granules, molecularly identical to plasma factor V), is activated to factor Va by thrombin, and serves as a cofactor for Xa, which converts prothrombin to thrombin. Factor Va is inactivated by activated protein C, which requires the cofactor protein S.

- Severe factor V deficiency manifests as typical hemophilia. The PT and PTT are prolonged, and the thrombin time is normal. The bleeding time may be prolonged because of a lack of platelet factor V.

Factor X Deficiency

- Deficiency of factor X is a rare autosomal recessive condition that results in a relatively severe bleeding disorder, with the majority experiencing large deep-seated hematomas, hemarthroses, gastrointestinal bleeding, or life-threatening bleeding from the umbilical stump.

- Factor X is synthesized in the liver as a vitamin K-dependent factor. In the circulation, it is activated either by the factor VIIa or the factor IXa-VIIIa complex. Russell viper venom (RVV) can activate factor X in vitro. Factor Xa converts prothrombin to thrombin.

- Factor X deficiency results in a prolonged PT, PTT, and dilute RVV time, with a normal TT and bleeding time.

- Like factor VII, the factor X gene is located at 13q. It consists of 8 exons in which a large number of mutations have been described, the majority in exon 8. Nearly all of these have been missense mutations, and interestingly no nonsense mutations have been described.

Factor XI Deficiency

- This condition is unique in many respects when compared with other isolated coagulation factor deficiencies. Factor XI deficiency is found mainly in Ashkenazi Jews, while most other deficiencies are dispersed widely among geographic and ethnic groups. In the Ashkenazim, the gene frequency may be as high as 5% to 10%. In addition, unlike the long list of unique mutations that give rise to other inherited factor deficiencies, 3 main types of mutation give rise to most cases of factor XI deficiency. Lastly, genotype-phenotype correlations are not strong, and even very low, factor XI levels may not result in a significant bleeding diathesis.

- Overall, the bleeding tendency tends to be mild. While knockout mice models in other factor deficiencies are usually incompatible with life, the knockout mouse in factor XI deficiency survives long enough to reproduce. Interestingly, deficiency in factor XII, the primary activator of factor XI, essentially never results in a bleeding diathesis.

- The factor XI gene is found at 4q32-q35 and is transcribed mainly in the liver. Genetic defects fall into 3 categories. Type I factor XI gene mutations affect the mRNA splice region in the last intron. Type II mutations are nonsense mutations (premature stop codons) in exon 5. Type III is a missense mutation (leucine substitution for phenylalanine at position 238) in exon 9. Together, type II and III mutations account for more than 95% of cases.

- Factor XI deficiency is a common finding in Noonan syndrome.

3: Disorders of Coagulation and Thrombosis

Hemophilia Caused by Coagulation Defects>Prothrombin Deficiency; Factor XIII Deficiency;
Inherited Combined Factor Deficiency; Fibrinogen Deficiency

Prothrombin Deficiency

- The prothrombin gene, consisting of 14 exons, is found on chromosome 11. Many of the identified mutations have been in the cleavage site for factor X, resulting in so-called dysprothrombinemia (decreased functional activity with normal antigenic levels). Mutations elsewhere result largely in concordant hypoprothrombinemia, in which antigen and activity level are similarly reduced.

Factor XIII Deficiency

- A severe bleeding diathesis results from deficiency of factor XIII. Unlike other autosomal recessive deficiencies, deep hematomas and hemarthroses are unusual; instead, life-threatening umbilical stump bleeding and intracranial bleeding are common. In heterozygotes, delayed bleeding, frequent miscarriages, defective wound healing, and the formation of hypertrophic scars are characteristic features.

- Factor XIII deficiency is rare. Inheritance is autosomal recessive, but while clinical abnormalities are most apparent in homozygotes, heterozygotes can have mild bleeding symptoms.

- Factor XIII deficiency is associated with essentially normal PT, PTT, and TT. The assay that detects factor XIII deficiency is the test of clot stability in 5 M mol/L of urea. Clots formed in vitro by factor XIII-deficient patients disperse, usually within a few minutes, in these conditions; normal clots, however, remain insoluble for 24 hours. Specific factor XIII assays can be used to confirm the diagnosis.

- Factor XIII consists of 2 catalytic A subunits (factor XIII-A) and 2 noncatalytic B subunits (factor XIII-B), encoded on 2 separate chromosomes (6p and 1q). Nearly all disease-causing mutations are found in the A subunit. In most cases of factor XIII deficiency, plasma levels of factor XIII-A are immeasurable, and levels of the factor XIII-B are moderately reduced.

- A factor XIII gene polymorphism (Val34Leu) is thought to be present in nearly half the population. It is believed to confer protection against deep venous thrombosis. The polymorphism is found somewhat more commonly in patients with intracranial hemorrhage than in the general population.

Inherited Combined Factor Deficiency T3.7

- While most single-factor deficiencies are caused by mutations in the gene that encodes the factor, there are mutations that affect genes involved in intracellular transport or posttranslational modification of clotting factors that can cause combined deficiency states.

- The most common inherited combined deficiency is the combined factor V and factor VIII deficiency. This is a very rare condition described in fewer than 100 patients and results in low levels of coagulant activity and antigen of both factors. Inheritance is autosomal recessive. It appears that a gene on 18q—the LMAN1 gene which encodes ERGIC-53—is responsible. ERGIC-53 is found in the rough endoplasmic reticulum and Golgi apparatus where it acts as a chaperone in the intracellular transport of factors V and VIII.

- Second most common is the combined deficiency of vitamin K-dependent factors. The syndrome of multiple deficiencies of vitamin K-dependent coagulation factors shows deficient factors II, VII, IX, X, and proteins C and S.

Fibrinogen Deficiency (Afibrinogenemia, Hypofibrinogenemia, and Dysfibrinogenemia)

- A cluster of 3 genes on chromosome 4q-fibrinogen alpha (*FGA*), fibrinogen beta (*FGB*), and fibrinogen gamma (*FGG*)—encode the protein fibrinogen. The fibrinogen molecule is a dimer, with each half composed of 3 polypeptide chains, Aα, Bβ, and γ. Disease-causing mutations are most often found in the Aα locus.

T3.7
Familial Combined Factor Deficiencies

Type	Deficiencies	Gene
I	V, VIII	LMAN1 (ERGIC-53)
II	VII, IX	Unknown
III	II, VII, IX, X, C, S	Vitamin K c arboxylase
IV	VII, VIII	Unknown
V	VIII, IX, XI	Unknown

3: Disorders of Coagulation and Thrombosis

Hemophilia Caused by Coagulation Defects>Fibrinogen Deficiency | Thrombophilia Caused by Platelet Disorders>
Thrombocytosis; Wien-Penzing Defect; Sticky Platelet Syndrome

- In the clotting cascade, fibrinogen is cleaved into fibrin by thrombin; fibrin then polymerizes noncovalently and finally is stabilized by covalent bonds mediated by factor XIIIa. In the formation of platelet thrombi, fibrinogen binds to platelet GPIIb/IIIa to mediate platelet aggregation.

- Fibrinogen abnormalities may be congenital or acquired, and in both instances may take the form of quantitative defects (afibrinogenemia, hypofibrinogenemia), qualitative defects (dysfibrinogenemia), or both (hypodysfibrinogenemia). The inherited quantitative defects afibrinogenemia and hypofibrinogenemias are autosomal recessive conditions arising from mutations that severely truncate the protein. Inherited dysfibrinogenemia (autosomal dominant) is caused by various missense mutations.

- Afibrinogenemia is associated with an immeasurably prolonged PT and PTT and a clinical bleeding disorder similar to moderate to severe hemophilia A.

- Hypofibrinogenemia may be congenital or acquired (disseminated intravascular coagulation [DIC], hepatic failure, and L-asparaginase therapy). Most hypofibrinogenemias manifest as a bleeding diathesis; however, some patients experience thrombosis. Still others whose basic defect is in the cellular secretion of fibrinogen develop cirrhosis as a result of intrahepatocytic fibrinogen accumulation, essentially behaving as a storage disorder. Bleeding occurs when the fibrinogen level falls below 50 mg/dL (1.47 μmol/L). Umbilical cord hemorrhage is often the first manifestation of inherited hypo- or afibrinogenemia, followed by a life-long bleeding diathesis.

- Dysfibrinogenemia may be congenital or acquired (liver disease, biliary disease, hepatocellular carcinoma, and renal cell carcinoma). Clinically, it may be asymptomatic (50%-60%), cause bleeding (30%-40%) or cause thrombosis (10%-20%), depending on the particular mutation. Recurrent miscarriages are a feature of dysfibrinogenemia (and factor XIII deficiency).

- The 3 separate genes encoding fibrinogen, Aα, Bβ, γ, are clustered in a region on chromosome 4q. The molecular defect in the hypo- and afibrinogenemias is most frequently found in the Aα gene. However, mutations in dysfibrinogenemia are more widespread throughout the several genes. Dysfibrinogenemia mutations associated with thrombosis tend to cluster in the γ gene. Direct DNA sequence analysis is available through a small number of laboratories at this time.

Thrombophilia Caused by Platelet Disorders

Thrombocytosis

- The risk of thrombotic events is known to be increased by thrombocytosis, but the relationship is not linear. Moreover, patients with *reactive* thrombocytosis generally do not display a significantly increased risk of thrombosis (the exception being patients with significant underlying atherosclerotic vascular disease). In contrast, thrombocytosis that is caused by a myeloproliferative disorder is strongly associated with both thrombosis and hemorrhage. This association is not limited to essential thrombocythemia; in fact, polycythemia vera has possibly the highest rate of thrombosis (see chapter 15).

- Inherited thrombocytosis (familial benign thrombocytosis) is extremely rare.

Wien-Penzing Defect

- An inherited deficiency of the lipoxygenase metabolic pathway, with compensatory increases in cyclooxygenase pathway products, including thromboxane, prostaglandin E2, and prostaglandin D2, has been described in extremely rare instances.

- A similar defect is seen much more often as an acquired feature of a myeloproliferative disorder.
- The defect is a cause of early myocardial infarction.

Sticky Platelet Syndrome (SPS)

- SPS is a cause of arterial thrombosis T3.8, recently described in a family experiencing premature myocardial infarction in the absence of coronary artery disease.

- Its exact incidence is unknown. However, testing for SPS has its maximum yield in young patients with cerebrovascular or myocardial infarction.

- The laboratory diagnosis relies on the demonstration of hyperaggregation patterns in platelet aggregation studies with epinephrine and ADP. Aggregation with thrombin, collagen, arachidonate, and ristocetin are normal. Aspirin treatment causes normalization of the aggregation patterns.

- Low-dose aspirin is the recommended treatment.

T3.8
Venous vs Arterial Thrombosis

Variable	Venous thrombosis	Arterial thrombosis
Presentation	Deep venous thrombosis	Stroke
	Pulmonary embolism	Myocardial infarction
	Mesenteric vein thrombosis	
	Budd-Chiari syndrome	
Causes (in order of decreasing incidence)	Factor V Leiden	Hyperhomocysteinemia
	Prothrombin 20210	Lupus anticoagulant
	MTHFR polymorphisms/hyperhomocysteinemia	Elevated PAI-1
	Lupus anticoagulant	Platelet glycoprotein polymorphisms
	Antithrombin deficiency	Factor XII deficiency
	Protein C deficiency	Wien-Penzing defect
	Protein S deficiency	Sticky platelet syndrome
	Dysfibrinogenemias	
	Heparin cofactor II (HCII) deficiency	

MTHFR = methylenetetrahydrofolate reductase; PAI-1 = plasminogen activator inhibitor 1.

Platelet Glycoprotein Polymorphisms

- Platelet glycoproteins are expressed on the platelet surface and have antigenic properties. Like the antigens on the surface of red cells (Kell, Kidd, ABO, etc), there may be several alleles (polymorphisms, isoforms) for any given platelet antigen.

- Glycoproteins IIb and IIIa are both encoded on chromosome 17q, and their gene products form a complex that act as a receptor for fibrinogen. In addition, this complex is the basis for the CD41/CD61 antigen.

  □ Glycoprotein IIIa (of the GPIIb/IIIa complex) has 2 alleles (polymorphisms) that are common in the population: PLA1 (HPA-1a, GPIIIa Leu33) and PLA2 (HPA-1b, GPIIIa Pro33). For example, antibodies against PLA2, formed in a person with only PLA1+ platelets, are commonly the basis for neonatal alloimmune thrombocytopenia and posttransfusion purpura. The difference between PLA1 and PLA2 is a single nucleotide (and a single

amino acid). PLA1, present in about 85% of the population, has a leucine at position 33 (Leu33), and PLA2, present in most of the remaining 15%, has a proline (Pro33). While still unclear, it appears that the Pro33 polymorphism may be associated with a mildly increased risk of thrombosis.

  □ Glycoprotein IIb (of the GPIIb/IIIa complex) has 2 common alleles: Baka (HPA-3a, GPIIb Ile843) and Bakb (HPA-3b, GPIIb Ser843). Again, a single nucleotide substitution separates these molecules. At amino acid position 843, an isoleucine is present in Baka, and a serine is present in Bakb. Thus far, a prothrombotic risk has not been found in either allele.

3: Disorders of Coagulation and Thrombosis

Thrombophilia Caused by Platelet Disorders>Platelet Glycoprotein Polymorphisms I
Thrombophilia Caused by Coagulation Disorders>Activated Protein C Resistance

- Glycoproteins Ib, V, and IX form a complex that acts as the platelet vWF receptor (and the CD42 antigen). The polymorphisms in this complex are mainly found within GPIb. Amino acid 145 determines whether the HPA2A (threonine) or HPA2B (methionine) antigen is expressed. HPA2A is present in about 90% of the population, and HPA2B in 10%. Furthermore, the PGIb protein normally has a certain number of leucine-rich repeats in its extracellular domain. The number of these can vary, resulting in additional polymorphisms (variable number of tandem repeats). The effect of these polymorphisms on thrombotic risk is unknown.

- The Ia/IIa complex forms a receptor for collagen. The Ia molecule, the product of a very large gene on 5q, has numerous polymorphisms. 1 of these, a threonine substitution at amino acid 807, is present in about 35% of the population and seems to be associated with thrombosis.

Thrombophilia Caused by Coagulation Disorders

Activated Protein C Resistance (Factor V Leiden)

- In the normal course of events, activated protein C (APC) degrades activated factors V and VIII by proteolytic cleavage, thus inhibiting coagulation. APC resistance is an autosomal dominant condition that is responsible for about 50% of the cases of hereditary thrombophilia. APC resistance usually results from heterozygosity for a mutant form of factor V called factor V Leiden. It is found in about up to 50% of those younger than 50 years who present with a thromboembolic event and in about 2% to 5% of unselected Caucasians. The factor V Leiden allele appears to be quite infrequent in those of sub-Saharan African, Chinese, Japanese, or Native American descent. Heterozygotes for factor V Leiden manifest a 5- to 8-fold increased risk of thrombosis, and the risk increases dramatically for homozygotes and compound heterozygotes having factor V Leiden and protein C deficiency or antithrombin III deficiency.

- The factor V gene is found on 1q (near the antithrombin gene). APC resistance is caused by a G to A point mutation at nucleotide 1691 in the factor V gene that results in a glutamine for arginine substitution at position 506 (FV R506Q) in the factor V protein. This change affects 1 of 3 APC cleavage domains. The result is a type of factor V (factor V Leiden) that is resistant to proteolytic cleavage by APC.

- Laboratory diagnosis relies on either a screening clotting assay (phenotypic analysis) and confirmatory DNA-based assay (genotypic analysis).

- The clotting assay, while more widely and quickly available, suffers from unreliability in the face of anticoagulation. The clotting assay is performed as follows: 2 activated partial thromboplastin time (aPTT) tests are performed, 1 with patient serum alone, and the other with patient serum in the presence of APC. The ratio of the clotting time with APC to the clotting time without APC (the resistance ratio) is calculated. A ratio more than 2 is normal, and lower ratios suggest APC resistance. This test is unreliable in patients undergoing anticoagulation. It otherwise correlates very well with the results of DNA testing. Discrepant results may be seen in compound heterozygotes having both the factor V Leiden mutation and a type I quantitative factor V deficiency, as well as in other rare scenarios. The overall sensitivity and specificity of this assay are around 85%. In a modification to this assay, plasma deficient only in factor V is added to the patient plasma (to control for any other factor deficiencies such as that due to warfarin therapy and to mitigate the effects of any lupus antiocoagulants), and a heparin neutralizer is added (to control for any heparin). This modified APC resistance assay has sensitivity and specificity higher than 95%.

- Molecular testing is most often available in the form of RFLP analysis. The factor V Leiden mutation results in the loss of a restriction endonuclease recognition site, permitting discernment of the mutated allele from the normal allele. The sensitivity is about 100%.

- 58% of APC-resistant patients had an associated risk factor at their first thrombotic event, and 1 very important risk factor is estrogen. Pregnancy and oral contraceptive use are associated with the first thrombotic episode in 35% and 30% of women, respectively. Furthermore, the factor V Leiden mutation is associated with a high risk of fetal loss and a high risk of thrombosis.

Prothrombin Variant (Prothrombin G20210A Mutation)

- A single nucleotide substitution—G to A—at position 20210 in the 3′-untranslated region of the prothrombin gene results in *elevated* levels of prothrombin. This mutation is believed to enhance prothrombin gene transcription and translation. The abnormal allele is transmitted as an autosomal dominant trait.

- The incidence of prothrombin 20210 approaches that of factor V Leiden—up to 4% of the general population and 20% of patients with thrombophilia. As such, the prothrombin variant is the second most common cause of inherited thrombophilia. The mutation is present in around 2% of those with European ancestry and about 0.5% of the black population. It is also interestingly present in up to 10% of those with the factor V Leiden mutation.

- While those harboring the 20210 mutation tend to have high levels of prothrombin (usually >115% of normal), the prothrombin activity is a poor (insensitive) screening test for the mutation.

- The mutation behaves as an autosomal dominant trait, substantially (about 3X) increasing the risk of thrombosis (by comparison, the relative risk in factor V Leiden is about 6). Venous events outnumber arterial ones. In particular, there appears to be a risk for cerebral vein thrombosis. This risk is compounded greatly by the concomitant use of oral contraceptives. Both the factor V Leiden and the prothrombin variant are associated with pregnancy complications, including a high risk of fetal loss and a high risk of thrombosis.

- Direct gene sequencing by polymerase chain reaction is clinically available to detect the prothrombin 20210 mutation. In fact, methods are now available to detect both the prothrombin G20210A mutation and factor V Leiden in the same reaction.

Hyperhomocysteinemia

- Probably the third most common cause of inherited thrombophilia overall, elevated levels of homocysteine are often associated with mutations in the *MTHFR* gene (see chapter 10).

Antithrombin Deficiency (Antithrombin III Deficiency)

- Antithrombin is produced in endothelial cells of the liver. When activated by heparin or heparan, antithrombin inhibits factors II, IXa, Xa, XIa, and XIIa.

- Antithrombin deficiency is an autosomal dominant disorder characterized by recurrent venous thrombosis. Heterozygotes have a 5- to 10-fold increased risk for venous thrombosis, and the homozygous state is considered incompatible with life. The age at onset of thrombosis is usually between 10 and 40 years. The prevalence of hereditary antithrombin deficiency appears to be around 1 in 2000. It is estimated to cause around 3% of unexplained venous thrombosis. Particular attention must be paid to antithrombin-deficient individuals during pregnancy (the combined antithrombin-lowering effect of pregnancy and the prothrombotic effect of pregnancy are a dangerous combination).

- Antithrombin deficiency may come to clinical attention by an apparent inability to achieve therapeutic responses to heparin therapy, as measured by the aPTT and Xa assays; *patients who are unresponsive to heparin should be tested for antithrombin deficiency.* Note that heparin therapy reduces the antithrombin activity, but never below 70%. Patients whose activity is tested below 60% should be considered antithrombin deficient. For antithrombin-deficient individuals, infusions of antithrombin concentrate will permit therapeutic heparinization.

Thrombophilia Caused by Coagulation Disorders>Antithrombin Deficiency; Heparin Cofactor II Deficiency; Protein C Deficiency and Protein S Deficiency

- With regard to laboratory diagnosis, the normal range for antithrombin is between 75% and 120%. Healthy newborns have levels in the 40% to 60% range. An antithrombin activity less than 60%, after the age of 6 months, even in heparinized patients, is abnormal. Heterozygotes generally have antithrombin levels between 40% and 70%. Also, note that about 70% of individuals with a recent deep vein thrombosis or pulmonary embolism have decreased levels of antithrombin before the initiation of anticoagulant therapy, because of the consumption of this factor. Estrogens may reduce antithrombin levels by about 15%.

- More than 100 disease-causing mutations have been identified in the antithrombin gene, *SERPINC1,* found on 1q23-q25 not far from the factor V gene. Because of the wide variety of mutations and murky genotype-phenotype correlations, antithrombin assays are preferable and molecular testing is not widely available. Nonetheless, there are 2 general classes of mutation: those resulting in the absence (quantitative) of antithrombin (type I), and those resulting in a dysfunctional (qualitative) form of antithrombin (type II). Heterozygotes for the type I mutation have decreased antithrombin, and homozygotes have no antithrombin. The type I mutations are either frameshift or complete gene deletions. Type II mutations are generally single-nucleotide point mutations and may be further subdivided into those affecting the heparin-binding domain and those affecting the thrombin-binding domain.

Heparin Cofactor II (HCII) Deficiency

- Thrombotic tendencies are associated with HCII levels less than 60%, but HCII deficiency appears to be an uncommon cause of thrombophilia (around 1% of all cases).

- -HCII, like antithrombin, is activated by heparin. In addition, like AT, it inhibits thrombin when activated but does not have antithrombin's widespread capacity to inactivate other clotting factors.

- HCII deficiency is inherited as an autosomal dominant trait.

Protein C Deficiency and Protein S Deficiency

- Protein C is activated in vivo by thrombin-thrombomodulin complexes. APC proteolytically cleaves factors such as Va and VIIIa into the inactive forms Vi and VIIIi. Protein S is the cofactor for protein C.

- The incidence of each condition in the general population is about 1 in 200, and each is responsible for 1% to 5% of thrombophilia. Both are autosomal dominant conditions in which heterozygotes have a 5- to 7-fold increased risk of thrombosis and are at risk for coumadin-induced skin necrosis. Homozygotes present as newborns with purpura fulminans, a rapidly fatal form of DIC that requires immediate treatment with anticoagulation and fresh frozen plasma.

- Both functional (coagulation based) and antigenic (immunologic) assays are available for proteins C and S.

- Deficiencies of protein C are classified as type I (quantitative) or type II (qualitative). Type I deficiency, in which both qualitative and quantitative results are low, is by far the most common. In type II deficiencies, the antigenic level of the protein is normal but with reduced activity; to detect the relatively uncommon type II deficiency it is widely recommended that a functional assay be used for screening. Protein C activity levels in healthy adults range from 70% to 140% and increase slightly with age. Protein C levels in heterozygous protein C deficiency usually fall below 55% but sometimes fall into an indeterminate zone between 55% and 70%. In these patients, it may be helpful to document 2 low levels on separate occasions. Protein C activity levels in newborns are normally around 20% to 40%.

- Normally about 60% of plasma protein S is bound to C4b-binding protein. Both free and total antigenic assays are available. Thus, 3 types of protein S deficiency states can be identified: type I is a quantitative defect, type II is a qualitative defect (the functional activity of protein S is decreased, but the antigen levels are normal), and type III is characterized by decreased free protein S (but a normal total protein S antigen). Type I is by far the most common. There is more overlap between normal and abnormal ranges for protein S than protein

- Because of a wide variety of disease-causing mutations, molecular testing is not widely available. Where available, direct DNA sequencing is required. The protein S gene is found on 3p11.1-q11.2. The protein C gene is on 2q13-q14.

3: Disorders of Coagulation and Thrombosis

Thrombophilia Caused by Coagulation Disorders>Paroxysmal Nocturnal Hemoglobinuria; Elevated Plasminogen Activator Inhibitor Type 1; Factor XII

Paroxysmal Nocturnal Hemoglobinuria (PNH)

- PNH is associated with thromboembolic events and, to a much lesser extent, bleeding. Despite this, when subjected to such measures of global platelet function as thromboelastography and aggregometry, a marked reduction of platelet reactivity is observed. This is compounded by the frequent development of thrombocytopenia. For these reasons, it is thought that the thrombotic tendency in PNH is based on some alteration in the coagulation system (see chapter 4).

Elevated Plasminogen Activator Inhibitor Type 1 (PAI-1 Gene Polymorphisms)

- PAI-1 is the major physiologic inhibitor of fibrinolysis (clot lysis). In the process of fibrinolysis, tissue plasminogen activator (tPA) converts plasminogen to plasmin, and plasmin degrades fibrin. PAI-1 inhibits tPA, and in the proper quantity it is a crucial part of the delicate balance between fibrin formation and fibrin degradation. Too much PAI-1 prevents fibrinolysis, promoting thrombophilia, and too little PAI-1 promotes bleeding.

- PAI-1 levels are under numerous influences, some of them genetic. Certain polymorphisms in the PAI-1 gene have been associated with increased blood concentrations. However, other influences on PAI-1 are clearly at work. Raised blood levels of insulin are associated with elevated PAI-1 levels, and patients with insulin resistance (eg, type 2 diabetes) tend to have increased PAI-1.

- Elevated PAI-1 causes a thrombophilic state, especially associated with arterial thrombotic events such as myocardial infarction.

- In the clinical laboratory, PAI-1 is usually measured with an immunoassay, but a functional assay is also available. Importantly, PAI-1 displays diurnal variation, with the highest plasma concentration seen in the morning (important for result interpretation but also possibly related to the early morning spike in myocardial infarctions). Further, PAI-1 is an acute-phase reactant and may be elevated after a thrombotic event. Low levels of PAI-1 suggest the very rare familial PAI-1 deficiency, a cause of hemophilia.

- The *SERPINE1* gene on chromosome 7q21.3-q22 encodes PAI-1.

Factor XII (Hagemann Factor) Deficiency

- Despite the fact that factor XII is active in the intrinsic clotting pathway, and deficiency in factor XII leads to tremendous prolongation in the aPTT, this condition virtually never causes a bleeding diathesis. Instead, patients with factor XII deficiency present with thrombosis, both arterial and venous. Factor XII-deficient patients have a 2% to 10% incidence of thrombosis, often with a presentation of myocardial infarctions in a young adult.

- The PTT is often more than 100 seconds, while the PT and TT are normal. When the 1:1 mix is performed, an initial correction is noted, which is followed by prolongation after a 10-minute incubation. The PTT can be corrected by exposure to glass.

- While factor XII initiates the intrinsic coagulation system in vitro, it is believed to be uninvolved in coagulation in vivo. Deficiencies in prekallikrein and high-molecular-weight kininogen are also not associated with clinical bleeding.

- There appear to be several disease-causing mutations in the factor XII gene. Most of them affect the serine protease domain.

References

References

Adcock DM. Factor VIII inhibitors in patients with hemophilia *A. Clin Hemost Rev* 2002; 16: 1.

Adcock DM, Fink L, Marlar RA. A Laboratory approach to the evaluation of hereditary hypercoagulability. *Am J Clin Pathol* 1997; 108: 434-449.

Anderson PD, Huizing M, Claassen DA, et al. Hermansky-Pudlak syndrome type 4 (HPS-4): clinical and molecular characteristics. *Hum Genet* 2003; 113: 10-17.

Andrew M, Paes B, Milner R, et al. Development of the human coagulation system in the full-term infant. *Blood* 1987; 70: 165-172.

Anikster Y, Huizing M, White J, et al. Mutation of a new gene causes a unique form of Hermansky-Pudlak syndrome in a genetic isolate of central Puerto Rico. *Nat Genet* 2001; 28: 376-380.

Antonarakis SE, Rossiter JP, Young M, et al. Factor VIII gene inversions in severe hemophilia A: results of an international consortium study. *Blood* 1995; 86: 2206-2212.

Anwar R, Miloszewski KJ. Factor XIII deficiency. *Br J Haematol* 1999; 107: 468-484.

Ariëns RA, Lai TS, Weisel JW, Greenberg CS, Grant PJ. Role of factor XIII in fibrin clot formation and effects of genetic polymorphisms. *Blood* 2002; 100: 743-754.

Asakai R, Chung DW, Davie EW, et al. Factor XI deficiency in Ashkenazi Jews in Israel. *N Engl J Med* 1991; 325(3): 153-158.

Baglin C, Brown K, Luddington R, et al. Risk of recurrent venous thromboembolism in patients with the factor V Leiden (FVR506Q) mutation: effect of warfarin and prediction by precipitating factors. *Br J Haematol* 1998; 100: 764-768.

Bagnall RD, Waseem N, Green PM, et al. Recurrent inversion breaking intron 1 of the factor VIII gene is a frequent cause of severe hemophilia A. *Blood* 2002; 99: 168-174.

Bayston TA, Lane DA. Antithrombin: molecular basis of deficiency. *Thromb Haemost* 1997; 78: 339-343.

Behrens WE. Mediterranean macrothrombocytopenia. *Blood* 1975; 46: 199-208.

Bernardi F, Marchetti G, Patracchini P, et al. Factor XII gene alteration in Hageman trait detected by TaqI restriction enzyme. *Blood* 1987; 69: 1421-1404.

Bick RL. Sticky platelet syndrome: a common cause of unexplained arterial and venous thrombosis. *Clin Appl Thromb Hemost* 1998; 4: 77-81.

Bolton-Maggs PH. Factor XI deficiency and its management. *Haemophilia* 2000; 6(suppl 1): 100-109.

Bolton-Maggs PH, Pasi KJ. Haemophilias A and B. *Lancet* 2003; 361: 1801-1809.

Bowen DJ. Haemophilia A and haemophilia B: molecular insights. *J Clin Pathol: Mol Pathol* 2002; 55: 127-144.

Brantly M, Avila NA, Shotelersuk V, et al. Pulmonary function and high-resolution CT findings in patients with an inherited form of pulmonary fibrosis, Hermansky-Pudlak syndrome, due to mutations in HPS-1. *Chest* 2000; 117: 129-136.

Casonato A, Pontara E, Sartorello F, et al. Identifying type Vicenza Von Willebrand Disease. *J Lab Clin Med* 2006; 147: 96-102.

Catto AJ, Kohler HP, Coore J, et al. Association of a common polymorphism in the factor XIII gene with venous thrombosis. *Blood* 1999; 93: 906-908.

Chace DH, Hillman SL, Millington DS, et al. Rapid diagnosis of homocystinuria and other hypermethioninemias from newborns' blood spots by tandem mass spectrometry. *Clin Chem* 1996; 42: 349-355.

Cunningham MT, Brandt JT, Laposata M, et al. Laboratory diagnosis of dysfibrinogenemia. *Arch Pathol Lab Med* 2002; 126: 499-505.

Cunningham MA, Pipe SW, Zhang B, et al. LMAN1 is a molecular chaperone for the secretion of coagulation factor VIII. *J Thromb Haemost* 2003; 1: 2360.

DeMoerloose P, Reber G, Perrier A, et al. Prevalence of Factor V Leiden and prothrombin G20210A mutations in unselected patients with venous thromboembolism. *Br J Haematol* 2000; 110: 125-129.

References

DeStefano V, Martinelli I, Mannucci PM, et al. The risk of recurrent deep venous thrombosis among heterozygous carriers of both factor V leiden and the G20210A prothrombin mutation. *N Engl J Med* 1999; 341: 801-806.

Doggen CJ, Cats VM, Bertina RM, et al. Interaction of coagulation defects and cardiovascular risk factors: increased risk of myocardial infarction associated with factor V Leiden or prothrombin 20210A. *Circulation* 1998; 97: 1037-1041.

Dossenbach-Glaninger A, Hopmeier P. Coagulation factor XI: A database of mutations and polymorphisms associated with factor XI deficiency. *Blood Coagul Fibrinolysis* 2005; 16: 231-238.

Eikenboom J, Van Marion V, Putter H, et al. Linkage analysis in families diagnosed with type 1 von Willebrand disease in the European study, molecular and clinical markers for the diagnosis and management of type 1 VWD. *J Thromb Haemost* 2006; 4 :774-782.

Elliot MA, Tefferi A. Thrombosis and haemorrhage in polycythemia vera and essential thrombocythaemia. *Br J Haematol* 2004; 128: 275-290.

Emmerich J, Rosendaal FR, Cattaneo M, et al. Combined effect of factor V Leiden and prothrombin 20210A on the risk of venous thromboembolism: pooled analysis of 8 case-control studies including 2310 cases and 3204 controls. *Thromb Haemost* 2001; 86: 809-816.

Fakharzadeh SS, Kazazian HH Jr. Correlation between factor VIII genotype and inhibitor development in hemophilia A. *Semin Thromb Hemost* 2000; 26: 167.

Favaloro EJ, Soltani S, McDonald J, et al. Reassessment of ABO blood group, sex, and age on laboratory parameters used to diagnose von Willebrand Disorder. *Am J Clin Pathol* 2005; 124: 910-917

Francis CW. Plasminogen activator inhibitor-1 levels and polymorphisms. *Arch Pathol Lab Med* 2002; 126: 1401-1404.

Furlan M, Robles R, Galbusera M, et al. Von Willebrand factor-cleaving protease in thrombotic thrombocytopenic purpura and the hemolytic-uremic syndrome. *N Engl J Med* 1998; 339: 1578-84.

Furlan M, Robles R, Solenthaler M, et al. Deficient activity of von Willebrand factor-cleaving protease in chronic relapsing thrombotic thrombocytopenic purpura. *Blood* 1997; 89: 3097-3103.

Gahl WA, Brantly M, Kaiser-Kupfer MI, et al. Genetic defects and clinical characteristics of patients with a form of oculocutaneous albinism (Hermansky-Pudlak syndrome). *N Engl J Med* 1998; 338: 1258-1264.

Gandrille S, Borgel D, Sala N, Espinosa-Parrilla Y, et al. Protein S deficiency: a database of mutations—summary of the first update. *Thromb Haemost* 2000; 84: 918.

Gerhardt A, Scharf RE, Beckmann MW, et al. Prothrombin and factor V mutations in women with a history of thrombosis during pregnancy and the puerperium. *N Engl J Med* 2000; 342: 374-380.

Gill JC. Diagnosis and treatment of Von Willebrand disease. *Hematol Oncol Clin North Am* 2004; 18: 1277-1299.

Gill JC, Endres-Brooks J, Bauer PJ, et al. The effect of ABO blood group on the diagnosis of von Willebrand's disease. *Blood* 1987; 69: 1691-1695.

Glueck CJ, Kupferminc MJ, Fontaine RN, et al. Genetic hypofibrinolysis in complicated pregnancies. *Obstet Gynecol* 2001; 97: 44-48.

Goodeve AC, Peake IR. The molecular basis of hemophilia A: genotype-phenotype relationships and inhibitor development. *Semin Thromb Hemost* 2003; 29: 23-30.

Griffin JH, Evatt B, Wideman C, et al. Anticoagulant protein C pathway defective in the majority of thrombophilic patients. *Blood* 1993; 82: 1989.

Gunay-Aygun M, Huizing M, Gahl WA. Molecular defects that affect platelet dense granules. *Semin Thromb Hemost* 2004; 30: 537-547.

Heath KE, Campos-Barros A, Toren A, et al. Nonmuscle myosin heavy chain IIA mutations define a spectrum of autosomal dominant macrothrombocytopenias: May-Hegglin anomaly and Fechtner, Sebastian, Epstein, and Alport-like syndromes. *Am J Hum Genet* 2001; 69: 1033-1045.

Heijboer H, Brandjes DP, Buller HR, et al. Deficiencies of coagulation-inhibiting and fibrinolytic proteins in outpatients with deep-vein thrombosis. *N Engl J Med* 1990; 323: 1512-1516.

References

Herrmann FH, Auerswald G, Ruiz-Saez A, et al. Factor X deficiency: clinical manifestation of 102 subjects from Europe and Latin America with mutations in the factor 10 Gene. *Haemophilia* 2006; 12: 479-489.

Herrmann FH, Wulff K, Auberger K, et al. Molecular biology and clinical manifestation of hereditary factor VII deficiency. *Semin Thromb Hemost* 2000; 26: 393-400.

Hoyer LW. Hemophilia A. *N Engl J Med* 1994; 330: 38-47.

Huizing M, Anikster Y, Gahl WA. Hermansky-Pudlak syndrome and Chediak-Higashi syndrome: disorders of vesicle formation and trafficking. *Thromb Haemost* 2001; 86: 233-245.

Inbal A, Freimark D, Modan B, et al. Synergistic effects of prothrombotic polymorphisms and atherogenic factors on the risk of myocardial infarction in young males. *Blood* 1999; 93: 2186-2190.

Kane WH, Davie EW. Blood coagulation factors V and VIII: structural and functional similarities and their relationship to hemorrhagic and thrombotic disorders. *Blood* 1988; 71: 539-555.

Kapiotis S, Quehenberger P, Jilma B, et al. Improved characteristics of APC-resistance assay: coatest APC resistance by predilution of samples with factor V deficient plasma. *Am J Clin Pathol* 1996; 106: 588-593.

Keeney S, Cummings AM. The molecular biology of von Willebrand disease. *Clin Lab Haematol* 2001; 23: 209-230.

Kelley MJ, Jawien W, Lin A, et al. Autosomal dominant macrothrombocytopenia with leukocyte inclusions (May-Hegglin anomaly) is linked to chromosome 22q12-13. *Hum Genet* 2000; 106: 557-564.

Kelley MJ, Jawien W, Ortel TL, et al. Mutation of MYH9, encoding non-muscle myosin heavy chain A, in May-Hegglin anomaly. *Nature Genet* 2000; 26: 106-108.

Kelly PJ, Furie KL, Kistler JP, et al. Stroke in young patients with hyperhomocysteinemia due to cystathionine beta-synthase deficiency. *Neurology* 2003; 60: 275-279.

Key NS, McGlennen RC. Hyperhomocysteinemia and thrombophilia. Arch Pathol Lab Med. 2002; 126: 1367-1374.

Kinoshita S, Yoshioka A, Park YD, et al. Upshaw-Schulman syndrome revisited: a concept of congenital thrombotic thrombocytopenic purpura. *Int J Hematol* 2001; 74: 101-108.

Kitchens CS. The contact system. *Arch Pathol Lab Med.* 2002; 126: 1382-1386.

Kottke-Marchant KK, Duncan A. Antithrombin deficiency: issues in laboratory diagnosis. *Arch Pathol Lab Med* 2002; 126: 1326-1336.

Kottke-Marchant KK, Corcoran G. The Laboratory diagnosis of platelet disorders: an algorithmic approach. *Arch Pathol Lab Med* 2002; 126: 133-146.

Kovalevsky G, Gracia CR, Berlin JA, et al. Evaluation of the association between hereditary thrombophilias and recurrent pregnancy loss: a meta-analysis. *Arch Intern Med* 2004; 164: 558-563.

Kwaan HC, Nabhan C. Hereditary and acquired defects in the fibrinolytic system associated with thrombosis. *Hematol Oncol Clin N Am* 2003; 17: 103-114.

Lak M, Sharifian R, Peyvandi F, et al. Symptoms of inherited factor V deficiency in 25 Iranian patients. *Br J Haematol* 1998; 103: 1067-1079.

Lederer DJ, Kawut SM, Sonett JR, et al. Successful bilateral lung transplantation for pulmonary fibrosis associated with the Hermansky-Pudlak syndrome. *J Heart Lung Transplant* 2005; 24: 1697-1699.

Leroyer C, Mercier B, Escoffre M, et al. Factor V Leiden prevalence in venous thromboembolism patients. *Chest* 1997; 111: 1603-1606.

Linnebank M, Homberger A, Junker R, et al. High prevalence of the I278T mutation of the human cystathionine beta-synthase detected by a novel screening application. *Thromb Haemost* 2001; 85: 986-988.

Liu ML, Nakaya S, Thompson AR. Non-inversion factor VIII mutations in 80 hemophilia A families including 24 with alloimmune responses. *Thromb Haemost* 2002; 87: 273-276.

Ljung R, Petrini P, Tengborn L, et al. Haemophilia B mutations in Sweden: a population-based study of mutational heterogeneity. *Br J Haematol* 2001; 113: 81-86.

References

McGlennen RC, Key NS. Clinical and laboratory management of the prothrombin G20210A mutation. *Arch Pathol Lab Med.* 2002; 126: 1319-1324.

McVey JH, Boswell E, Mumford AD, et al. Factor VII deficiency and the FVII mutation database. *Hum Mutat* 2001; 17: 3-17.

Mammen EF. Ten years experience with the sticky platelet syndrome. *Clin Appl Thromb Hemost* 1995; 1: 66-72.

Mammen EF. Sticky platelet syndrome. *Semin Thromb Hemost* 1999; 25: 361-365.

Mannucci PM, Duga S, Peyvandi F. Recessively inherited coagulation disorders. *Blood* 2004; 104: 1243-1252.

Mannucci PM, Tuddenham EG. The hemophilias: from royal genes to gene therapy. *N Engl J Med* 2001; 344: 1773-1779.

Mannucci PM, Vigano S. Deficiencies of protein C, an inhibitor of blood coagulation. *Lancet* 1982; 2: 463.

Mariani G, Herrmann FH, Dolce A, et al. Clinical phenotypes and factor VII genotype in congenital factor VII deficiency. *Thromb Haemost* 2005; 93: 481-487.

Martinelli I, Taioli E, Cetin I, et al. Mutations in coagulation factors in women with unexplained late fetal loss. *N Engl J Med* 2000; 343: 1015-1018.

Michelson AD. Platelet function in the newborn. *Semin Thromb Hemost* 1998; 24: 507-512.

Middeldorp S, Meinardi JR, Koopman MM, et al. A prospective study of asymptomatic carriers of the factor V Leiden mutation to determine the incidence of venous thromboembolism. *Ann Intern Med* 2001; 135: 322-327.

Mikkola H, Palotie A. Gene defects in congenital factor XIII deficiency. *Semin Thromb Hemost* 1996; 22: 393-398.

Miletich J, Sherman L, Broze G Jr. Absence of thrombosis in subjects with heterozygous protein C deficiency. *N Engl J Med* 1987; 317: 991-996.

Miller JL. Platelet-type von Willebrand's disease. *Thromb Haemost* 1996; 75: 865-869.

Moake JL. Thrombotic thrombocytopenia purpura and the hemolytic uremic syndrome. *Arch Pathol Lab Med.* 2002; 126: 1430-1433.

Nair S, Ghosh K, Kulkarni B, et al. Glanzmann's thrombasthenia: updated. *Platelets* 2002; 13: 387-393.

Neerman-Arbez M, de Moerloose P, Bridel C, et al. Mutations in the fibrinogen Aα gene account for the majority of cases of congenital afibrinogenemia. *Blood* 2000; 96: 149-152.

Nurden AT, Nurden P. Inherited defects of platelet function. *Rev Clin Exp Hematol* 2001; 54: 314-334.

Pamukcu B, Oflaz H, Nisanci Y. The role of platelet glycoprotein IIIa polymorphism in the high prevalence of in vitro aspirin resistance in patients with intracoronary stent restenosis. *Am Heart J* 2005; 149: 675-680.

Poort SR, Michiels JJ, Reitsma PH, et al. Homozygosity for a novel missense mutation in the prothrombin gene causing a severe bleeding disorder. *Thromb Haemost* 1994; 72: 819.

Poort SR, Rosendaal FR, Reitsma PH, et al. A common genetic variation in the 3'-untranslated region of the prothrombin gene is associated with elevated plasma prothrombin levels and an increase in venous thrombosis. *Blood* 1996; 88: 3698-3703.

Press RD, Bauer KA, Kujovich JL, et al. Clinical utility of factor V Leiden (R506Q) testing for the diagnosis and management of thromboembolic disorders. *Arch Pathol Lab Med* 2002; 126: 1304-1308.

Preston FE, Rosendaal FR, Walker ID, et al. Increased fetal loss in women with heritable thrombophilia. *Lancet* 1996; 348: 913-916.

Rees DC, Cox M, Clegg JB. World distribution of factor V Leiden. *Lancet* 1995; 346: 1133-1134.

Reiner AP, Siscovick DS, Rosendaal FR. Platelet glycoprotein gene polymorphisms and risk of thrombosis: facts and fancies. *Rev Clin Exp Hematol* 2001; 53: 262-287.

Reitsma PH, Bernardi F, Doig RG, et al. Protein C Deficiency: A database of mutations, 1995 update—on behalf of the Subcommittee on Plasma Coagulation Inhibitors of the Scientific and Standardization Committee of the ISTH. *Thromb Haemost* 1995; 73: 876-889.

Rodeghiero F, Tosetto A. The epidemiology of inherited thrombophilia. *Thromb Haemost* 1997; 78: 636-640.

References

Roelse J, Koopman R, Büller H, et al. Association of idiopathic venous thromboembolism with single point-mutation at Arg506 of factor V. *Lancet* 1994; 343: 1535-1539.

Rožman P. Platelet antigens: the role of human platelet alloantigens (HPA) in blood transfusion and transplantation. *Transplant Immunol* 2002; 10: 165-181.

Rubbia-Brandt L, Neerman-Arbez M, Rougemont A, et al. Fibrinogen gamma375 Arg-Trp mutation (fibrinogen Aguadilla) causes hereditary hypofibrinogenemia, hepatic endoplasmic reticulum storage disease and cirrhosis. *Am J Surg Pathol* 2006; 30: 906-911.

Ruggeri ZM, Pareti FI, Mannucci PM, et al. Heightened interaction between platelets and factor VIII/von Willebrand factor in a new subtype of von Willebrand's disease. *N Engl J Med* 1980; 302: 1047-1051.

Schinella RA, Greco MA, Cobert BL, et al. Hermansky-Pudlak syndrome with granulomatous colitis. *Ann Intern Med* 1980; 92: 20-23.

Schloesser M, Zeerleder S, Lutze G, et al. Mutations in the human factor XII gene. *Blood* 1997; 90: 3967-3977.

Schrijver I, Koerper MA, Jones CD, et al. Homozygous factor V splice site mutation associated with severe factor V deficiency. *Blood* 2002; 99: 3063-3065.

Seligsohn U, Lubetsky A. Genetic susceptibility to venous thrombosis. *N Engl J Med* 2001; 344:1222-1231.

Seri M, Cusano R, Gangarossa S, et al. Mutations in MYH9 result in the May-Hegglin anomaly, and Fechtner and Sebastian syndromes. *Nat Genet* 2000; 26: 103-105.

Simioni P, Prandoni P, Lensing AW, et al. The risk of recurrent venous thromboembolism in patients with an Arg506-Gln mutation in the gene for factor V (factor V Leiden). *N Engl J Med* 1997; 336: 399-403.

Simioni P, Prandoni P, Lensing AW, et al. Risk for subsequent venous thromboembolic complications in carriers of the prothrombin or the factor V gene mutation with a first episode of deep-vein thrombosis. *Blood* 2000; 96: 3329-3333.

Sinzinger H, Kaliman J, O'Grady J. Platelet lipooxygenase defect (Wien-Penzing defect) in two patients with myocardial infarction. *Am J Hematol* 1991; 36: 202-205.

Svensson PJ, Dahlback B. Resistance to activated protein C as a basis for venous thrombosis. *N Engl J Med* 1994; 330: 517-522.

Tans G, Rosing J. Structural and functional characterization of factor XII. *Semin Thromb Hemost* 1987; 13: 1-14.

Thompson AR. Structure and function of the factor VIII gene and protein. *Semin Thromb Hemost* 2003; 29: 11-22.

Tollefson DM. Heparin cofactor II deficiency. *Arch Pathol Lab Med* 2002; 126: 1394-1400.

Tsai HM, Lian EC. Antibodies to von Willebrand factor-cleaving protease in acute thrombotic thrombocytopenic purpura. *New Engl J Med* 2002; 339: 1585-1594.

Uprichard J, Perry DJ. Factor X deficiency. *Blood Rev* 2002; 16: 97-110.

Weiss EJ, Bray PF, Tayback M, Schulman SP, et al. The platelet glycoprotein IIIa polymorphism PLA2 : an inherited platelet risk factor for coronary thrombotic events. *N Engl J Med* 1996; 334: 1090-1094.

White JG, Key NS, King RA, Vercellotti GM. The White platelet syndrome: a new autosomal dominant platelet disorder. *Platelets* 2004; 15: 173-184.

Wiener-Megnagi Z, Ben-Shlomo I, Goldberg Y, et al. Resistance to activated protein C and the leiden mutation: high prevalence in patients with abruptio placentae. *Am J Obstet Gynecol* 1998; 179: 1565-1567.

Wiman B. Plasminogen activator inhibitor-1 (PAI-1) in plasma: its role in thrombotic disease. *Thromb Haemost* 1995; 74: 71-76.

Zotz RB, Winkelmann BR, Nauck M, et al. Polymorphism of platelet membrane glycoprotein IIIa: Human platelet antigen 1b (HPA-1b/PLA2) is an inherited risk factor for premature myocardial infarction in coronary artery disease. *Throm Haemost* 1998; 79: 731-735.

Chapter 4

Nonneoplastic Hematologic Disorders

4: Nonneoplastic Hematologic Disorders

Red Blood Cell Cytoskeletal Disorders>Hereditary Spherocytosis; Hereditary Elliptocytosis/Hereditary Ovalocytosis; Hereditary Stomatocytosis

Red Blood Cell Cytoskeletal Disorders

Hereditary Spherocytosis (HS)

- HS manifests clinically as chronic hemolysis, jaundice, and splenomegaly. In the United States, the incidence is about 1 in 5000; in parts of Northern Europe, the incidence approaches 1 in 1000.

- While most families display autosomal dominant inheritance, about 1 in 4 show an autosomal recessive pattern. This variation derives from the fact that the HS phenotype can be caused by any 1 of several defects in cytoskeletal proteins T4.1, including band 3 (AE1), protein 4.2, spectrin, and ankyrin. The most commonly affected gene is the *ANK1* (ankyrin) gene located on 8p (about 60% of cases), followed by the band 3 (AE1) and spectrin β chain genes.

- The plurality of underlying molecular defects contributes to clinical heterogeneity, with phenotypes ranging from mild to severe, with some cases presenting at birth with neonatal jaundice. While the hemolytic anemia in some cases is quite severe, in most cases it is mild and well-compensated. Some patients require splenectomy, which usually results in clinical remission.

- The most characteristic complete blood count (CBC) abnormality is an *increased mean corpuscular hemoglobin concentration (MCHC)*. The mean corpuscular volume (MCV) and mean corpuscular hemoglobin (MCH) are usually normal but variable. The peripheral blood film shows numerous spherocytes, lacking in central pallor. The reticulocyte count is usually elevated. Typical of extravascular hemolysis, the lactate dehydrogenase (LDH) and bilirubin levels are elevated. Either the osmotic fragility or autohemolysis test may be used for screening.

T4.1
Red Cell Cytoskeletal Proteins

Cytoskeletal component	Associated diseases
Ankyrin (ANK1)	Hereditary spherocytosis
Band 3 (AE1)	Hereditary spherocytosis Southeast Asian ovalocytosis
Spectrin	Hereditary spherocytosis Hereditary elliptocytosis
Protein 4.2	Guanosine monophosphate (GMP)

Hereditary Elliptocytosis (HE)/Hereditary Ovalocytosis

- Like HS, HE is a phenotype that can result from several genotypes. By definition, more than 25% of circulating red cells are elliptocytes, defined as cells twice as long as they are wide.

- The incidence of HE, like that of glucose-6-phosphate dehydrogenase (G6PD) deficiency appears to vary with the historical incidence of malaria; presumably, these anomalies confer some survival advantage in malaria-ridden areas. The incidence varies from 1 in 2500 (United States) to 1 in 100 (parts of Africa).

- HE is usually inherited as an autosomal dominant disorder and most commonly caused by mutations in the spectrin α chain, resulting in defective formation of spectrin tetramers. However, many cases have been described in association with mutations in band 3 protein and protein 4.1.

- 3 types of HE are seen.

  □ The common type is found mostly in African Americans; the heterozygotes have mild or no hemolysis, while the homozygotes have moderate to severe anemia. A variant of common HE is hereditary pyropoikilocytosis (HPP), which is characterized by unusual sensitivity of red cells to heat. Most commonly HPP is a transient finding in neonates with common HE; HPP as a permanent aberration is rare.

  □ The spherocytic type results from double heterozygosity for HS and HE.

  □ The stomatocytic type, also known as Southeast Asian Ovalocytosis (SAO), is a common finding in Malaysia. It is caused by a specific band 3 protein defect (a 27 base-pair gene deletion resulting in a 9 amino-acid deletion resulting in a 9 amino-acid deletion) and confers protection against *Plasmodium vivax* malaria.

Hereditary Stomatocytosis

- Hereditary stomatocytosis is a group of autosomal dominant disorders in which red cells have an elongated, mouthlike, central pallor, in association with abnormal sodium and potassium permeability.

4: Nonneoplastic Hematologic Disorders

Red Blood Cell Cytoskeletal Disorders>Hereditary Stomatocytosis I Red Blood Cell Enzyme Disorders>Glucose-6-Phosphate Dehydrogenase Deficiency

- There are at least 2 main types: a more severe hydrocytotic (overhydrated) type in which red cells take on extra water, and a less severe xerocytosis type in which they lose water. Significant stomatocytosis, macrocytosis, moderate to severe hemolysis, and a low mean corpuscular hemoglobin concentration (MCHC) characterize the hydrocytosis syndromes. The membrane protein stomatin is decreased. The xerocytosis syndromes have normocytic red cells characterized morphologically by spiculated dessicocytes, mild stomatocytosis, and target cells. The gene for xerocytic hereditary stomatocytosis has been mapped to 16q23-q24.

- Hereditary stomatocytosis syndromes have a marked tendency toward thrombosis after splenectomy, so therapeutic splenectomy is generally avoided (and usually unnecessary).

- Stomatocytosis is also a feature of the Rhnull red cell phenotype.

Red Blood Cell Enzyme Disorders

- Red blood cell enzyme defects may cause chronic (eg, pyruvate kinase [PK] deficiency) or episodic (G6PD deficiency) hemolysis. Because these disorders are not associated with a spherocytic red cell shape, they are sometimes called chronic nonspherocytic hemolytic anemias.

Glucose-6-Phosphate Dehydrogenase (G6PD) Deficiency

- Even in normal circumstances, G6PD deteriorates over time such that reticulocytes have significantly more G6PD activity than older red cells. The most common forms of G6PD deficiency are associated with an accentuation of this pattern, in which red cell G6PD is exceptionally fragile and short-lived. G6PD is involved in the production of NADPH (the reduced form of nicotinamide adenine dinucleotide phosphate) through the hexose monophosphate shunt, which maintains glutathione, and consequently other proteins, in the reduced state when erythrocytes are subjected to an oxidant stress. When hemoglobin becomes oxidized, it precipitates as Heinz bodies. When red cells bearing Heinz bodies pass through the spleen, they are targeted by sinusoidal macrophages.

- G6PD-deficient red cells are therefore hypersensitive to sources of oxidant stress, such as certain medications, fava beans (hemolysis associated with ingestion of fava beans is called favism), and infection. Following oxidant exposure, the peripheral smear shows poikilocytosis, spherocytosis, Heinz bodies (with supravital dyes such as methyl violet, crystal violet, or brilliant cresyl blue), bite cells, and blister cells.

- There is a high prevalence of G6PD deficiency in Africa, southern Europe, the Middle East, Southeast Asia, and Oceania. Because G6PD deficiency is an X linked disorder, the main clinical manifestations are seen in males. In areas where G6PD deficiency is prevalent, homozygous females will also be affected.

- The gene for G6PD is found on the X chromosome. Several polymorphic and mutant alleles are prevalent in the population. These include the functionally normal alleles G6PD^B (the wild-type) and G6PD^A (a normal variant common in Africa and African Americans), as well as several abnormal alleles including G6PD^{A-} (common in Africans and African Americans), G6PD^{Med} (Sephardic Jews, Sicilians, Greeks), and G6PD^{Canton} (Asians). These mutants differ in severity, with G6PD^{Med} being most severe (even very young red cells are depleted of G6PD and steady-state enzyme activity is around 10% of normal) and G6PD^{A-} least severe (young red cells maintain adequate G6PD levels and the steady-state G6PD activity is in the range of 20%-60%).

- The consequences of these allelic differences are: (1) the rise in enzyme concentrations caused by reticulocytosis may cause G6PD activity to appear to be within the normal range if the G6PD^{A-} patient is tested while actively releasing reticulocytes (immediately after a hemolytic episode), but this effect is not seen in G6PD^{Med}, (2) the presence of young red cells imposes a limitation on the extent of hemolysis in G6PD^{A-}, a limitation that is not available to those with G6PD^{Med}, and (3) favism is a feature only of G6PD^{Med}. G6PD deficiency affects 12% of African Americans, most of whom have the milder G6PD^{A-} allele.

- Other inherited enzyme deficiencies involving the hexose monophosphate shunt are rare, including GSH synthetase deficiency, glutathione reductase deficiency, and gamma-glutamyl cysteine synthetase deficiency. These cause syndromes similar to G6PD deficiency.

Pyruvate Kinase (PK) Deficiency

- PK deficiency is usually a recessively inherited condition. The disease is rare but worldwide in distribution. There is a relatively high frequency in Northern Europeans and Pennsylvania Amish.

- PK catalyzes the rate-limiting step in the Embden-Meyerhoff (glycolysis) pathway, which is the main generator of adenosine triphosphatase (ATP) in red cells (which lack mitochondria). ATP depletion leads to impaired ion pumps, red cell dehydration, and finally hemolysis.

- PK deficiency is not the only known inherited glycolytic pathway enzyme defect, but it is the most common. Others, such as aldolase deficiency, hexokinase (glucokinase) deficiency, and glucose-6-isomerase deficiency have autosomal recessive patterns of inheritance; phosphofruktokinase deficiency is X-linked recessive.

- PK deficiency causes chronic hemolysis at a relatively constant rate, producing the usual manifestations of chronic hemolysis, such as gallstones, jaundice, and splenomegaly; the severity, however, differs from 1 patient to the next. Echinocytes (dessicocytes) are the classic peripheral smear finding, but these appear in large numbers only after splenectomy. The benefit of splenectomy is well established.

- 2 separate genes, *PKLR* (expressed in liver and red blood cells) on 1q21 and *PKM* (expressed in muscle and leukocytes) on 15q22, encode pyruvate kinase. *PKLR* transcription is under the control of 2 separate promoters, each resulting in a distinct transcript. 1 leads to translation of the R isoenzyme (present in mature red cells), and the other leads to the L isoenzyme (liver). Mutation of the *PKLR* gene results in a labile form of PK, leading to PK deficiency (unlike the anucleate red cell, the liver can compensate by making more PK).

Pyrimidine 5′ Nucleotidase Deficiency

- Red cell pyrimidine 5′ nucleotidase is responsible for the degradation of RNA that is present within reticulocyte (this degradation changes the tinctorial features of reticulocytes to resemble those of a mature erythrocyte).

- Unmetabolized pyrimidines precipite within the cell, recognizable as basophilic stippling, and cause hemolysis. Incidentally, lead inhibition of pyrimidine 5′ nucleotidaseis is the source of the basophilic stippling observed in lead poisoning.

Hemoglobin Disorders

Hemoglobin is a tetramer **T4.2** composed of 2 α chains and two β chains. The α genes are located on chromosome 16, and β genes are located on chromosome 11p15.5. There is 1 copy of the β gene on each chromosome 11, for a total of 2 productive genes in normal cells. In adult life, the capacity to produce β chain substitutes (δ and γ) is preserved; thus, diminished production of β can be partially compensated by increased production of HbA2 and HbF. There are 2 copies of the α genes on each chromosome 16, for a total of 4 alpha chain-producing gene loci in each normal cell. Even at birth, the capacity to produce α chain substitutes is lost; thus, there is no transcriptional way to compensate for α chain defects.

Hemoglobinopathy refers to the production of a structurally abnormal globin chain. Thalassemia refers to a quantitative abnormality of structurally normal globin chain synthesis. Thalassemia is most prevalent in the Mediterranean, Africa, and Southeast Asia, paralleling the prevalence of malaria.

Hemoglobin S

- The S allele has a valine in place of glutamate at position 6 of the hemoglobin β chain (β6glu→val). The S allele has persisted in parts of the world in which falciparum malaria is prevalent **T4.5**. In the United States, the vast majority of those carrying the gene are African-American.

- Sickle cell disease

T4.2
Normal Hemoglobins

Hemoglobin	Components	Role
Hb A	α2β2	Major adult Hb
Hb A2	α2δ2	Minor adult Hb
Hb F	α 2γ2	Major late fetal Hb
Hb Gower1	ζ2ε2	Major early fetal Hb
Hb Gower2	α 2 ε 2	Minor early fetal Hb

□ Results from inheritance of 2 S alleles (homozygous HbS, genotype SS). Sickled red blood cells result from the abnormal polymerization **T4.3** of deoxygenated hemoglobin S. These cells have a shortened survival in the blood, with an average lifespan of 17 days (compared with a normal lifespan of 120 days). The peripheral smear shows numerous sickled cells. Theoretically, sickled cells should return to their normal shape on exposure to atmospheric oxygen; thus, sickled forms on the peripheral blood smear are by definition irreversibly sickled cells (ISCs). The percentage of ISC is more or less constant in an individual and does not appear to predict or reflect episodic crises; however, it does seem to be correlated inversely with that patient's red cell survival.

□ Laboratory screening tests include the metabisulfite sickling test and the dithionate solubility test. The metabisulfite sickling test is based on the principle that metabisulfite promotes hemoglobin deoxygenation. The dithionate solubility test result is positive; in this test, lysed red cells are incubated with dithionate, which precipitates hemoglobin S. The diagnosis can be confirmed with electrophoresis, which shows more than 80% hemoglobin S, 1% to 20% hemoglobin F, 1% to 4% hemoglobin A2, and 0% hemoglobin A.

□ The clinical manifestations **T4.4** associated with sickle cell disease are not limited to those with the SS genotype, being more or less similar in sickle cell β^0 thalassemia, sickle cell disease (hemoglobin SC), and sickle cell β^+ thalassemia.

T4.4
Abnormal Hemoglobin Genotypes: Clinical Severity

Severity	Genotype
Clinically normal	AC, AS, AE, AG, AD, DD, S-α thal
Mild	EE, CC, OO
Moderate	SC, SD
Severe	SS, SO, S-β thal

□ Hemoglobin F, present at birth, has an inhibitory effect on hemoglobin S polymerization; thus, the manifestations of sickle cell disease are not apparent until hemoglobin S levels increase beyond 40%, usually at about 6 months of age. Likewise, in patients with combined sickle cell disease and hereditary persistence of fetal hemoglobin (SS-HPFH), clinical manifestations are milder than in SS. The lower intraerythrocyte concentrations of hemoglobin S associated with α thalassemia also lessen the hematologic and clinical manifestations of disease.

■ Sickle cell trait results from the inheritance of 1 S allele and 1 normal A allele (HbSA). The prevalence of sickle cell trait is about 10% among African Americans. SA is usually asymptomatic, but may manifest as mild isosthenuria and/or splenic infarcts at high altitudes, and a risk for renal medullary carcinoma. The peripheral blood smear shows no sickle cells. Results of the metabisulfite sickling test and dithionate solubility test are positive. The electrophoresis shows 35% to 45% hemoglobin S,

T4.3
Abnormal Hemoglobins: Functional Impact

Functional Impact	Predominant Findings	Examples
Polymerization	Hemolysis Crystals	Hb S, Hb C
Oxidation (precipitation/unstable hemoglobins)	Hemolysis Heinz bodies	Hb Köln, Hb Hasharon, Hb Zurich, Hb Hammersmith
Oxidation (methemoglobins)	Cyanosis	Hb M Boston, M Iwate, M Saskatoon, Hyde Park, Milwaukee
High oxygen affinity	Erythrocytosis	Hb Chesapeake, Hb Ypsilanti, Hb Denver
Low oxygen affinity	Cyanosis	Hb Kansas and Hb Beth Israel
Ineffective erythropoiesis	Thalassemia Microcytosis	HbE, Hb Lepore, Hb CS, α-thal, β-thal
None	None	Hb G

Hemoglobin Disorders>Hemoglobin S; Hemoglobin C; Hemoglobin E; Hemoglobin D & G; Hemoglobin Lepore; Hemoglobin Constant Spring

T4.5
β-Chain Variants

Variant	Amino Acid Alteration	Geography
S	6 Glu→Val	Africa
C	6 Glu→Lys	Africa
C-Harlem	6 Glu→Val and 73 Asp→Asn	Africa
E	26 Glu→Lys	Asia
D (D-Los Angeles, D-Punjab)	121 Glu→Gln	Europe, India
O-arab	121 Glu→Lys	Africa

less than 1% hemoglobin F, 1% to 3% hemoglobin A2, and 50% to 55% hemoglobin A. The roughly 60:40 ratio of A:S is caused by a greater affinity of α chains for βA chains over βS chains.

- S-α thalassemia (coinheritance of 1 α-thalassemia allele and 1 S allele) results in decreased hemoglobin S (compared with SA). The degree to which hemoglobin S is decreased is relative to the number of α-globin genes deleted. A single gene alpha gene deletion (-α/αα) results in about 30% to 35% hemoglobin S, while 2 alpha gene deletions (--/αα or -α/-α) result in 25% to 30% hemoglobin S.

- S-β thalassemia (coinheritance of 1 β thalassemia allele and 1 S allele) results in an increased proportion of HbS (S usually >50%). Disease manifestations can be quite severe, depending on the type of β thalassemia defect.

- SC disease (double heterozygosity for the S allele and C allele) results in about 50% hemoglobin S and clinical manifestations intermediate in severity between SS and SA. Red cells with hemoglobin SC have an average lifespan of 27 days (compared with 17 days for SS and 120 days for normal red cells). The peripheral smear is remarkable for mild sickling and abundant target cells.

Hemoglobin C (β6glu→lys)

- Hemoglobin C trait (heterozygous AC) has about 40% to 50% of hemoglobin in the in C band (HbA2 + HbC). C trait is generally asymptomatic, but the peripheral smear has scattered target cells.

- Hemoglobin C disease (homozygous CC) manifests 90% hemoglobin C, 7% hemoglobin F, 3% hemoglobin

A2, 0% hemoglobin A. There is mild hemolytic anemia, splenomegaly, and numerous target cells. Hexagonal or rod-shaped crystals may be found in the red cells, especially after splenectomy.

Hemoglobin E (β26glu→lys)

- Hemoglobin E is common in Southeast Asia. The complete blood count shows thalassemic indices and the peripheral smear contains numerous target cells.

Hemoglobin D & G

- Hemoglobin D and hemoglobin G are best considered polymorphisms of the β globin and α globin genes, respectively, because those with hemoglobin D or G are clinically normal.

- Cellulose acetate shows a band that runs with hemoglobin S and runs with hemoglobin A on citrate.

Hemoglobin Lepore

- Lepore is common near the Mediterranean, especially Italy.

- It produces a band that runs with S on routine electrophoresis (suspect hemoglobin Lepore whenever less than 30% hemoglobin S on electrophoresis). Actual hemoglobin S is rarely present in this quantity unless aggressively transfused. Hemoglobin Lepore is inefficiently produced so that it only comprises 8% to 15% of total hemoglobin .

- Hemoglobin Lepore is the result of a fusion between δ and β genes.

- Hemoglobin F may be as high as 20%.

Hemoglobin Constant Spring (CS)

- Hemoglobin CS causes thalassemic-type red cell indices. It results from a mutation in the α gene stop codon, producing an abnormally long transcript that is unstable. The αcs gene is thus inefficient, producing thalassemia.

- The termination codon TAA is mutated to CAA which, instead of indicating the cessation of transcription, encodes the amino acid glutamine. This mutation is common in Southeast Asia. If it arises in association with α-globin gene deletion (on the homologous chromosome), hemoglobin H disease can result.

4: Nonneoplastic Hematologic Disorders

Hemoglobin Disorders>Hemoglobin Constant Spring; Altered Oxygen Affinity Hemoglobins; Unstable Hemoglobins; Methemoglobin; β Thalassemia

- In the heterozygote, the hemoglobins produced are α-β (HbA), αcs-β (HbCS), α-δ (HbA2), αcs-δ (4 bands are seen in the adult on cellulose acetate electrophoresis). In the newborn, α-γ (HbF), and αχσ-γ are also seen.

Altered Oxygen Affinity Hemoglobins

- A group of hemoglobins with left-shifted (high oxygen affinity) or right-shifted (low oxygen affinity) oxygen dissociation curves.

- Examples of high affinity variants include hemoglobin Chesapeake, hemoglobin Ypsilanti, and hemoglobin Denver. Examples of low affinity variants include hemoglobin Kansas and hemoglobin Beth Israel.

- Most of these cannot be resolved on either gel electrophoresis or high-pressure liquid chromatography (HPLC), but the clue to their diagnosis is the common finding of erythrocytosis (high affinity) or cyanosis (low affinity). The Hb02 dissociation curve (P50) is diagnostic.

Unstable Hemoglobins

- A group of hemoglobins that are associated with characteristic peripheral smear findings of Heinz bodies and bite cells. Oxidative stresses may precipitate hemolytic crisis.

- Screening for unstable hemoglobins is carried out by incubating lysed red cells with 17% isopropanol which causes precipitation of unstable hemoglobins.

- Examples include hemoglobin Hasharon, Koln, and Zurich, but only hemoglobin Hammersmith is associated with severe hemolysis.

Methemoglobin (Hi, Hemiglobin)

- Methemoglobin (Hi) is the form of hemoglobin in which iron is in the oxidized ferric (Fe^{+++}) state instead of the usual ferrous (Fe^{++}), often resulting from oxidation of hemoglobin. It is incapable of combining with oxygen.

- Under normal circumstances, a small degree of hemoglobin oxidation occurs, and up to 1.5% of total hemoglobin is normally methemoglobin. The small amount of methemoglobin that normally forms is reduced in the erythrocyte by the NADH-dependent methemoglobin reductase system. Cyanosis results when methemoglobin reaches 10% of total hemoglobin or around 1.5 g/dL; at this concentration of methemoglobin, the blood is chocolate-brown on gross examination.

- Hereditary methemoglobinemia can result from either (1) deficiency in the methemoglobin reductase system, or (2) inheritance of an abnormal hemoglobin (HbM) on which this enzyme cannot act.

  □ The most common cause of a defective methemoglobin reductase system is inherited cytochrome b5R deficiency. This is inherited in an autosomal recessive manner and is particularly common in Navajo Indians and the Yakutsk of Siberia. Type I deficiency is mild, with cyanosis only, and type II deficiency is severe, causing neurologic deficits.

  □ Hemoglobin M is actually a group of hemoglobins that, because of various amino acid substitutions, prefer the ferric (methemoglobin) state, which binds oxygen poorly. Examples of hemoglobin M include hemoglobin M_{Iwate}, hemoglobin M_{Boston}, hemoglobin $M_{Hyde Park}$, and hemoglobin $M_{Saskatoon}$. Cyanosis appears at 6 months of age (for beta chain hemoglobin M) or at birth (for alpha chain hemoglobin M or those affecting a fetal hemoglobin). Most M hemoglobins run with A on routine gels.

β Thalassemia

- There is 1 copy of the β gene on each chromosome 11, for a total of 2 productive genes in normal cells. The β-globin (HBB) gene is regulated by an upstream (5') promoter sequence and an upstream regulatory gene known as the locus control region (LCR). Nearby (in the HBB gene cluster) are the genes for the delta globin chain, gamma globin chains, and a pseudo-HBB gene. A large number of possible abnormal alleles exist at the HBB gene locus (>200). The vast majority of these consist of point mutations. Large deletions are a feature of α thalassemia but are rarely seen in β thalassemia.

- Based on their impact on β globin chain production, these abnormal alleles can be categorized as βo alleles (result in complete absence of β chain production, usually the result of nonsense or frameshift mutations), β+ alleles (diminished β chain production, resulting from mutations in the promoter sequence, LCR, or 5' untranslated region), silent alleles (almost no impact on chain production because of mutation of the promoter's CACCC box or the 5' untranslated region), and complex alleles (fusion δ-β- and γ-δ-β-chains resulting from deletion of noncoding intervening segments of the HBB gene cluster). β^+Mediterranean tends to be more severe than β^+American seen in American blacks.

- Because of the large number of possible mutations, β thalassemia may be difficult to detect with targeted mutation analysis. Within any given ethnic group, however, particular molecular defects will be more or less common. Knowledge of ethnicity can guide the use of appropriate primers for amplification or dot-blot analysis. Failing this, direct sequence analysis can be undertaken.

- β thalassemia syndromes

  □ β thalassemia is most common in Mediterranean populations, and manifestations do not become evident until 6 to 9 months of age.

  □ β thalassemia minor **T4.6** typically results from inheritance of 1 abnormal β gene, either β^+ or β^0. On hemoglobin electrophoresis, one sees high hemoglobin A2 (<2.5%, usually 4%-8%) and normal hemoglobin F. Iron-deficiency anemia can mask these findings.

  □ In δ-β thalassemia (deletion of both the δ and β genes) the level of hemoglobin A2 is normal and hemoglobin F is elevated (5% to 20%); in heterozygous hemoglobin Lepore

(fusion of δ and β) the level of hemoglobin A2 is normal, hemoglobin F is slightly elevated, and a band in the S region comprises 6% to 15% hemoglobin (Hb Lepore).

  □ β thalassemia major results from inheritance of 2 abnormal β genes such as $\beta^0\beta^0$, $\beta+^{med}\beta+^{med}$, or $\beta^0\beta+^{med}$. Individuals are not anemic at birth but develop anemia within 1 year. The hemoglobin electrophoresis shows increased hemoglobin F (50%-95%), normal to elevated hemoglobin A2, and little to no hemoglobin A. β thalassemia intermedia and major (Cooley anemia) are distinguished by the dependence of the latter on transfusions.

α Thalassemia

- Each chromosome 16 carries 2 copies of the alpha gene, for a total of 4 alpha chain-producing gene loci in each normal cell. α-thalassemia syndromes usually result from a large structural deletion in the translated portion of the gene, but occasionally result from a point mutation in the untranslated region (eg, hemoglobin CS).

- 1 potential allotype, α thalassemia 2 (α^+ thalassemia) refers to a copy of chromosome 16 that has 1 normal and 1deleted alpha gene (-α/). This is the most common genotype in African Americans with thalassemia. Another allotype, α thalassemia 1 (α^o thal) refers to a copy of chromosome 16 that has 2 deleted alpha genes (--/). This is prevalent in Asians.

- Reduced synthesis of alpha chains results in decreased total hemoglobin production, leading to hypochromasia and microcytosis.

- Continued synthesis of a normal quantity of beta chains leads to its relative abundance and precipitation of these chains in the red cell, reducing the cell's lifespan. In α thalassemia, β4 tetramers (HbH) and γ4 tetramers (Hb Barts) form.

- α-thalassemia syndromes **T4.7**

  □ CBC findings typical of thalassemia ("thalassemic indices") include an elevated RBC count ($>5.5\times10^{12}$/L in men, $>5.0\times10^{12}$/L in women), low MCV (65 to 75 fL in α thalassemia, 55 to 65 fL in β thalassemia), low hematocrit, and normal to slightly increased red cell distribution width.

T4.6
β-Thalassemia Syndromes

Syndrome	Genotype
β thalassemia minor	α α α α α β/β⁺
	α α α α α β/β°
β thalassemia major	α α α α α β/β°
	α α α α α β⁺/β⁺
	α α α α α β⁺ / β°

T4.7
α-Thalassemia Syndromes

Syndrome	Genotype	Complete blood count	Electrophoresis
normal person	αα/αα	Normal	normal
silent carrier	-α/αα	Normal	normal
thal trait	-α/-α or --/αα	Thalassemic	normal
Hb H disease	--/-α or --/αCSα	Thalassemic Heinz bodies	fast-migrating Hb H Hb H = b4 tetramers.
Hb Barts disease (hydrops fetalis)	--/--	HypochromianRBCs	fast-migrating Hb Barts. Hb Barts = γ4 tetramers.

□ Peripheral smear findings include microcytic hypochromic anemia with occasional target cells (more in β thalassemia than α thalassemia), and basophilic stippling.

□ Double heterozygosity for β thalassemia and a structurally abnormal beta chain results in *increased* percentage of the abnormal beta chain, eg, in S-β thalassemia, hemoglobin S is more than 50% with hemoglobin F levels of 1% to 15%. α thalassemia leads to decreased percentage of abnormal beta chains, eg, in S-α thalassemia hemoglobin S is 30% to 35% with 1 alpha gene deletion, and 25% to 30% with 2 alpha gene deletions.

□ α thalassemia is most common in those of sub-Saharan African and southeast Asian descent. The α thalassemia 1 gene is prevalent only in Asians, who are at risk for the very severe kinds of α thalassemia (hemoglobin Bart and hemoglobin H diseases). The α thalassemia 2 gene is most prevalent in blacks.

□ Persons with single gene deletion α thalassemia are entirely asymptomatic, have normal CBC, and normal findings on electrophoresis. Though they are of interest clinically for genetic counseling, the hematology laboratory is of little use in identifying these individuals.

□ Persons with 2 gene deletions (α thalassemia trait) manifest a CBC with thalassemic indices and an electrophoresis with normal A and A2 bands. Hemoglobin A2 is not increased. In the absence of iron deficiency, this can be interpreted as consistent with α thalassemia trait. Unlike β thalassemia, the manifestations of α thalassemia are present at birth.

■ Most cases of thalassemia can be diagnosed in the hematology laboratory, with a combination of CBC data and electrophoresis (or HPLC). Genetic testing is available in reference laboratories. Most assays are aimed at identifying several of the most common deletions.

α-Thalassemia/Mental Retardation Syndrome

■ Mutations in the *ATRX* gene, a transcription regulator gene, are associated with a spectrum of syndromes, all sharing a component of X-linked mental retardation.

■ Other *ATRX*-related conditions are the Smith-Fineman-Myers syndrome, Carpenter-Waziri syndrome, Juberg-Marsidi syndrome, and the α-thalassemia myelodysplasia syndrome (ATMDS). Direct gene sequencing is available on a limited basis to detect mutations in the *ATRX* gene.

4: Nonneoplastic Hematologic Disorders

Hemoglobin Disorders>Hereditary Persistence of Fetal Hemoglobin | Disorders of Hematopoietic Cell Proliferation and Maturation>Pure Red Cell Aplasia/Blackfan-Diamond Syndrome; Fanconi Anemia

Hereditary Persistence of Fetal Hemoglobin

- HPFH results from a delayed switch from γ to β or δ chains.

- This can result from deletion of the beta and delta genes.

- Hemoglobin F is present in a pancellular distribution.

- HPFH by itself causes no clinical consequences. The main importance of HPFH is its ameliorating impact on other hemoglobinopathies. For example, combined sickle cell-HPFH is found in about 1 in 100 of those with homozygous HbSS. In these cases, hemoglobin F is about 25% and neither anemia nor vasoocclusive episodes are seen.

- An adult hemoglobin electrophoresis with hemoglobin S, F, and A2 has 2 possible causes: combined sickle cell-HPFH and combined sickle cell-β-thalassemia. These can be distinguished by the pancellular distribution in the former and heterocellular in the latter.

Disorders of Hematopoietic Cell Proliferation and Maturation

This group of disorders may result from inherited (germline) genomic abnormalities or acquired (somatic) abnormalities. Some of the latter group (eg paroxysmal nocturnal hemoglobinuria) are discussed here, others (eg, myelodysplastic syndromes) are discussed in chapter 15.

Furthermore, this group of disorders may concern a single cell line (eg, congenital neutropenia) or all cell lines (the many causes of aplastic anemia **T4.8**). In many cases, a disorder that initially affects 1 cell line progresses eventually to involve all cell lines (eg, Fanconi anemia); alternatively, many of these disorders may present as myelodysplasia (MDS), acute leukemia (usually acute myelogenous leukemia [AML]), or as a proclivity to solid tumors.

While it is common for these disorders to come to clinical attention at a young age, some (eg, Fanconi anemia) may present initially as aplastic anemia or MDS in an adult. Subtle physical anomalies, a family history, or a tendency to develop solid tumors may be the only clues at this point.

Pure Red Cell Aplasia (PRCA)/ Blackfan-Diamond Syndrome

- PRCA may be acquired (eg, in thymoma and infection with parvovirus B19) or congenital (the Blackfan-Diamond syndrome).

- Congenital PRCA is a rare, constitutional, red cell aplasia with an incidence of about 1 in 200,000. The median age at diagnosis is 3 months, with nearly all cases becoming evident by 5 years of age. Leukocytes and platelets are typically unaffected.

- Erythroid precursors in the marrow are typically sparse or absent.

- The i antigen is overexpressed on red cells, erythrocyte adenosine deaminase (ADA) is increased, and the hemoglobin F level is increased.

- About 75% of patients respond to corticosteroid therapy.

- Mutations in the *RPS19* gene (19q1.32) are found in about 25% of cases. Another locus, 8p23.2, appears to harbor a second disease-associated gene.

Fanconi Anemia

- Fanconi anemia is an inherited (autosomal recessive) chromosomal breakage syndrome (see chapter 9) in which, over time, aplastic anemia develops, usually by the age of 10 years. Often macrocytic anemia (or thrombocytopenia) exists in isolation for a period before pancytopenia emerges.

- Those who do not succumb to the complications of marrow failure may develop clonal hematopoietic defects, including MDS and AML. The predominant type of AML has monocytic differentiation (M4 or M5). The incidence of epithelial malignancies is increased as well, including cutaneous malignancies (squamous cell carcinoma), hepatocellular carcinoma, gastric carcinoma, and others.

- Associated findings include absent thumbs or radii, microcephaly, renal anomalies, short stature, café au lait spots, and elevated hemoglobin F.

- In several genes, certain mutations have been identified in association with Fanconi anemia, among which *FANCA, FANCC,* and *FANCG* account for the great majority of cases. Additional genes, such as *FANCB, FANCD1, FANCD2, FANCE, FANCF,* and *BRCA2,* have been reported, each accounting for about 1% of cases. If all genes are included, it is estimated that 1 in 300 Americans are carriers. The overall incidence is about 1 in 100,000, and particularly high incidence is present in descendants of white South Africans.

T4.8
Causes of Aplastic Anemic

Syndrome	Gene (chromosome)	Inheritance	Physical findings	Hematologic findings
Fanconi anemia	FANCA (16q24)	Autosomal recessive	Café-au-lait spots, thumb and radial anomalies, short stature, microcephaly	Initially anemia or thrombocytopenia, increased HbF, macrocytosis
	FANCC (9q22)			
	FANCG (9p13)			
Blackfan-Diamond syndrome	DBA1 / RPS19 (19q13.2)	Autosomal dominant	Thumb and radial anomalies, short stature, cardiac septal defects	Initially anemia, increased HbF
Dyskeratosis congenita	DKC1 (Xq28)	X-linked recessive	Nail dystrophy, reticulated skin pigmentation, oral leukoplakia, lacrimal duct atresia, testicular atrophy	Increased HbF, macrocytosis
	TERC			
Kostmann syndrome	ELA2 (19p)	Autosomal dominant	Severe infections, beginning in infancy	Initially neutropenia, uncommonly progresses to aplastic anemia
Congenital amegakaryocytic thrombocytopenia (CAMT)	CMPL (1p34)	Autosomal recessive	Thumb and radial anomalies	Initially thrombocytopenia
Schwachman-Diamond syndrome	SBDS (7q11)	Autosomal recessive	Pancreatic exocrine insufficiency, short stature	Increased HbF, macrocytosis
Reticular dysgenesis		Autosomal recessive	See chapter 9	
Down syndrome	Trisomy 21	Sporadic	See chapter 2	

- The screening test is based on the known hypersensitivity of Fanconi anemia cells to DNA cross-linking agents (mitomycin C, diepoxy butane, cisplatin). Cells grown in culture are exposed to 1 of these agents and their metaphase spreads examined. Increased chromosomal breaks, gaps, radials, and rearrangements are consistent with a diagnosis of Fanconi anemia.

Dyskeratosis Congenita (Zinsser-Engman-Cole Syndrome)

- Dyskeratosis congenita may initially present with leukopenia, anemia, or thrombocytopenia, but invariably these isolated cytopenias progress to pancytopenia.

4: Nonneoplastic Hematologic Disorders

Disorders of Hematopoietic Cell Proliferation and Maturation>Dyskeratosis Congenita; Congenital Dyserythropoietic
Anemia; Congenital Sideroblastic Anemia

- Other findings, many of which may precede cytopenias, include reticulated skin hyperpigmentation, nail dystrophy, oral leukoplakia, lacrimal duct atresia (causing overflow lacrimation), and testicular atrophy.

- Dyskeratosis congenita appears to have more than 1 genetic basis: both X-linked (most common) and autosomal (recessive and dominant) forms exist. In fact, dyskeratosis congenita has been associated with mutations in several genes, the common thread being telomere maintenance. *DKC1* (Xq28) encodes the protein dyskerin and is responsible for X-linked cases, while most autosomal cases are related to mutations in the *TERC* gene. Telomeres function in the stabilization of chromosome during DNA replication. They are composed of hexanucleotide repeats (TTAGGG) that are associated with a set of proteins (including telomerase) and nucleic acids whose function is to maintain the telomere. These include TERC (an untranslated RNA molecule), TERT (a reverse transcriptase), and the proteins dyskerin, GAR1, NHP2, and NOP10. Paucity or impaired function of telomerase leads to progressive shortening of telomeres with each round of cell division. At a critical length, the cell is signaled to stop dividing. Telomere shortening has been noted in patients with dyskeratosis congenita. Telomerase expression in tissue is proportional to the rate of proliferation; thus, it is high in hematopoietic cells (and many malignant cells).

- Anticipation, the finding of increased severity or younger age at onset in successive generations, usually thought of as a feature of trinucleotide repeat disorders, is found in many families with dyskeratosis congenita. This is believed to be the result of inheritance of progressively shorter telomeres (in addition to inheritance of the mutant allele).

Congenital Dyserythropoietic Anemia (CDA)

- CDA type II is by far the most common in this uncommon group of red cell disorders. It is recessively inherited and characterized by multinucleate erythroid precursors and a positive acidified serum test, hence the alternate designation of hereditary erythroblast multinuclearity with positive acidified serum (HEMPAS).

- There is an important distinction between the positive acidified serum (Ham's) test in CDA type II and that seen in paroxysmal nocturnal hemoglobinuria (PNH). In CDA type II, lysis is observed in heterologous serum only, whereas in PNH, lysis is seen in autologous

and heterologous serum. The positive Ham's test result in CDA II is because of an exceptionally high density of i antigen present on the surface of the red cells.

- The disease appears to be genetically heterogeneous, and to date no specific genetic test is available.

Congenital Sideroblastic Anemia

- The term *sideroblastic anemia* denotes a group of disorders unified by the presence of anemia and ringed sideroblasts in the bone marrow aspirate. The peripheral blood usually shows a hypochromic anemia that is microcytic, normocytic, or macrocytic. Microcytic presentations and the classically described bimodal red cell volume distribution are more common in inherited forms of sideroblastic anemia, while macrocytosis more often is seen in acquired forms. A type of basophilic stippling caused by iron-containing Pappenheimer bodies may be observed.

- In addition to ringed sideroblasts, the bone marrow shows increased iron stores and erythroid hyperplasia. A degree of dyserythropoiesis may be present. The serum iron concentration is elevated, percentage of transferrin saturation is high, and ferritin is high. Often, because of intramedullary hemolysis associated with ineffective erythropoiesis, there is hyperbilirubinemia, high LDH, and a drop in the serum haptoglobin.

- Sideroblastic anemia, particularly hereditary forms, must be distinguished from hereditary hemochromatosis, because both produce a clinical picture of iron overload. The low hemoglobin (and low MCV) should help in this distinction.

- Inherited sideroblastic anemia is rare and usually displays x-linked recessive inheritance. Some inherited sideroblastic anemias can be overcome with large doses of pyridoxine (B6). The responsible gene is most often *ALAS2*, found on the X chromosome, in which a large number of different mutations have been found. Inherited sideroblastic anemia usually manifests initially in childhood, and while organ dysfunction may occur because of iron overload in any of the sideroblastic anemias, it is particularly common in this form.

4: Nonneoplastic Hematologic Disorders

Disorders of Hematopoietic Cell Proliferation and Maturation>Paroxysmal Nocturnal Hemoglobinuria; Congenital Amegakaryocytic Thrombocytopenia; Thrombocytopenia with Absent Radii Syndrome; Pearson Syndrome; Isolated Neutropenia

Paroxysmal Nocturnal Hemoglobinuria

- PNH is an acquired clonal red cell disorder. The defect is acquired at the level of a hematopoietic stem cell, and the affected clone manifests a set of intrinsic defects on the cell membrane. Over time, this clone expands to dominate the red cell population and variable proportions of the white cell and platelet populations.

- In classic cases, patients are described as having episodic hemolysis, especially at night. Affected individuals more commonly develop a chronic normocytic, normochromic anemia. Over time, transient thrombo- and leukopenias develop. The bone marrow is hypercellular in early PNH, but evolution to aplastic anemia and/or AML is common.

- The affected red cells display a set of characteristic abnormalities, including diminished cell-surface decay-accelerating factor (DAF, CD55), decreased membrane inhibitor of reactive lysis (MIRL, CD59), decreased acetylcholinesterase (AchE), decreased CD16, and decreased CD48.

- Affected red cells are hypersensitive to complement-mediated lysis, as demonstrated in the sucrose hemolysis test the acidified serum (Ham's) test. The leukocyte alkaline phosphatase (LAP) score is decreased. Flow cytometry can demonstrate diminished CD59 and CD55 on the surfaces of leukocytes and platelets as well as red cells. When patients are studied serially using flow cytometry, the abnormal red cell population may initially be small in proportion. It expands with successive studies as the disease progresses.

- All of the phenotypic anomalies intrinsic to this clone appear to spring from a single molecular defect, decreased glycosyl phosphatidyl inositol (GPI) anchors. The GPI anchor is a protein whose function is to attach an array of proteins to the cell surface. Many of the GPI-anchored proteins function to deflect destruction by the immune system. The initial step in GPI synthesis is encoded by the phosphatidyl inositol glycan class A (*PIG-A*) gene located on the X chromosome. PNH is currently thought to be the result of various *PIG-A* mutations.

- Cytogenetic anomalies have been reported in some cases, without a single consistent finding. It is possible also to screen for *PIG-A* mutations, but this test is not currently widely available.

Congenital Amegakaryocytic Thrombocytopenia (CAMT)

- An autosomal recessive disorder that often presents in neonates with severe thrombocytopenia and the absence of megakaryocytes in the marrow.

- Progressive thrombocytopenia proceeds to pancytopenia by the second decade of life.

- Mutations of the thrombopoietin receptor (*MPL*) gene are the cause of CAMT.

Thrombocytopenia with Absent Radii (TAR) Syndrome

- TAR syndrome includes defective development of the bilateral radii and severe thrombocytopenia.

- Thrombocytopenia is most profound at birth and becomes *less* severe during the first year of life. TAR syndrome does not proceed to aplastic anemia.

- The molecular origin of TAR syndrome remains unknown.

Pearson Syndrome

- An extremely rare entity characterized by chronic pancreatitis, autosomal dominant inheritance, and marrow failure.

- The marrow shows sideroblastic anemia with vacuolization of precursors, and the pancreas shows fibrosis typical of chronic pancreatitis.

- The molecular defect is a microdeletion in the mitochondrial DNA.

Isolated Neutropenia

- Cyclic neutropenia, Kostmann syndrome (severe congenital neutropenia), Shwachman-Diamond syndrome, Dyskeratosis congenita, Chediak-Higashi syndrome, Myelokathexis (WHIM syndrome), and Fanconi anemia (chapter 9).

References

References

Al Fadhli S, Kaaba S, Elshafey A, et al. Molecular characterization of glucose-6-phosphate dehydrogenase gene defect in the Kuwaiti population. *Arch Pathol Lab Med* 2005; 129: 1144-1147.

Alter BP. Bone marrow failure syndromes in children. *Pediatr Clin N Am* 2002; 49: 973-988.

Alter BP. Molecular medicine and bone marrow failure syndromes. *J Pediatr* 2000; 136: 275-276.

Atweh GF, DeSimone J, Saunthararajah Y, et al. Hemoglobinopathies. *Hematology* 2003: 14-39.

Bagby GC, Lipton JM, Sloand EM, et al. Marrow failure. *Hematology* 2004; 318-336.

Bhardwaj U, Zhang Y, Jackson DS, et al. DNA diagnosis confirms hemoglobin deletion in newborn screen follow-up. *J Pediatr* 2003; 142: 346-348.

Baronciani L, Beutler E. Analysis of pyruvate kinase-deficiency mutations that produce nonspherocytic hemolytic anemia. *Proc Natl Acad Sci U S A* 1993; 90: 4324-4327.

Bender MA. Sickle cell disease. Available at www.GeneTests.org. Accessed March 7, 2006.

Benz EJ. Hemoglobin variants associated with hemolytic anemia, altered oxygen affinity, and methemoglobin-emias. In: Hoffman R, Silberstein LE, Benj EJ, et al, eds. *Hematology: Basic Principles and Practice*. 4th ed. Philadelphia, Pa: Elsevier Health Sciences, 2005.

Berliner N, Horwitz M, Loughran TP. Congenital and acquired neutropenia. *Hematology Am Soc Hematol Educ Program* 2004; 63-79.

Beutler E, Waalen J. The definition of anemia: what is the lower limit of normal of the blood hemoglobin concentration? *Blood* 2006; 107: 1747-1750.

Bizzarro MJ, Colson E, Ehrenkranz RA. Differential diagnosis and management of anemia in the newborn. *Pediatr Clinics North Am* 2004; 51: 1087.

Boxer LA, Stein S, Buckley D, et al. Strong evidence for autosomal dominant inheritance of severe congenital neutropenia associated with ELA2 mutations. *J Pediatr* 2006; 148: 633-636.

Brodsky RA, Jones RJ. Aplastic anemia. *Lancet* 2005; 365: 1647-1656.

Cao A, Rosatelli MC, Monni G, et al. Screening for thalassemia: a model of success. *Obstet Gynecol Clin North Am* 2002; 29: 305-328.

Carella M, Stewart G, Ajetunmobi JF, et al. Genomewide search for dehydrated hereditary stomatocytosis (hereditary xerocytosis): mapping of locus to chromosome 16 (16q23-qter). *Am J Hum Genet* 1998; 63: 810-816.

Chen FE, Ooi C, Ha SY, Cheung BM, et al. Genetic and clinical features of hemoglobin H disease in Chinese patients. *N Engl J Med* 2000; 343: 544-550.

Chen S, Warszawski J, Bader-Meunier B, et al. Diamond-Blackfan anemia and growth status: The French registry. *J Pediatr* 2005; 147: 669-673.

Clark BE, Thein SL. Molecular diagnosis of haemoglobin disorders. *Clin Lab Haematol* 2004; 26: 159-176.

Colosimo A, Guida V, De Luca A, et al. Reliability of DHPLC in mutational screening of beta-globin (HBB) alleles. *Hum Mutat* 2002; 19: 287-295.

D'Andrea AD, Grompe M. The Fanconi anaemia/BRCA pathway. *Nat Rev Cancer* 2002; 3: 23-34.

Delaunay J. The hereditary stomatocytoses: genetic disorders of the red cell membrane permeability to monovalent cations. *Semin Hematol* 2004; 41: 165-172.

Del Giudice EM, Francese M, Nobili B, et al. High frequency of de novo mutations in ankyrin gene (ANK1) in children with hereditary spherocytosis. *J Pediatr* 1998; 132: 117-120.

Dinauer MC, Coates TD. Disorders of phagocyte function and number. In Hoffman R, Silberstein LE, Benj EJ, et al, eds. *Hematology: Basic Principles and Practice*. 4th ed. Philadelphia, Pa: Elsevier Health Sciences, 2005.

Dokal I. Dyskeratosis congenita in all its forms. *Br J Haematol* 2000; 110: 768-779.

References

Dokal I, Vulliamy T. Dyskeratosis congenita: its link to telomerase and aplastic anaemia. *Blood Rev* 2003; 17: 217-225.

Drachman JG. Inherited thrombocytopenia: when a low platelet count does not mean ITP. *Blood* 2004; 103: 390-398.

Dror Y, Sung L. Update on childhood neutropenia: molecular and clinical advances. *Hematol Oncol Clin North Am* 2004; 18: 1439-1458.

Fibbe WE. Telomerase mutations in aplastic anemia. *N Engl J Med* 2005; 352: 1481-1483.

Gallagher PG. Red cell membrane disorders. *Hematology Am Soc Hematol Educ Program* 2005: 13-18

Gallagher PG, Jarolim P. Red blood cell membrane disorders. In: Hoffman R, Silberstein LE, Benj EJ, et al, eds. *Hematology: Basic Principles and Practice.* 4th ed. Philadelphia, Pa: Elsevier Health Sciences, 2005.

Gregg XT, Prchal JT. Red blood cell enzymopathies. In: Hoffman R, Silberstein LE, Benj EJ, et al, eds. *Hematology: Basic Principles and Practice.* 4th ed. Philadelphia, Pa: Elsevier Health Sciences, 2005.

Heimpel H, Anselstetter V, Chrobak L, et al. Congenital dyserythropoietic anemia type II: epidemiology, clinical appearance, and prognosis based on long-term observation. *Blood* 2003; 102 (13): 4576-4581.

Iolascon A, De Mattia D, Perrotta S, et al. Genetic heterogeneity of congenital dyserythropoietic anemia type II [letter]. *Blood* 1998; 92: 2593-2594.

Jeng MR, Vichinsky E. Hematologic problems in immigrants from Southeast Asia. *Hematol Oncol Clin North Am* 2004; 18: 1405-1422.

Kacena MA, Kirk J, Chou ST, et al. GATA1-related X-linked cytopenia. Available at: www.GeneTests.org. Accessed March 30, 2007.

Kiss TL, Ali MAM, Livine M, et al. An algorithm to aid in the investigation of thalassemia trait in multicultural populations. *Arch Pathol Lab Med* 2000; 124: 1320-1323.

Landmann E, Bluetters-Sawatzki R, Schindler D, et al. Fanconi anemia in a neonate with pancytopenia. *J Pediatr* 2004; 145: 125-127.

Marrone A, Dokal I. Dyskeratosis congenita: molecular insights into telomerase function, ageing and cancer. *Expert Rev Mol Med* 2004; 6: 1-23.

Marwaha RK, Bansal D, Trehan A, et al. Congenital dyserythropoietic anemia: clinical and hematological profile. *Indian Pediatr* 2003; 40: 551-555.

Mason PJ, Wilson DB, Bessler M. Dyskeratosis congenita: a disease of dysfunctional telomere maintenance. *Curr Mol Med* 2005; 5 (2): 159-170.

Prchal JT, Gregg XT. Red cell enzymes. *Hematology Am Soc Hematol Educ Program* 2005: 19-23.

Needleman H. Lead poisoning. *Annu Rev Med* 2004; 55: 209-222.

Pissard S, De Montalembert M, Bachir D, et al. Pyruvate kinase (PK) deficiency in newborns: the pitfalls of diagnosis. *J Pediatr* 2007; 150: 443-445.

Rosenberg PS, Huang Z-G, Alter BP. Individualized risks of first adverse events in patients with Fanconi anemia. *Blood* 2004; 104: 350-355.

Sgro M, Campbell D, Shah V. Incidence and causes of severe neonatal hyperbilirubinemia in Canada. *CMA J* 2006; 175: 587-590.

Steinberg MH, Benz EJ Jr, Adewoye HA, et al. Pathobiology of the human erythrocyte and its hemoglobins. In: Hoffman R, Silberstein LE, Benj EJ, et al, eds. *Hematology: Basic Principles and Practice.* 4th ed. Philadelphia, Pa: Elsevier Health Sciences, 2005.

Strippoli P, Savoia A, Iolascon A, et al. Mutational screening of thrombopoietin receptor gene (c-MPL) in patients with congenital thrombocytopenia and absent radii (TAR). *Br J Haematol* 1998; 103: 311-314.

Taniguchi T. Fanconi anemia (Fanconi pancytopenia). Available at: www.GeneTests.org. Accessed June 22, 2007.

Tischkowitz M, Dokal I. Fanconi anemia and leukemia: clinical and molecular aspects. *Br J Haematol* 2004; 126: 176-191.

References

Van Wijk R, Van Solinge WW. The energy-less red blood cell is lost: erythrocyte enzyme abnormalities of glycolysis. *Blood* 2005; 106: 4034-4042.

Vulliamy T, Marrone A, Dokal I, et al. Association between aplastic anaemia and mutations in telomerase RNA. *Lancet* 2002; 359: 2168-2170.

Yaghmai R, Kimyai-Asadi A, Rostamiani K, et al. Overlap of dyskeratosis congenita with the Hoyeraal-Hreidarsson syndrome. *J Pediatr* 2000; 136: 390-393.

Chapter 5

Renal Diseases

5: Renal Diseases

Inherited Nephritic Syndromes (Collagen IV-Related Nephropathies)>Alport Syndrome; Benign Familial Hematuria I
Inherited Nephrotic Syndromes>Congenital Nephrotic Syndrome of the Finnish Type

Inherited Nephritic Syndromes (Collagen IV-Related Nephropathies)

Alport Syndrome

- A spectrum of disease associated with derangements in collagen type IV ranges from Alport syndrome to thin basement membrane disease. Alport syndrome consists of glomerulonephritis, sensorineural hearing loss, and multiple ocular lesions (corneal, lenticular, and macular). It usually presents first with hematuria, a manifestation of glomerulonephritis that will progress eventually to end-stage renal disease.

- Several patterns of inheritance are seen, including X-linked recessive (80%), autosomal recessive (15%), and autosomal dominant (5%). In the most common X-linked recessive form, males manifest the full syndrome, while female carriers experience largely asymptomatic hematuria.

- The simplest way of making the diagnosis is through examination of skin or renal biopsies. The absence of immunohistochemical staining for the α5 chain of type IV collagen, α5(IV), supports the diagnosis. In fact, immunohistochemical staining of kidneys often shows complete absence of α3, α4, and α5 chains of type IV collagen. The immunohistochemical tests are imperfect, with normal staining seen in up to 20% of cases. Glomerular examination with electron microscopy (EM) shows a thin, disrupted, and inhomogeneous lamina densa, sometimes appearing multilaminar, that entraps rounded electron-dense bodies. EM may show scalloping of the epithelial aspect of the glomerular basement membrane.

- Unaffected family members of those with Alport syndrome have a high incidence of thin glomerular basement membranes and a clinical phenotype similar to that of benign familial hematuria.

- 3 genes, *COL4A3, COL4A4,* and *COL4A5,* have been associated with the collagen IV–related nephropathies. X-linked Alport syndrome is caused by mutations in *COL4A5,* on Xq22.3, which encodes the α5 chain of type IV collagen. Autosomal cases are caused by mutations in *COL4A3* and *COL4A4,* both on 2q36-q37, encoding the α3 and α4 chains of type IV collage, respectively.

- Alport syndrome with diffuse leiomyomatosis is an association for which several reports now exist. This appears to result from large deletions that span the adjacent *COL4A5* and *COL4A6* genes.

Benign Familial Hematuria (Thin Basement Membrane Disease)

- Thin basement membrane disease manifests as persistent hematuria, without proteinuria or progression to renal failure. It appears to represent a benign or heterozygous variant of Alport syndrome.

- Unlike Alport, there is normal staining for α3, α4, and α5 chains.

- Glomerular EM displays the diffuse uniform thinning of glomerular basement membranes that defines this entity.

Inherited Nephrotic Syndromes

Nephrotic syndrome is a common pediatric illness characterized by massive proteinuria, edema, hypoalbuminemia, and hyperlipidemia, and has numerous causes. The most common cause of nephrotic syndrome in the pediatric population is an *acquired* glomerular disease, minimal change disease, which usually arises between the ages of 1 and 10 years. Minimal change disease is exquisitely sensitive to steroids. As a result, children with nephrotic syndrome are often treated empirically with steroids, and improvement is taken as presumptive evidence of minimal change disease. In those who do not improve, other possibilities are considered, and a biopsy may be undertaken.

Congenital nephrotic syndrome T5.1, defined as nephrotic syndrome detected before 3 months of age, is less likely to be caused by minimal change disease. Congenital nephrotic syndrome may present just after birth but often begins in utero. Typical findings include dependent edema (dorsum for a neonate), abdominal distension, and a large placenta. Proteinuria (nephrotic-range), hypoalbuminemia, and hyperlipidemia are marked. The differential diagnosis must include certain perinatal infections (rubella, toxoplasmosis, syphilis, cytomegalovirus) and a group of inherited disorders (inherited nephrotic syndromes).

Congenital Nephrotic Syndrome of the Finnish Type

- The gene responsible for congenital nephrotic syndrome of the Finnish type is *NPHS1* (19q13.1), which encodes the protein nephrin, a key component of the glomerular slit diaphragm.

Inherited Nephrotic Syndromes>Congenital Nephrotic Syndrome of the Finnish Type; Pierson Syndrome; Nail-Patella Syndrome; Denys-Drash Syndrome; Familial Autosomal Dominant Focal Segmental Glomerulosclerosis

- Affected children are born in association with a markedly enlarged placenta. Massive proteinuria begins in utero, and the nephrotic syndrome is fully manifested by 1 month of age.

- EM is notable for an abnormal variation in the size of the slit pores (the space between podocyte foot processes) and rarefaction of the slit diaphragms.

Pierson Syndrome

- Nephrotic syndrome presents soon after birth and is associated with microcoria (fixed, narrow, pupils). Nephrotic syndrome results in death within several months.

- Renal biopsy shows mesangial sclerosis and crescents.

- Pierson syndrome is caused by mutations in *LAMB2* (3p21), a gene encoding β2 laminin, which is a component of the glomerular basement membrane.

Nail-Patella Syndrome

- Autosomal dominant disorder manifesting with skeletal and ocular anomalies, abnormalities of the nails, and renal disease. Renal involvement is variable, with some patients having nephrotic syndrome and others having none.

- The renal biopsy shows basement membrane expansion by what ultrastructurally appear as fibrillary collagen deposits.

- Nail-patella syndrome is caused by mutations in the *LMX1B* gene (9q34.1), which encodes a transcription factor (which regulates transcription of *COL4A3* and others).

Denys-Drash Syndrome

- The Denys-Drash syndrome is caused by a germline *WT1* gene (11p13) mutation and is associated with a high rate of Wilms tumors, male pseudohermaphroditism, and rapidly progressive renal failure. Glomerulonephropathy becomes apparent by several months of age and progresses to end-stage renal disease by the age of 3 years. The renal biopsy shows mesangial sclerosis.

- A related syndrome, also caused by mutations in *WT1*, is Frasier syndrome. In it, patients are predisposed to gonadoblastomas and progression to renal failure occurs more slowly.

Familial Autosomal Dominant Focal Segmental Glomerulosclerosis

- Mutations in *ACTN4* (α-actinin) are responsible for familial focal segmental glomerulosclerosis type 1, and mutations in the *TRPC6* (transient receptor potential cation channel 6) gene cause type 2.

- Onset of nephrotic syndrome in adolescence or young adulthood.

T5.1
Inherited Nephrotic Syndrome

Disease	Inheritance	Gene (Chromosome)	Comments
Congenital nephrotic syndrome, Finnish type	Autosomal recessive	NPHS1 (19q)	Nephrin gene
Pierson syndrome	Autosomal recessive	LAMB2 (3p)	Laminin β2 gene
Nail-patella syndrome	Autosomal dominant	LMX1B (9q)	LMX1B gene encodes a transcription factor that controls expression of nephrin and podocin
Denys-Drash	Autosomal dominant	WT1 (11p)	WT1 transcription factor gene
Familial FSGS	Autosomal dominant	ACTN4 (19q), TRPC6 (11q)	
Corticosteroid-resistant nephrotic syndrome	Autosomal recessive	NPHS2 (1q)	Podocin gene

5: Renal Diseases

Inherited Nephrotic Syndromes>Familial Autosomal Recessive Corticosteroid-Resistant Nephrotic Syndrome I Inherited Tubular Disorders>Renal Fanconi Syndrome I Autoimmune Renal Disease>Goodpasture Syndrome I PKD>ARPKD

Familial Autosomal Recessive Corticosteroid-Resistant Nephrotic Syndrome

- This syndrome is characterized by the onset of proteinuria in early childhood.

- The renal biopsy findings initially resemble mimimal change disease but often transform into focal segmental glomerulosclerosis.

- The disease is caused by mutations in the *NPHS2* gene which encodes podocin.

Inherited Tubular Disorders

A number of rare inherited diseases produce an isolated defect in tubular reabsorption. These may result in selective bicarbonate wasting (renal tubular acidosis), amino acid wasting (eg, cystinuria), and glycosuria.

Renal Fanconi Syndrome

- Renal Fanconi syndrome is a term that refers to a generalized defect in proximal renal tubular absorption, and its causes are numerous.

- Generalized proximal tubular dysfunction manifests as glycosuria, amino aciduria, phosphaturia, hypokalemia, and metabolic acidosis (bicarbonate wasting). Phosphaturia can cause rickets in children and osteomalacia in adults.

- Causes of *acquired* renal Fanconi syndrome include mainly toxic insults to the proximal tubule (myeloma kidney, urate nephropathy, and heavy metals). *Hereditary* diseases that cause renal Fanconi syndrome **T5.2** are of 2 types: (1) those that produce toxic insults to the proximal tubule (similar to acquired forms), and (2) those that are primarily defects in the proximal tubule (idiopathic renal Fanconi syndrome).

- Dent disease (X-linked recessive hypophosphatemic rickets) is caused by mutations in the *CLCN5* gene (Xp11.22), which encodes a chloride channel called ClCn-5.

Autoimmune Renal Disease

Goodpasture Syndrome

- Like many autoimmune conditions, Goodpasture syndrome displays a tendency to cluster within families. It does not display Mendelian inheritance, however, and has the markings of a multigenic disorder.

T5.2
Inherited Diseases that Cause Renal Fanconi Syndrome

Cystinosis (autosomal recessive)

Tyrosinemia type I (autosomal recessive)

Galactosemia (autosomal recessive)

Wilson disease (autosomal recessive)

Glycogen storage disease (autosomal recessive)

Idiopathic renal Fanconi syndrome (autosomal dominant)

Dent disease (X-linked recessive)

- Goodpasture syndrome most commonly affects young males, classic cases presenting with hemoptysis, hematuria, and proteinuria (non-nephrotic range). Hemoptysis predominantly affects *smokers* with Goodpasture syndrome, and it may be severe enough to require transfusion. Antiglomerular basement membrane (anti-GBM) antibodies can be detected in the serum.

- Renal biopsy shows segmental necrotizing/crescentic glomerulonephritis with the highly characteristic *linear* reaction of anti-IgG.

- The targeted antigen in Goodpasture syndrome is the α3 domain of type IV collagen. Such antibodies are sometimes produced after transplantation in Alport syndrome (because these patients are naïve to this epitope), causing a posttransplant Goodpasture syndrome.

- There is strong association between HLA-DR haplotypes and Goodpasture syndrome. Increased susceptibility is seen with the HLA-DRB1*1501 and DRB1*1502 alleles in particular. HLA-DR7 and HLA-DR1 appear to be protective.

Polycystic Kidney Diseases T5.3

Autosomal Recessive Polycystic Kidney Disease (ARPKD)

- ARPKD, also called infantile polycystic kidney disease, often first manifests as oligohydramnios. Echogenic cysts can be detected on prenatal ultrasound. Hypertension and respiratory distress are often present at birth, the latter a result of pulmonary hypoplasia as part of the oligohydramnios sequence. At birth, the kidneys are enlarged (palpable) by radially oriented "cysts" composed of ectatic collecting ducts, but the kidneys retain their reniform shape. This is in contrast to the large rounded macrocysts of the autosomal dominant variant. More than half of all cases progress to end-stage renal disease, usually within the first decade of life.

- Hepatic involvement is present to some degree in nearly all cases, but this becomes problematic only in those who survive into adulthood. The morphologic features are those of typical biliary plate malformations (see chapter 8): ectatic portal bile ducts, circumferential proliferation of ductules, and periportal fibrosis.

- Mutations in the *PKHD1* gene (6p) are responsible for ARPKD. Mutation scanning by denaturing HPLC identifies a mutation in more than 95% of cases. The large size of the *PKHD1* gene, however, makes direct gene sequencing impractical, and most mutations appear to be private (limited to a single kindred).

Autosomal Dominant Polycystic Kidney Disease (ADPKD)

- ADPKD, also called adult polycystic kidney disease, is the most common of the inherited polycystic disorders, with an estimated prevalence at birth of 1 in 500.

- Penetrance is essentially 100% by the 5th decade. Even before symptoms emerge, the kidneys display an impaired concentrating capacity (isosthenuria). Hypertension is ubiquitous, resulting from a reduction in renal blood flow, and may be the initial manifestation. Flank pain is common and may be

caused by cyst hemorrhage, cyst infection, intracystic tumor, and renal stones (the prevalence of renal stones is 20%, usually in the form of calcium oxalate or urate stones). About half of all cases progress to end-stage renal disease by the age of 60 years.

- In the kidneys, cysts arise from multiple parts of the nephron, are cortical and medullary, and highly variable in size. On gross examination, the kidneys are enlarged, with at least vague retention of the basic reniform shape.

- There has been debate regarding susceptibility to renal cell carcinoma (long-term dialysis–associated cystic disease is the only condition unequivocally associated with an increased risk), but tumors occur at a younger-than-usual age, are often multicentric and/or bilateral, and are very difficult to detect.

- Extrarenal manifestations affect primarily the liver, which is involved in 75% of cases (polycystic liver disease). Mitral valve prolapse is identified in up to 25% of cases, pancreatic cysts in about 10%, and intracranial berry aneurysms in 10% to 20%. Other findings include seminal vesicle cysts, arachnoid cysts, and dilation of the aortic root.

- In 85% of those with ADPKD, the cause is a mutation in *PKD1* (16p13). *PKD1* is located immediately adjacent to the *TSC2* gene of tuberous sclerosis, and "contiguous gene" syndromes with overlapping features of ADPKD and TS have been reported. The remaining 15% have mutations in *PKD2* (4q). *PKD1* and *PKD2* encode polycystins 1 and 2, respectively.

T5.3
Inherited Cystic Kidney Disease

Disease	Inheritance	Genes (Chromosome)	Proteins	Notes
Autosomal dominant (adult) polycystic kidney disease	Autosomal dominant	*PKD1* (16p) *PKD2* (4q)	Polycystin-1 Polycystin-2	Enlarged polycystic kidneys Hepertension Hepatic cysts Intracranial berry aneurysms
Autosomal recessive (infantile) polycystic kidney disease	Autosomal recessive	*PKHD1* (6p)	Fibrocystin	Enlarged polycystic kidneys Hepatic fibrosis
Nephronophthisis (medullary sponge kidney)	Autosomal recessive	*NPH1* (2q) *NPH2* (9q) *NPH3* (3q)	Nephrocystin	Medullary cysts

- The diagnosis can be confirmed with imaging studies alone, for which specific criteria exist; however, these findings are often not fully penetrant until about the age of 30 to 50, so molecular testing may be needed if earlier diagnosis is desired. When sufficient relatives are available and willing to be tested, the diagnosis can be made with linkage analysis. Informative microsatellites are adjacent to the *PKD1* and *PKD2* genes, which can be exploited for this purpose. Direct sequencing of the large *PKD1* and *PKD2* genes is difficult but can detect up to 85% of disease-causing mutations.

Glomerulocystic Kidney Disease (GCKD)

- GCKD is a rare disorder that presents in the neonatal period with large palpable flank masses. It may be very difficult to distinguish, clinically and radiographically, from ARPKD; however, it appears to be related genotypically more to ADPKD.

- Microscopic examination shows dilation of Bowman capsule and renal dysplasia.

Cystic Renal Dysplasia (Multicystic Dysplastic Kidney)

- This is a fairly common cause of flank masses in infants. It is apparently a noninherited disorder that may result from in utero obstruction.

- Kidneys are distinctly nonreniform in shape and contain a mixture of cartilage, cysts, and mesenchyme. Sometimes the disease affects only a segment of the kidney, but usually the entire kidney is involved, and occasionally it is bilateral.

Nephronophthisis (Juvenile Nephronophthisis, Medullary Sponge Kidney)

- Nephronophthisis is an autosomal recessive condition in which cysts arise at the corticomedullary junction.

- Various genotypic forms of the disease exist, leading to phenotypes that differ mainly in age at presentation.

- The *NPHP1* gene, on 2q, is mutated in juvenile-onset forms of the disease. These present in children as a renal tubular defect (Fanconi renal syndrome, impaired renal concentrating capacity, polyuria, polydipsia), sometimes in association with extrarenal anomalies (hepatic fibrosis, retinal degeneration). The *NPHP2* and *NPHP3* genes are mutated in adult-onset disease. Adult-onset cases have a similar presentation, without the extrarenal features.

Meckel-Gruber Syndrome

- The Meckel-Gruber syndrome is a rare autosomal recessive disorder that is associated with a wide and variable range of anomalies. The syndrome is uniformly fatal as a result of pulmonary hypoplasia or renal failure. The most consistent of these are polycystic kidney disease, polydactyly, and occipital encephalocele. Variable features of Meckel-Gruber syndrome include cleft palate, ductal plate malformations of the liver, and cardiac abnormalities. The incidence is about 1 in 100,000.

- An associated locus has been identified on chromosome 17q, named MKS1.

Potter Sequence

- Potter sequence refers to the numerous, often lethal, effects of low urine output in utero. Urine is important for maintaining an adequate volume of amniotic fluid, and it is the inhalation and exhalation of amniotic fluid that promotes growth and differentiation of the lungs. Furthermore, amniotic fluid protects the developing fetus from compression by the surrounding uterus. Thus, anything that markedly reduces urine volume can lead to a syndrome characterized by pulmonary hypoplasia and a typical physical appearance, known as Potter sequence (or Potter syndrome).

- The most common causes of Potter sequence include bilateral renal agenesis, urine outflow obstruction (posterior urethral valves), prune belly syndrome, and autosomal recessive polycystic kidney disease. Aside from ARPKD, these disorders are largely sporadic or multifactorial.

Bilateral Renal Agenesis

- Bilateral renal agenesis occurs with a frequency of about 1 in 3000 births, and it is the cause of about 1 in 5 cases of the Potter sequence. It is quickly fatal, largely because of pulmonary hypoplasia.

- Bilateral renal agenesis is often suspected when fetal ultrasound (performed for evaluation of oligohydramnios) fails to visualize a bladder (contracted because of lack of urine) or kidneys.

- It is thought to result from an event that interrupts development of the renal bud during the first trimester. Some cases have been associated with mutations in transcription factors or homozygosity for severely deleterious mutations in *WT-1*. Some cases occur in families with a high rate of other urologic anomalies, including unilateral renal agenesis.

Prune Belly Syndrome (Eagle-Barrett Syndrome)

- Prune belly syndrome is the triad of abdominal wall muscle flaccidity, urinary tract dilation, and bilaterally undescended testes. Though the genetic basis is unknown, it is thought that prune belly syndrome is an inherited disorder.

- Prune belly syndrome is rare and affects mostly males. It is believed that a severe urethral obstruction occurs early in fetal life, possibly because of the transient existence of an obstructing urethral membrane that subsequently recanalizes. Early obstruction is thought to impair the development of the abdominal wall musculature. Reestablishment of urinary outflow permits the development of adequate (though hypoplastic) lungs and kidneys. Nonetheless, the kidneys have some degrees of dysplasia, the prostatic urethra, bladder, and ureters are massively dilated, and the testes are usually intraabdominal. The bladder empties incompletely because its muscle, like that of the abdominal wall, is relatively flaccid.

Posterior Urethral Valves

- This is the most common cause of severe urinary obstruction in the neonate, affecting predominantly males. Posterior urethral valves are membranous cusps of tissue that form in the prostatic urethra and, while having a slitlike aperture, cause obstruction.

- Ultimately, this leads to hydronephrosis and/or renal dysplasia, in addition to the other features of Potter sequence.

References

Adeva M, El-Youssef M, Rossetti S, et al. Clinical and molecular characterization defines a broadened spectrum of autosomal recessive polycystic kidney disease (ARPKD). *Medicine* 2006; 85: 1-21.

Ariyurek Y, Lantinga-van Leeuwen I, Spruit L, et al. Large deletions in the polycystic kidney disease 1 (PKD1) gene. *Hum Mutat* 2004; 23: 99.

Belz MM, Fick-Brosnahan GM, Hughes RL, et al. Recurrence of intracranial aneurysms in autosomal-dominant polycystic kidney disease. *Kidney Int* 2003; 63: 1824-1830.

Bergmann C, Senderek J, Kupper F, et al. PKHD1 mutations in autosomal recessive polycystic kidney disease (ARPKD). *Hum Mutat* 2004; 23: 453-463.

Bergmann C, Senderek J, Schneider F, et al. PKHD1 mutations in families requesting prenatal diagnosis for autosomal recessive polycystic kidney disease (ARPKD). *Hum Mutat* 2004; 23: 487-495.

Bergmann C, Senderek J, Windelen E, et al. Clinical consequences of PKHD1 mutations in 164 patients with autosomal-recessive polycystic kidney disease (ARPKD). *Kidney Int* 2005; 67: 829-848.

Bonnardeaux A, Bichet DG. Inherited disorders of the renal tubule. In: Brenner BM, ed. *Brenner & Rector's The Kidney*. Philadelphia, Pa: Elsevier, 2004.

Buzza M, Dagher H, Wang YY, et al. Mutations in the COL4A4 gene in thin basement membrane disease. *Kidney Int* 2003; 63: 447-453.

Dell KM, Avner ED. Autosomal recessive polycystic kidney disease. Available in: www.GeneTests.org. Accessed March 21, 2006.

Dische FE, Weston MJ, Parsons V. Abnormally thin glomerular basement membranes associated with hematuria, proteinuria or renal failure in adults. *Am J Nephrol* 1985; 5: 103-109.

References

Falk RJ, Jennette JC, Nachman PH. Primary glomerular disease. In: Brenner BM, ed. *Brenner & Rector's The Kidney*. Philadelphia, Pa: Elsevier, 2004.

Ghiggeri GM, Caridi G, Magrini U, et al. Genetics, clinical and pathological features of glomerulonephrites associated with mutations of nonmuscle myosin IIA (Fechtner syndrome). *Am J Kidney Dis* 2003; 41: 95-104.

Guay-Woodford LM, Desmond RA. Autosomal recessive polycystic kidney disease: the clinical experience in North America. *Pediatrics* 2003; 111: 1072-1080.

Gubler MC, Knebelmann B, Beziau A, et al. Autosomal dominant Alport syndrome: immunohistochemical study of type IV collagen chain distribution. *Kidney Int* 1995; 47: 1142-1147.

Haas M. Thin glomerular basement membrane nephropathy: incidence in 3471 consecutive renal biopsies examined by electron microscopy. *Arch Pathol Lab Med* 2006; 130: 699-706.

Harris PC, Torres VE. Autosomal dominant polycystic kidney disease. Available in: www.GeneTests.org. Accessed June 6, 2006.

Hateboer N, Dijk MA, Bogdanova N, et al. Comparison of phenotypes of polycystic kidney disease types 1 and 2. *Lancet* 1999; 353: 103-107.

Hudson BG, Tryggvason K, Sundaramoorthy M, et al. Alport's syndrome, Goodpasture's syndrome, and type IV collagen. *N Engl J Med* 2003; 348: 2543-2556.

Johnson CA, Gissen P, Sergi C. Molecular pathology and genetics of congenital hepatorenal fibrocystic syndromes. *J Med Genet* 2003; 40: 311-319.

Kamath BM, Piccoli DA. Heritable disorders of the bile ducts. *Gastroenterol Clin North Am* 2003; 32: 857-875.

Kashtan CE. Alport syndrome: an inherited disorder of renal, ocular, and cochlear basement membranes. *Medicine* 1999; 78: 338-360.

Kashtan CE. Diagnosis of Alport syndrome. *Kidney Int* 2004; 66: 1290-1291.

Knebelmann B, Breillat C, Forestier L, et al. Spectrum of mutations in the COL4A5 collagen gene in X-linked Alport syndrome. *Am J Hum Genet* 1996; 59: 1221-1232.

Lilova M, Kaplan BS, Meyers KE. Recombinant human growth hormone therapy in autosomal recessive polycystic kidney disease. *Pediatr Nephrol* 2003; 18: 57-61.

Nagel M, Nagorka S, Gross O. Novel COL4A5, COL4A4, and COL4A3 mutations in Alport syndrome. *Hum Mutat* 2005; 26.

Ong AC, Harris PC. Molecular pathogenesis of ADPKD: the polycystin complex gets complex. *Kidney Int* 2005; 67: 1234-1247.

Qian Q, Li A, King BF, Kamath PS, et al. Clinical profile of autosomal dominant polycystic liver disease. *Hepatology* 2003; 37: 164-171.

Ramasamy R, Haviland M, Woodard JR, et al. Patterns of inheritance in familial prune belly syndrome. *Urology* 2005; 65: 1227.e26-1227.e27.

Ramirez-Seijas F, Granado-Villar D, Cepero-Akselrad A, et al. Congenital nephrotic syndrome. *Int Pediatr* 2000; 15: 121-122.

Ravine D, Gibson RN, Walker RG, et al. Evaluation of ultra-sonographic diagnostic criteria for autosomal dominant polycystic kidney disease 1. *Lancet* 1994; 343: 824-827.

Reynolds DM, Falk CT, Li A, et al. Identification of a locus for autosomal dominant polycystic liver disease, on chromosome 19p13.2-13.1. *Am J Hum Genet* 2000; 67: 1598-1604.

Rossetti S, Chauveau D, Kubly V, et al. Association of mutation position in polycystic kidney disease 1 (PKD1) gene and development of a vascular phenotype. *Lancet* 2003; 361: 2196-2201.

Rossetti S, Chauveau D, Walker D, et al. A complete mutation screen of the ADPKD genes by DHPLC. *Kidney Int* 2002; 61: 1588-1599.

Rossetti S, Strmecki L, Gamble V, et al. Mutation analysis of the entire PKD1 gene: Genetic and diagnostic implications. *Am J Hum Genet* 2001; 68: 46-63.

References

Rossetti S, Torra R, Coto E, et al. A complete mutation screen of PKHD1 in autosomal-recessive polycystic kidney disease (ARPKD) pedigrees. *Kidney Int* 2003; 64: 391-403.

Sampson JR, Maheshwar MM, Aspinwall R, et al. Renal cystic disease in tuberous sclerosis: role of the polycystic kidney disease 1 gene. *Am J Hum Genet* 1997; 61: 843–851.

Tiebosch AT, Frederik PM, van Breda Vriesman PJ, et al. Thin-basement-membrane nephropathy in adults with persistent hematuria. *N Engl J Med* 1989; 320: 14–18.

Torres VE, Wilson DM, Hattery RR, et al. Renal stone disease in autosomal dominant polycystic kidney disease. *Am J Kidney Dis* 1993; 22: 513–519.

Tryggvason K, Patrakka J, Wartiovaara J. Hereditary proteinuria syndromes and mechanisms of proteinuria. *N Engl J Med* 2006; 354: 1387–1401.

Van De Voorde R, Witte D, Kogan J, Goebel J. Pierson syndrome: a novel cause of congenital nephrotic syndrome. *Pediatrics* 2006; 118; e501–e505.

Wilson PD. Mechanisms of disease: polycystic kidney disease. *N Engl J Med* 2004; 350: 151–164.

Chapter 6

Cardiovascular Disease

6: Cardiovascular Disease

Cardiac Conduction Disorders (Cardiac Channelopathies)>Brugada Syndrome; Arrhythmogenic Right Ventricular Dysplasia; The Long QT Syndromes

Cardiac Conduction Disorders (Cardiac Channelopathies)

Brugada Syndrome

- In Southeast Asia, where Brugada syndrome is most prevalent, it has been called by various names: the "sleep death" (Laos), "sudden and unexpected death in sleep" (Japan), and "to rise and moan in sleep" (Philippines). Also called SUDS (sudden unexpected nocturnal death syndrome), Brugada syndrome occurs in young, healthy men in whom death occurs suddenly (with a moan), usually during sleep. An autosomal dominant pattern of inheritance is noted in affected kindreds, and the incidence is higher in males.

- Those affected have a very high risk of ventricular arrhythmias and may present with electrocardiographic (ECG) abnormalities, cardiac rhythm disturbances, or sudden cardiac death (SUDS). While most cases are diagnosed in adults, the syndrome may present as sudden infant death syndrome (SIDS).

- A characteristic ECG pattern includes right bundle branch block with ST segment elevation in the right chest leads V1-V3.

- The *SCN5A* gene, on 3p21, encodes a subunit of the sodium channel. Mutations in this gene are the cause of about 1 in 4 cases, the remaining cases having as yet undetermined causes. Direct sequence analysis is clinically available for this gene. Interestingly, mutations in *SCN5A* are also responsible for 1 type of the long QT syndrome (LQT type 3).

Arrhythmogenic Right Ventricular Dysplasia (ARVD, Uhl Anomaly)

- Another suspect in the sudden cardiac death scenario is ARVD, characterized by cardiac conduction disturbances in association with the histologic findings of fatty and fibrous replacement of the right ventricular wall. While the dominant features are arrhythmia and right-sided anatomic findings, it is now clear that heart failure and left-sided disease can occur.

- Clinically, ARVD typically affects young adult males. Most cases are diagnosed between the ages of 15 and 40 years, most commonly as a result of sudden cardiac death, syncope, right heart or biventricular failure, or an episode of ventricular tachycardia. A right bundle branch block and/or T-wave inversion in leads V1-V3 are common during episodes of ventricular

tachycardia. These features have led to comparisons with Brugada syndrome and some to conjecture that these represent a single entity.

- ARVD accounts for up to 20% of sudden cardiac deaths in young adults, especially those occurring during physical activity. This association with physical activity and the finding of histologic abnormalities in the right ventricle are 2 key differences with Brugada syndrome.

- The clinical diagnosis of ARVD often begins with ECG and 24-hour Holter monitoring. In addition, some advocate formal invasive electrophysiological (EP) testing, magnetic resonance imaging (MRI), and/or right ventricular endomyocardial biopsy.

- Several genes have been associated with ARVD: *RYR2* (ARVD2) on 1q, that encodes the cardiac ryanodine receptor protein; *DSP* (ARVD8) on 6p, that encodes desmoplakin; and *PKP2* (ARVD9) also on 6p, that encodes plakophilin-2. Molecular genetic testing is available in the form of direct sequence analysis of the *RYR2, DSP,* and *PKP2* genes.

- An autosomal recessive form of ARVD that is associated with cutaneous findings and wooly hair has been called Naxos disease (after the Greek island in which it was first discovered).

- It seems that a clinicopathologic picture similar to inherited ARVD can be caused by Coxsackievirus B3.

The Long QT Syndromes (LQTS)

- The QT interval is the section on the ECG tracing between the QRS complex (a reflection of left ventricular contraction) and the T wave (cardiac repolarization). The length of the QT interval is somewhat variable from person to person and within an individual over time. The QT interval increases with decreasing heart rate as well, and the QT interval must be corrected for heart rate (QTc). Those with a persistently prolonged QT interval are prone to develop ventricular arrhythmias, including the type of ventricular tachycardia known as torsade de pointes. Ventricular arrhythmias may manifest as syncope or sudden cardiac death.

- A long QT interval occurs **T6.1** because of either a defect in ion balance or a defect in ion channels, and this defect may be acquired or inherited. The *inherited* long QT syndromes have traditionally been divided, according to clinical presentation, into the *Romano-Ward syndrome* (autosomal dominant,

Cardiac Conduction Disorders (Cardiac Channelopathies)>The Long QT Syndromes

no hearing loss) and the *Jervell Lange-Nielsen syndrome* (autosomal recessive, with hearing loss). A very rare type of long QT syndrome is the *Anderson-Tawil syndrome*. More recently, there has been a tendency to classify them according to their genotype: LQTS1 through LQTS7.

- Despite autosomal inheritance there is a 2:1 female predominance in clinically significant long QT syndrome. Even in normal adults, the QT interval is somewhat longer in women than in men. Furthermore, estrogen appears to downregulate the implicated channels on cardiac myocytes. Thus, the disease has greater *penetrance* in females. An additional factor appears to be operative in the form of so-called transmission distortion (positive selection of the mutated allele in females); however, the mechanism for this is not known.

- Romano-Ward is the most common form of inherited long QT syndrome, with autosomal dominant inheritance and an estimated prevalence of 1:7000. The diagnosis can be made with relative confidence when there is a prolonged QT interval, particularly when a familial autosomal dominant pattern can be established, in the *absence* of sensorineural hearing loss.

- Jervell and Lange-Nielsen syndrome (JLNS), in contrast, is autosomal recessive and associated with bilateral sensorineural hearing loss. Classic cases of JLNS present with congenital hearing loss in a child who experiences syncopal episodes during periods of stress, often ending in sudden cardiac death at a young age.

- At least 6 gene loci are known to be associated with LQTS: LQT1 to LQT7. In general, heterozygous mutations in these genes cause Romano-Ward syndrome, and homozygous (or compound heterozygous) mutations cause JLNS.

  □ LQT1 (the *KCNQ1* gene) is located at 11p15.5. It encodes a portion of a voltage-gated potassium channel. While this is the most commonly mutated gene in the long QT syndrome, most specific mutations are "private" (confined to a single kindred).

  □ LQT2 (*KCNH2*, previously called *HERG*) is located at 7q35-36. It encodes a second voltage-activated potassium channel and is the second most commonly affected gene in LQTS.

  □ LQT3 (*SCN5A*) is located at 3p21-25. It encodes a sodium channel.

  □ LQT4 (*ANKB* or Ankyrin-B gene) is located at 4q25-27. Its gene product appears to anchor ion channels.

  □ LQT5 (*mink* or *KCNE1*) is located at 21q22.1. It encodes a small protein that associates noncovalently with transmembrane ion channels (KCNQ1, KCNH2, etc) and appears to be necessary for their proper function.

  □ LQT6 (*MiRP1* or *KCNE2*) encodes a channel-associated product similar to minK. It is thought to be located close to mink on 21q22.1.

- Interestingly, the trigger for a fatal arrhythmia in those with LQT1 mutations is quite predictably exercise, *especially swimming*. The LQT2 gene is associated most commonly with auditory stimuli or emotional stress as the triggering stimulus. LQT3 patients most often suffer their fatal arrhythmia at sleep. All genes appear to encode portions of a voltage-gated transmembrane potassium channel protein.

T6.1
Differential Diagnosis: Long QT Interval

Inherited	Acquired
Romano-Ward syndrome (LQTS1 – LQTS5)	Hypokalemia
Jervell Lange Nielsen syndrome	Hypomagnesemia
	Hypercalcemia
Andersen-Tawil syndrome	Medications (tricyclic antidepressants, phenothiazines, macrolide antibiotics, class IA antiarrhytmics, class III antiarrhythmics)

6: Cardiovascular Disease

Cardiac Conduction Disorders (Cardiac Channelopathies)>Catecholamine-Induced Polymorphic Ventricular Tachycardia I
Myocardial Disorders>Dilated Cardiomyopathy; Hypertrophic Cardiomyopathy; Restrictive Cardiomyopathy

- Lastly, mutations in *KCNJ2* (LQT7), a gene encoding portions of a channel shared with skeletal muscle have been identified in patients with Andersen-Tawil syndrome, which is composed of a clinical triad including episodic (periodic) paralysis of the skeletal muscles, long QT interval, and dysmorphic features.

Catecholamine-Induced Polymorphic Ventricular Tachycardia (CPVT)

- CPVT is characterized by syncope occurring during exercise or acute emotional stimuli.

- Mutations in either the *CASQ2* or *RYR2* gene result in this clinical phenotype. *CASQ2* mutations cause autosomal recessive disease, and RYR2 mutations cause disease with autosomal dominant inheritance.

- Calsequestrin 2 is a calcium-binding protein located in the sarcoplasmic reticulum in cardiac myocytes. It is encoded by the *CASQ2* gene on chromosome 1.

- The cardiac ryanodine receptor channel is encoded by *RYR2*, also on chromosome 1. This should be distinguished from *RYR1*, which is associated with malignant hyperthermia.

Myocardial Disorders T6.2

Dilated Cardiomyopathy

- Historically, dilated cardiomyopathy was attributed to 1 of 4 etiologies: myocarditis (coxsackie B, Chagas disease, diphtheria, human immunodeficiency virus [HIV], sarcoidosis), toxin (alcohol, adriamycin), pregnancy, and idiopathic. Many previously idiopathic cases are now known to result from several molecular defects, together accounting for about 30% of cases.

- Dilated cardiomyopathy presents with congestive heart failure and a progressively dwindling ejection fraction. Most patients die within 5 years, from either decompensated heart failure or arrhythmia.

- In About 30% of cases there is a family history. Most such cases display an autosomal dominant inheritance pattern. X-linked dilated cardiomyopathy has been linked to mutations in the dystrophin gene. The same gene is implicated in Duchenne and Becker muscular dystrophy, syndromes in which heart failure is common in those who survive to adulthood. Autosomal dominant dilated cardiomyopathy has been associated with a large number of mutations, most commonly in the *MYH7* gene encoding β-myosin heavy chain (also involved in some cases of hypertrophic cardiomyopathy).

Hypertrophic Cardiomyopathy (Idiopathic Hypertrophic Subaortic Stenosis)

- Sudden death is a frequent presentation of hypertrophic cardiomyopathy, and this is 1 of the most common causes of sudden death in young adults. The overall incidence is estimated by ultrasound studies to be 1 in 500. The pattern of inheritance is autosomal dominant.

- Examination of the heart reveals myocardial hypertrophy with disproportionate thickening of the ventricular septum compared with the left ventricular free wall (asymmetric septal hypertrophy). In some cases, however, hypertrophy is symmetrical. The sonographic and gross anatomic findings can be closely mimicked by amyloidosis and hypertensive heart disease. Histologically, hypertrophic cardiomyopathy displays myocyte hypertrophy, myofiber disarray with prominent myocyte branching, and interstitial fibrosis.

- Hypertrophic cardiomyopathy may result from any 1 of several mutations, usually in genes that encode sarcomeric proteins. The large number of affected proteins and the variety of mutations in the encoding genes accounts for a great deal of clinical diversity. The most commonly implicated mutation is the R403Q mutation in the *MYH7* (β-myosin heavy chain) gene found on 14q. Other mutations involve cardiac troponin T, cardiac troponin I, tropomyosin, myosin, and actin.

Restrictive Cardiomyopathy

- This pattern of myocardial disease is usually acquired, common causes including radiation fibrosis, amyloidosis, sarcoidosis, and metastatic tumor. Inherited causes are rare and include inborn errors of metabolism and endocardial fibroelastosis.

- Endocardial fibroelastosis is a very rare condition in which there is diffuse thickening of the left ventricular endocardium. This results in decreased compliance and impaired diastolic function (restrictive cardiomyopathy). The disease often presents in infants, in whom postmortem examination finds excessive subendocardial deposition of collagen and elastic fibers. The most common form displays X-linked recessive inheritance.

T6.2
Myocardial Disorders

Features	Dilated	Restrictive	Hypertrophic
Etiologies	Ischemia Myocarditis Toxin (alcohol, adriamycin) Sarcoidosis Hemochromatosis Pregnancy Inherited (30%)	Amyloidosis Sarcoidosis Endomyocardial fibrosis Loeffler's endomyocarditis Endocardial fibroelastosis Radiation	Inherited (>50%)
Manifestations	Congestive heart failure 4-chamber dilation Mural thrombi	Diastolic dysfunction	Angina, Sudden death Atrial fibrillation
Ejection fraction	Low	Low to normal	High
Ventricular wall	Thin	Normal	Thick, with disproportionate septal thickening
Cardiomegaly	Marked	Mild	Moderate (globular heart)

- Endocardial fibroelastosis should be distinguished from the entity known as endomyocardial fibrosis. The latter is principally a disease of children living in tropical areas. It is characterized by fibrosis of the ventricular endocardium and superficial myocardium which characteristically begins at the apex and spreads toward the base. The causes are unknown.

Familial Cardiac Amyloidosis (Transthyretin Amyloidosis, Familial Amyloid Polyneuropathy)

- In the past, tissue biopsy or immunometric techniques were employed to detect transthyretin amyloid. Molecular assays capable of detecting nearly 100% of disease-causing alleles are now available for mutations in the *TTR* gene.

- Familial cardiac amyloidosis usually presents in the third or fourth decade with a combination of peripheral neuropathy (dysautonomic and sensorimotor), cardiomyopathy, and cardiac conduction blocks.

Nephropathy, leptomeningeal amyloidosis, and vitreous opacities may also be seen. Some individuals have solely cardiac or leptomeningeal involvement, without any other features. In the past, the isolated cardiac variety has been referred to as *senile cardiac amyloidosis*, and it has been associated with specific *TTR* gene mutations. Likewise, isolated leptomeningeal type has been called *cerebral amyloid angiopathy*, and it has been linked to specific *TTR* mutations.

- Transthyretin amyloidosis displays autosomal dominant inheritance. The disease shows pockets of high prevalence in Portugal, Sweden, Japan, and parts of Africa. The frequency of TTR amyloidosis is about 1 in 500 in northern Portugal. In the United States, it is about 1 in 100,000 among Caucasians, but estimated to be much higher in African-Americans.

- The *TTR* gene is located on 18q and encodes transthyretin. Targeted mutation analysis for the most common V30M mutation, can detect about 30% to 45% of affected persons. Direct sequence analysis can detect nearly 100%.

6: Cardiovascular Disease

Myocardial Disorders>Skeletal Muscle Disorders | Coronary Artery Disorders>eNOS Deficiency; Inherited Conditions that Promote Atherosclerosis and Thrombosis | Structural Disorders>Single-Gene Disorders Resulting in Structural Cardiac Defects

Skeletal Muscle Disorders

- Several of the diseases customarily thought of as skeletal muscle disorders also affect the myocardium (see chapter 11).

Coronary Artery Disorders

Endothelial Nitric Oxide Synthase (eNOS) Deficiency

- Nitric oxide is a paracrine agent that induces vasodilation.
- A deficiency in nitric oxide has been associated with coronary vascular disease.
- A mutation in the *eNOS* gene results in decreased synthesis of nitric oxide and an increased risk for coronary artery disease (thought to be on the basis of coronary spasm).

Inherited Conditions that Promote Atherosclerosis

- See chapter 10

Inherited Conditions that Promote Thrombosis

- See chapter 3

Structural Disorders

Single-Gene Disorders Resulting in Structural Cardiac Defects

- *NKX2-5* mutations
  - The *NKX2-5* gene on chromosome 5q34 encodes a transcription factor that is expressed very early in cardiogenesis and appears to be responsible for activating transcription of most genes involved in the process.
  - Mutations in *NKX2-5* have been identified in patients with a large variety of structural malformations.
- *GATA-4* mutations
  - *GATA-4,* a gene located on 8p, encodes a transcription factor that is important in cardiac embryogenesis.
  - Rare kindreds have been identified that carry germline *GATA-4* mutations and have

autosomally inherited septal defects, especially ostium secundum atrial septal defects.

- *TBX-5* mutations: Holt-Oram syndrome (heart-hand syndrome)
  - An autosomal dominant disorder combining characteristic heart and upper limb anomalies. Upper limb malformations may involve the radius, thumb phalanges, or carpal bones, and they range from severe (phocomelia) to minimal (carpal bone deformities, present in nearly all patients). These are usually bilateral and symmetrical, and if asymmetrical, the left is more severely affected.
  - Cardiac malformations most commonly take the form of septal defects, especially secundum atrial septal or muscular ventricular septal defects.
  - Mutations in the *TBX5* (T-box) gene (on 12q) are responsible for about 70% of cases. Direct DNA sequencing of the *TBX5* gene is clinically available.
- *TBX-1* mutations: DiGeorge syndrome
  - *TBX-1* is found on 22q and is contained within the region commonly deleted in DiGeorge syndrome (See Chapter 2).
- *PTPN11* mutations: Noonan syndrome
  - In Noonan syndrome, once referred to as *male Turner syndrome* (See Chapter 2), congenital heart disease is right-sided (unlike the left-sided defects in Turner syndrome), including most commonly pulmonic stenosis. Hypertrophic cardiomyopathy is the second most common finding. Lymphatic malformations are also common.
  - While the incidence of Noonan syndrome in the population is only about 1 in 1500, the incidence in children with congenital heart disease may be as high as 1 in 100.
  - Prolonged coagulation times are frequently observed because of a wide range of defects (von Willebrand disease phenotypes, factor V deficiency, and factor VIII deficiency).
  - Noonan syndrome is inherited in an autosomal dominant manner, but many cases are sporadic because of *de novo* mutations. It is caused by mutations in either the *PTPN11* gene (12q) or the *KRAS* gene (12p: K-ras). Direct sequence analysis is clinically available for these loci. *PTPN11* has also been implicated in some examples of LEOPARD syndrome and juvenile myelomonocytic leukemia.

6: Cardiovascular Disease

Structural Disorders>Single-Gene Disorders Resulting in Structural Cardiac Defects; Chromosomal Disorders Associated with Structural Cardiac Anomalies; Multifactorial Structural Cardiac Disorders

- *JAG1* mutations: Alagille syndrome (see chapter 8)

  □ Best known for its association with bile duct paucity, Alagille syndrome (arteriohepatic dysplasia) is also a disease of blood vessels and the heart.

  □ Cardiovascular anomalies are seen in nearly 100% of cases. Most commonly affected is the pulmonary circulation, in the form of pulmonary artery stenosis. Other defects include tetralogy, atrial septal defects, ventricular septal defects, aortic stenosis, and coarctation.

  □ Alagille syndrome is an autosomal dominant condition caused by mutations in the *JAG1* gene.

Chromosomal Disorders Associated with Structural Cardiac Anomalies

- Chromosomal anomalies (see chapter 2).

  □ Down syndrome is associated with structural cardiac anomalies in over half of cases. The classic association is malformation of the endocardial cushion, resulting most commonly in a membranous ventricular septal defect. This is followed in frequency by patent ductus arteriosus, atrial septal defect, and atrioventricular septal defect.

  □ Cardiac anomalies are present in up to 50% of those with Turner syndrome. Bicuspid aortic valve is the most common defect, followed by coarctation of the aorta. Aortic root dilation is common and may lead to aortic dissection.

- Microdeletions and sequences

  □ The 22q11 microdeletion syndrome (DiGeorge syndrome, velocardiofacial syndrome, Shprintzen

syndrome) is the most common of these, and among its most common manifestations are cardiac anomalies. Structural cardiac anomalies are present in about 75% of affected individuals, especially the conotruncal malformations. These include tetralogy of Fallot, interrupted aortic arch, ventricular septal defects, and truncus arteriosus. Among the several genes wiped out by this microdeletion, *TBX1* is believed to be responsible for the cardiac and anomalies (see chapter 2).

  □ Williams syndrome is the result of a microdeletion of 7q11.23 and is characterized by dysmorphic facial features, mental retardation, short stature, hypercalcemia, abnormalities of connective tissue (hernias, diverticula, joint laxity, skin laxity) and structural cardiac and vascular defects. The most distinctive cardiac anomaly is supravalvar aortic stenosis (hourglass stenosis). Many of the findings in Williams syndrome can be attributed to deletion of the elastin gene.

Multifactorial Structural Cardiac Disorders

- The vast majority of structural cardiac anomalies have traditionally been considered "multifactorial" in origin. That is, while a mendelian pattern of inheritance is inapparent and a specific genetic defect has not been found, there is a certain clustering of these findings within families and around particular exposures. Furthermore, it is known that offspring of consanguineous parents are strongly predisposed to structural cardiac anomalies.

- Cardiac anomalies are prominent among the multifactorial disorders, others being pyloric stenosis, cleft lip, and cleft palate.

References

References

Abbott GW, Sesti F, Splawski I, et al. MiRP1 forms IKr potassium channels with HERG and is associated with cardiac arrhythmia. *Cell* 1999; 97: 175-187.

Ackerman MJ, Siu BL, Sturner WQ, et al. Postmortem molecular analysis of SCN5A defects in sudden infant death syndrome. *JAMA* 2001; 286: 2264-2269.

Adams D, Samuel D, Goulon-Goeau C, et al. The course and prognostic factors of familial amyloid polyneuropathy after liver transplantation. *Brain* 2000; 123: 1495-1504.

Ahmad F, Li D, Karibe A, et al. Localization of a gene responsible for arrhythmogenic right ventricular dysplasia to chromosome 3p23. *Circulation* 1998; 98: 2791-2795.

Alcalai R, Metzger S, Rosenheck S, et al. A recessive mutation in desmoplakin causes arrhythmogenic right ventricular dysplasia, skin disorder, and woolly hair. *J Am Coll Cardiol* 2003; 42: 319-327.

Ando Y, Nakamura M, Araki S. Transthyretin-related familial amyloidotic polyneuropathy. *Arch Neurol* 2005; 62: 1057-1062.

Antzelevitch C, Brugada P, Brugada J, et al. Brugada syndrome 1992-2002: a historical perspective. *J Am Coll Cardiol* 2003; 41: 1665-1671.

Barhanin J, Lesage F, Guillemare E, et al. KVLQT1 and IsK (minK) proteins associate to form the IKs cardiac potassium current. *Nature* 1996; 384: 78-80.

Bernstein D. Congenital heart disease. In: *Nelson Textbook of Pediatrics.* 17th ed. Philadelphia, Pa: WB Saunders, 2004.

Barua RS, Ambrose JA, Eales-Reynolds LJ, et al. Dysfunctional endothelial nitricoxide biosynthesis in healthy smokers with impaired endothelium-dependent vasodilatation. *Circulation* 2001; 104(16): 1905-1910.

Basson CT, Cowley GS, Solomon SD, et al. The clinical and genetic spectrum of the Holt-Oram syndrome (heart-hand syndrome). *N Engl J Med* 1995; 330: 885-891.

Bernier FP, Spaetgens R. The geneticist's role in adult congenital heart disease. *Cardiol Clin* 2006; 24: 557-569.

Bowles NE, Ni J, Marcus F, et al. The detection of cardiotropic viruses in the myocardium of patients with arrhythmogenic right ventricular dysplasia/cardiomyopathy. *J Am Coll Cardiol* 2002; 39: 892-895.

Brugada P, Brugada J. Right bundle-branch block, persistent ST segment elevation and sudden cardiac death: a distinct clinical and electrocardiographic syndrome: a multicenter report. *J Am Coll Cardiol* 1992; 20: 1391-1396.

Brugada J, Brugada R, Brugada P. Determinants of sudden cardiac death in individuals with the electrocardiographic pattern of Brugada syndrome and no previous cardiac arrest. *Circulation* 2003; 108: 3092-3096.

Chen Q, Zhang D, Gingell RL, et al. Homozygous deletion in KVLQT1 associated with Jervell and Lange-Nielsen syndrome. *Circulation* 1999; 99: 1344-1347.

Corrado D, Basso C, Schiavon M, et al. Screening for hypertrophic cardiomyopathy in young athletes. *N Engl J Med* 1998; 339: 364-369.

Curran ME, Splawski I, Timothy KW, et al. A molecular basis for cardiac arrhythmia: HERG mutations cause long QT syndrome. *Cell* 1995; 80: 795-803.

Fontaine G, Fontaliran F, Frank R. Arrhythmogenic right ventricular cardiomyopathies: clinical forms and main differential diagnoses. *Circulation* 1998; 97: 1532-1535.

Garcia-Castro M, Reguero JR, Batalla A, et al. Hypertrophic cardiomyopathy: low frequency of mutations in the myosin heavy chain (MYH7) and cardiac troponin T (TNNT2) genes among Spanish patients. *Clin Chem* 2003; 49: 1279-1285.

Garg V, Kathiriya IS, Barnes R, et al. GATA4 mutations cause human congenital heart defects and reveal an interaction with TBX5. *Nature* 2003; 424: 443-447.

Gerull B, Heuser A, Wichter T, et al. Mutations in the desmosomal plakophilin-2 are common in arrhythmogenic right ventricular cardiomyopathy. *Nat Genet* 2004; 36: 1162-1164.

Ghilardi G, Biondi ML, DeMonti M, et al. Independent risk factor for moderate to severe internal carotid artery stenosis: T786C mutation of the endothelial nitric oxide synthase gene. *Clin Chem* 2002; 48: 989-993.

References

Grumbach IM, Heim A, Vonhof S, et al. Coxsackie virus genome in myocardium of patients with arrhythmogenic right ventricular dysplasia/cardiomyopathy. *Cardiology* 1998; 89: 241-245.

Hattori T, Takei Y, Koyama J, et al. Clinical and pathological studies of cardiac amyloidosis in transthyretin type familial amyloid polyneuropathy. *Amyloid* 2003; 10: 229-239.

Holt M, Oram S. Familial heart disease with skeletal malformations. *Br Heart J* 1960; 22: 236-242.

Hong K, Brugada J, Oliva A, et al. Value of electrocardiographic parameters and ajmaline test in the diagnosis of Brugada syndrome caused by SCN5A mutations. *Circulation* 2004; 110: 3023-3027.

Huang FD, Chen J, Lin M, et al. Long-QT syndrome-associated missense mutations in the pore helix of the HERG potassium channel. *Circulation* 2001; 104: 1071-1075.

Hulot JS, Jouven X, Empana JP, et al. Natural history and risk stratification of arrhythmogenic right ventricular dysplasia/cardiomyopathy. *Circulation* 2004; 110: 1879-1884.

Imboden M, Swan H, Denjoy I, et al. Female predominance and transmission distortion in the long-QT syndrome. *N Engl J Med* 2006; 355: 2744-2751.

Jacobson DR, Pastore RD, Yaghoubian R, et al. Variant-sequence transthyretin (isoleucine 122) in late-onset cardiac amyloidosis in black Americans. *N Engl J Med* 1997; 336: 466-473.

Jervell A, Lange-Nielsen F. Congenital deaf-mutism, functional heart disease with prolongation of the Q-T interval and sudden death. *Am Heart J* 1957; 54: 59-68.

Kamisago M, Sharma SD, DePalma SR, et al. Mutations in sarcomere protein genes as a cause of dilated cardiomyopathy. *N Engl J Med* 2000; 343: 1688-96.

Keating MT, Atkinson D, Dunn C, et al. Linkage of a cardiac arrhythmia, the long QT syndrome, and the Harvey ras-1 gene. *Science* 1991; 252: 704-706.

Laitinen PJ, Brown KM, Piippo K, et al. Mutations of the cardiac ryanodine receptor (RyR2) gene in familial polymorphic ventricular tachycardia. *Circulation* 2001; 103: 485-490.

Li H, Chen Q, Moss AJ, et al. New mutations in the KVLQT1 potassium channel that cause long QT syndrome. *Circulation* 1998; 97: 1264-1269.

Lin AE, Herring AH, Scharenberg K. Cardiovascular malformations:changes in prevalence and birth status, 1972-1990. *Am J Med Genet* 1999; 84: 102.

Ng B, Connors LH, Davidoff R, et al. Senile systemic amyloidosis presenting with heart failure: a comparison with light chain-associated amyloidosis. *Arch Intern Med* 2005; 165: 1425-1429.

Piippo K, Swan H, Pasternack M, et al. A founder mutation of the potassium channel KCNQ1 in long QT syndrome: implications for estimation of disease prevalence and molecular diagnostics. *J Am Coll Cardiol* 2001; 37: 562-568.

Priori SG, Napolitano C, Giordano U, et al. Brugada syndrome and sudden cardiac death in children. *Lancet* 2000; 355: 808-809.

Priori SG, Napolitano C, Tiso N, et al. Mutations in the cardiac ryanodine receptor gene (hRyR2) underlie catecholaminergic polymorphic ventricular tachycardia. *Circulation* 2002; 102: r49-r53.

Protonotarios N, Tsatsopoulou A, Anastasakis A, et al. Genotype-phenotype assessment in autosomal recessive arrhythmogenic right ventricular cardiomyopathy (Naxos disease) caused by a deletion in plakoglobin. *J Am Coll Cardiol* 2001; 38: 1477-1484.

Pyeritz RE. Genetics and cardiovascular disease. In: *Braunwald's Heart Disease: A Textbook of Cardiovascular Medicine*, 7th ed. Philadelphia, Pa: Elsevier Saunders, 2005.

Rampazzo A, Nava A, Malacrida S, et al. Mutation in human desmoplakin domain binding to plakoglobin causes a dominant form of arrhythmogenic right ventricular cardiomyopathy. *Am J Hum Genet* 2002; 71: 1200-1206.

References

Richardson P, McKenna W, Bristow M, et al. Report of the 1995 World Health Organization/International Society and Federation of Cardiology Task Force on the Definition and Classification of Cardiomyopathies. *Circulation* 1996; 93: 841-842.

Rossi GP, Cesari M, Zanchetta M, et al. The T786C endothelial nitric oxide synthase genotype is a novel risk factor for coronary artery disease in Caucasian patients of the GENICA study. *J Am Coll Cardiol* 2003; 41: 930-937.

Sanguinetti MC, Curran ME, Zou A, et al. Coassembly of KvLQT1 and minK (IsK) proteins to form cardiac IKs potassium channel. *Nature* 1996; 384: 80-83.

Schwartz PJ, Priori SG, Spazzolini C, et al. Genotype-phenotype correlation in the long-QT syndrome: gene-specific triggers for life-threatening arrhythmias. *Circulation* 2001; 103: 89-95.

Splawski I, Shen J, Timothy KW, et al. Spectrum of mutations in long-QT syndrome genes: KVLQT1, HERG, SCN5A, KCNE1, and KCNE2. *Circulation* 2000102: 1178-1185.

Tabib A, Loire R, Chalabreysse L, et al. Circumstances of death and gross and microscopic observations in a series of 200 cases of sudden death associated with arrhythmogenic right ventricular cardiomyopathy and/or dysplasia. *Circulation* 2002; 108: 3000-3005.

Tiso N, Stephan DA, Nava A, et al. Identification of mutations in the cardiac ryanodine receptor gene in families affected with arrhythmogenic right ventricular cardiomyopathy type 2 (ARVD2). *Hum Mol Genet* 2001; 10: 189-194.

Towbin JA. Molecular genetic basis of sudden cardiac death. *Pediatr Clin North Am* 2004; 51: 1229-1255.

Trudeau MC, Warmke J, Ganetzky B, et al. HERG, a human inward rectifier in the voltage-gated potassium channel family. *Science* 1995; 269: 92-95.

Vatta M, Dumaine R, Varghese G, et al. Genetic and biophysical basis of sudden unexplained nocturnal death syndrome (SUNDS), a disease allelic to Brugada syndrome. *Hum Mol Genet* 2002; 11: 337-345.

Viitasalo M, Oikarinen L, Vaananen H, et al. Differentiation between LQT1 and LQT2 patients and unaffected subjects using 24-hour electrocardiographic recordings. *Am J Cardiol* 2002; 89: 679-685.

Wang Q, Curran ME, Splawski I, et al. Positional cloning of a novel potassium channel gene: KVLQT1 mutations cause cardiac arrhythmias. *Nat Genet* 1996; 12: 17-23.

Wang DW, Viswanathan PC, Balser JR, et al. Clinical, genetic, and biophysical characterization of SCN5A mutations associated with atrioventricular conduction block. *Circulation* 2002; 105: 341-346.

Wilde AA, Antzelevitch C, Borggrefe M, et al. Proposed diagnostic criteria for the Brugada syndrome. *Circulation* 2002; 106: 2514-2519.

Yoshimura M, Nakayama M, Shimasaki Y, et al. A T786C mutation in the 5'-flanking region of the endothelial nitric oxide synthase gene and coronary arterial vasomotility. *Am J Cardiol* 2000; 85: 710-714.

Zareba W, Moss AJ, Schwartz PJ, Vincent GM, et al. Influence of genotype on the clinical course of the long-QT syndrome. *N Engl J Med* 1998; 339: 960-965.

Chapter 7

Endocrine Disorders

Steroid Hormones

Congenital Adrenal Hyperplasia (CAH)

- CAH is a group of autosomal recessive disorders in which the deficiency of an enzyme involved in the synthesis of cortisol leads to an excess in the production of androgens which results in virilization. Several enzymes are involved in the biosynthesis of cortisol from cholesterol, each of which may be congenitally deficient. Many of these deficiencies can lead to the CAH phenotype. The reduced synthesis of cortisol leads to markedly elevated adrenocorticotrophic hormone (ACTH), leading to adrenal hyperplasia. Some affected individuals also manifest salt wasting (because of decreased mineralocorticoid activity). The main clinical presentations are (1) a female who is virilized at birth or becomes virilized shortly thereafter, (2) a female with precocious puberty, and (3) a male with pseudoprecocious puberty (the external appearance of puberty), and (4) an infant with salt-losing crisis (similar to an Addisonian crisis).

- 17-hydroxyprogesterone (17-OHP) is elevated in all forms of CAH; this forms the basis for diagnosis in many cases. 17-OHP can be measured by immunoassay, which can be performed on dried blood spots for neonatal screening. Because some neonates may present in the first days of life with an adrenal insufficiency crisis, early knowledge of the diagnosis can be extremely beneficial.

- 21-hydroxylase deficiency is the most common cause of CAH. It is responsible for about 90% of cases and has an estimated incidence of 1 in 10,000 to 1 in 25,000.

- The range of clinical severity can best be understood based on three principles. First, mild enzyme deficiency affects mainly the production of cortisol, while severe deficiency impairs both cortisol and mineralocorticoid (aldosterone) production. Thus, mild deficiencies result in the so-called simple virilizing form of the disease, while severe enzyme deficiencies result in the salt-wasting form of disease. Second, the most profound consequences of hypocortisolism for the developing fetus is not the paucity of cortisol itself but rather the very high ACTH that drives the build-up of androgens (and other cortisol precursors such as 17-OHP). Third, males and females have differing reactions to androgen.

- An elevated serum 17-OHP, which is a precursor in the cortisol biosynthetic pathway, is indicative of CAH, including that caused by 21-hydroxylase deficiency.

This test forms the basis for neonatal screening programs. Concomitant elevation in plasma renin activity (PRA) is consistent with the salt-wasting form of the disease. Serum progesterone and androstenedione are also increased in 21-hydroxylase deficiency.

- 21-hydroxylase (also called CYP21A2 and P450C21) is a cytochrome P-450 enzyme found in the smooth endoplasmic reticulum. Its function is the hydroxylation of C21 on steroid precursors, and its main physiologic role is in the steroid hormone biosynthetic pathway where it catalyzes (1) the conversion of 17-OHP to 11-deoxycortisol, a precursor of cortisol, and (2) the conversion of progesterone to deoxycorticosterone, a precursor of aldosterone.

- The gene encoding 21-hydroxylase is *CYP21*. *CYP21* is located at 6p21 and is thus within the HLA locus, adjacent to genes that encode complement protein C4. Nearby is a gene known as *CYP21P*, a pseudogene (nontranscribed gene) with more than 95% homology with *CYP21* but rendered nonfunctional by virtue of several nucleotide differences.

- The most common disease-causing mutations are (1) large *CYP21* gene deletions and (2) gene conversions—recombinations between *CYP21* and *CYP21P*, converting CYP21 into a nonfunctional allele. Several additional point mutations have been desribed. Different mutations have different phenotypic effects, with some causing complete enzyme deficiency and others causing only impaired enzyme activity.

- Molecular testing of the CYP21 gene is available. Directed mutation analysis for a set of common mutations can detect more than 95% of abnormal alleles. 1 common approach is the use of Southern blot analysis with restriction enzymes. Restriction enzymes produce predictable digestion fragments that can be compared to known standards and to an internal standard *(CYP21P)*. Polymerase chain reaction (PCR) is problematic because of simultaneous amplification of *CYP21P*.

- Prenatal diagnosis of 21-hydroxylase is possible with molecular testing of material obtained through chorionic villus sampling or amniocentesis. This may permit prenatal treatment through the administration of corticosteroids, leading to suppression of ACTH secretion.

- 11-hydroxylase deficiency is the second most common cause of CAH (5%-7% of cases). It is caused by mutations in the *CYP11B1* gene located on chromosome 8q24 and is especially prominent in North African Jews. Unlike 21-hydroxylase deficiency, a salt-wasting form of 11-hydroxylase deficiency is very uncommon; however, hypertension is much more commonly seen in 11-hydroxylase deficiency. Findings indicative of androgen excess are equally common in both conditions.

■ About 2% of cases are caused by 3β-hydroxysteroid dehydrogenase (3β-HSD) deficiency.

■ About 1% of cases are caused by 17-hydroxylase deficiency.

Adrenoleukodystrophy

■ This is a syndrome of combined adrenal cortical deficiency and central nervous system demyelination.

■ See chapter 11.

Androgen Insensitivity Syndrome (Testicular Feminization)

■ Androgen insensitivity is an X-linked recessive (XLR) disorder, affecting 46,XY males. Depending on the degree of insensitivity, it may present as feminization of the external genitalia at birth, abnormal secondary sexual development found in puberty, and/or infertility in adulthood. This spectrum of disease severity has resulted in a classification system including complete, partial, and mild androgen insensitivity syndromes.

■ Often a mass is detected in the inguinal canal, representing undescended testes. Usually rudimentary Müllerian structures are present (ovary, fallopian tubes, uterus), and serum testosterone levels are normal to elevated, conversion of testosterone to dihydrotestosterone is normal, and serum leutenizing hormone (LH) level is normal or elevated. In complete androgen insensitivity, the external genitalia resemble that of a female, while at the opposite end of the spectrum the external genitalia may be ambiguous or male-appearing.

■ Initially, a karyotype is needed to begin sorting out these findings. A 46,XY karyotype must be present to entertain the diagnosis of androgen insensitivity. Following this, direct sequencing of the androgen receptor (AR) gene may be undertaken, with the finding of a mutation providing definitive diagnosis. Mutations in the *AR* gene, found on Xq11-12, are found in more than 95% of males with complete insensitivity and only about 40% of those with partial or mild insensitivity.

Steroid Sulfatase Deficiency (X-Linked Ichthyosis)

■ It is the function of steroid sulfatase to remove sulfate moieties from steroid sulfates (including cholesterol sulfate), thus permitting either their biologic activity or their conversion into biologically active forms.

■ Steroid sulfatase deficiency may present first as prolonged or nonprogressive labor, unresponsive to oxytocin. After birth, cholesterol sulfate begins to accumulate in the blood and in tissues such as the cornea and skin. In skin, it appears to prevent the dissolution of desmosomal attachments (desquamation), leading to the X-linked ichthyosis (scaly skin) phenotype. X-linked ichthyosis is 1 of several types of ichthyosis, including ichthyosis vulgaris (inherited as an autosomal dominant trait), congenital ichthyosiform erythroderma (autosomal recessive), lamellar ichthyosis (autosomal recessive), and acquired forms of ichthyosis (often paraneoplastic). Ichthyosis becomes apparent shortly after birth. Corneal opacities develop somewhat later. Males have a high incidence of cryptorchidism, which leads to a higher incidence of germ cell tumors.

■ The gene for steroid sulfatase (*STS*) is located on the short arm of the X chromosome (Xp22.3). In nearly 90% of cases, steroid sulfatase deficiency is the result of a complete *STS* gene deletion, sometimes including the entire distal short arm of the X-chromosome. Most of the remaining patients have single point mutations in the *STS* gene.

■ The diagnosis may be made in several ways. The enzyme may be specifically assayed in samples of peripheral blood leukocytes or skin. Elevated cholesterol sulfate levels may be demonstrated in serum or skin. Lastly, the gene deletion may be demonstrated by fluorescence in situ hybridization (FISH).

Hermaphroditism and Pseudohermaphroditism

■ This is an extremely complicated topic about which only a few general comments will be made here. *Genotypic sex* is determined by the status of the Y chromosome—the presence of a single Y chromosome (regardless of the number of X chromosomes)—is definitive of a genotypic male. The *gonadal sex* depends on the histologic nature of the gonads. The Y chromosome, in particular the *SRY* gene, influences the genital primoridium to develop into testes; in the

7: Endocrine Disorders and Disorders of Skeletal Growth

Steroid Hormones>Hermaphroditism and Pseudohermaphroditism I Pituitary>Multiple Pituitary Hormone Deficiency/ Pituitary Hypoplasia and Aplasia; Kallmann Syndrome; Isolated Growth Hormone Deficiency; Ataxia-Telangiectasia

absence of a Y chromosome, the gonadal primordium will develop into ovaries. *Phenotypic sex* refers to the status of the external genitalia.

- The term *true hermaphrodite* implies the presence of both ovarian and testicular tissue, either separately or in the same gonadal structure (ovotestis). This is an extremely rare condition in which the genotype is usually 46,XX but transposed *SRY* gene material can nearly always be found with FISH. In some cases, in fact, true hermaphroditism is associated with 46,XX/46,XY mosaicism. A 46,XY genotype is not associated with true hermaphroditism.

- Pseudohermaphroditism refers to a discordance between the phenotypic sex and the gonadal/ genotypic sex. The presumed sex is that indicated by the histologic features of the gonads; thus, male pseudohermaphrodites have a Y chromosome and testes, but the external genitalia (and often the genital ducts) are either ambiguous or feminized. Various causes are responsible, the most common of which are the androgen insensitivity syndromes (testicular feminization). Female pseudohermaphrodites have no Y chromosome (usually 46,XX), ovaries, and external genitalia that are either ambiguous or male-appearing (virilized). Female pseudohermaphroditism is caused by excessive exposure to androgens during fetal development, most commonly because of CAH.

Pituitary

Multiple Pituitary Hormone Deficiency/ Pituitary Hypoplasia and Aplasia

- Several genes are involved in the normal formation of the pituitary gland, and as would be expected, there are several genetic types of inherited panhypopituitarism.

- While some of these manifest as isolated hypopituitarism and pituitary hypoplasia, others are associated with multiple anomalies outside the pituitary. In particular, cleft lip, cleft palate, and solitary maxillary central incisor (single front tooth) are findings with a high likelihood of associated pituitary hypoplasia.

- Transcription factor genes involved in pituitary formation and in which disease-causing mutations have been described include *TPIT, SOX2, SOX3, HESX1, LHX3, LHX4, PROP1,* and *POU1F1 (PIT1).*

Kallmann Syndrome

- This is a syndrome that affects primarily males, consisting of hypogonadotropic hypogonadism and anosmia. The olfactory lobes are absent or poorly formed, there is deficiency of LH-releasing hormone, small testes, small penis, gynecomastia, and a failure to enter puberty.

- Kallmann syndrome may be inherited as an X-linked, autosomal dominant, or autosomal recessive trait. The *KAL1* gene, found at Xp22.3, is responsible for most X-linked cases and about 15% of cases overall. It encodes a protein called anosmin-1.

Isolated Growth Hormone (GH) Deficiency

- Several types of isolated GH deficiency have been described, including autosomal recessive, autosomal dominant, and XLR forms. These may be caused by mutations in the GH-releasing hormone (*GHRH*) gene, usually transmitted as an autosomal recessive trait, mutations in the *GH1* gene, usually autosomal dominant, or mutations in the *BTK* gene on the X chromosome. This latter gene is also involved in causing Bruton agammaglobulinemia, and indeed many affected individuals are also immunocompromised.

- These defects lead to short stature but failure of puberty and growth plate closure, with continued growth into the mid-30s. Like patients with hemophilia, many develop anti-GH antibodies after GH therapy.

- Some patients display end-organ GH resistance, caused either by mutations in the gene encoding the GH receptor (Laron syndrome) or mutations in the gene encoding insulinlike growth factor-I (*IGF-I*), the major effecter of GH action.

Ataxia-Telangiectasia (A-T)

- See Chapter 9.

- Patients with A-T have pleomorphic, bizarre cytologic changes in their pituitary glands.

- This does not appear to be associated with pituitary dysfunction or pituitary neoplasia.

Parathyroid

Inherited Hypoparathyroidism

- Hypoparathyroidism is most often inherited as part of the DiGeorge syndrome (see chapter 2). Neonatal hypocalcemia, often associated with tetany, occurs in most cases.

- Isolated hypoparathyroidism is rarely inherited as an XLR trait, typically presenting as infantile seizures (not associated with fever).

- Kearns-Sayre syndrome, 1 of the mitochondrial disorders, is associated with hypoparathyroidism (see chapter 10).

- Lastly, as part of the syndrome of hypoparathyroidism, sensorineural hearing loss, and renal anomalies, hypoparathyroidism may be inherited as an autosomal recessive trait. This has been attributed to mutations in the *GATA3* gene found on 10p14.

Albright Hereditary Osteodystrophy (Pseudohypoparathyroidism Type IA)

- *Pseudohypoparathyroidism* is a term encompassing multiple diseases in which there is peripheral resistance to parathyroid hormone (PTH). Infantile tetany is often the presenting feature. Older children display short stature, a round face, dimpling of the dorsum of the hand, brachydactyly (characteristically, the second digit is spared, such that it is longer than the third), dystrophic soft tissue calcification, and heterotopic ossification. The biochemical features include hypocalcemia and *elevated PTH*.

- The confusing term *pseudo-pseudohypoparathyroidism* has been applied to partially affected individuals only manifesting elevated PTH with normal calcium levels.

- Albright hereditary osteodystrophy is an autosomal dominant disorder caused by mutations in the *GNAS1* gene, a guanine nucleotide (G-protein)–encoding gene located on chromosome 20q13.2. Specifically, *GNAS1* encodes the α subunit of the G protein ($G_{S\alpha}$). The protein is critical for transmembrane signaling when PTH is bound to its receptor. Furthermore, there appears to be a degree of imprinting involved in inheritance, with paternal transmission of mutations leading to a simple form of pseudo-pseudohypoparathyroidism and maternal transmission leading to the more fully developed syndrome.

- G protein mutations

  - Peptide hormone receptors often exert their intracellular effects through a G protein, and mutations in G protein genes form the basis for a variety of diseases **T7.1**.

  - Cell surface receptors that use a G protein are called G protein coupled receptors (GPCRs). When GPCRs bind agonist, they activate the linked G protein to exchange GTP for GDP. This exchange is mediated by the α subunit of the stimulatory domain of the G protein ($G_{S\alpha}$). This domain has GTPase activity; thus, it is rapidly deactivated when GTP is hydrolyzed back to GDP. The effect of G protein activation is the activation of adenylate cyclase and the generation of cyclic AMP.

  - Some mutations in the $G_{S\alpha}$ lead to reduced activity of the subunit (loss-of-function mutations), and other mutations lead to enhanced activity (gain-of-function). Since G proteins were elucidated in the 1970s, it is interesting that 2 diseases whose description is attributed in part to Fuller Albright in the 1930s—Albright hereditary osteodystrophy and McCune-Albright syndrome—are caused by these opposing mutations. Activating (gain-of-function) mutations, particularly involving Arg201, are found in the McCune-Albright syndrome (and endocrine neoplasms); alternatively, loss-of-function mutations lead to Albright hereditary osteodystrophy.

T7.1

Inherited G Protein Coupled Receptor–Associated Diseases

Albright hereditary osteodystrophy
Pseudohypoparathyroidism type 1a
Pseudohypoparathyroidism type 1b
X-linked nephrogenic diabetes insipidus (renal vasopressin resistance)
Congenital night blindness
Familial hypocalciuric hypercalcemia
Hirschsprung disease
Fibrous dysplasia
McCune-Albright syndrome

McCune-Albright Syndrome

- McCune-Albright syndrome is caused by gain-of-function mutations in the *GNAS1* gene. An interesting feature of these mutations is that they must exist as mosaicisms to be compatible with life. Thus, all mutations necessarily arise at some point after fertilization (ie, all mutations are somatic rather than germline). Furthermore, widely disparate clinical syndromes, ranging from fully developed McCune-Albright syndrome to isolated fibrous dysplasia, can result from this single mutation, depending on the stage of development at which the mutation occurs. Early mutations lead to the full syndrome; somewhat later mutations lead to polyostotic fibrous dysplasia; late mutations, some even arising postnatally, lead to isolated fibrous dysplasia, endocrine hyperfunction, or endocrine neoplasms.

- McCune-Albright syndrome is characterized by café-au-lait spots, polyostotic fibrous dysplasia, precocious puberty, and other endocrine anomalies. Precocious puberty is a feature mainly of females with the syndrome, with many achieving puberty by the age of 3 years. Levels of LH and follicle-stimulating hormone are low. Hyperthyroidism often arises, with reduced levels of thyroid-stimulating hormone (TSH), and in some patients, Cushing syndrome or gigantism develops, again with low levels of ACTH and GH. Lastly, many experience phosphaturia with low serum phosphate levels. All of these are manifestations of end-organ hypersensitivity to hormone, because of constitutively activated G proteins. The skin hyperpigmentation is felt to be because of the action of receptors for melanocyte-stimulating hormone.

Familial Hypocalciuric Hypercalcemia

- This is a largely asymptomatic disorder (also called *familial benign hypercalcemia*), inherited as an autosomal dominant trait, in which hypercalcemia is usually discovered incidentally. The parathyroid glands are of normal size or minimally hypertrophic, and importantly, subtotal parathyroidectomy has no effect on calcium levels.

- The serum PTH is normal (inappropriately so, compared with the calcium level). Serum magnesium is normal to slightly elevated. Urine calcium is low, as is the ratio of urinary calcium clearance to urinary creatinine clearance.

- This has been attributed to a mutation of a G-protein gene located at 3q2, resulting in parathyroid insensitivity to elevated calcium levels. Thus, the normal feedback loop is interrupted. 1 of the actions of PTH is to enhance renal tubular reabsorption of calcium, explaining the low urinary calcium.

Thyroid Hormones

Congenital Hypothyroidism

- The effects of fetal hypothyroidism are mitigated by a maternal supply of thyroid hormone; however, postnatal hypothyroidism can have profound consequences, particularly on the development of the brain, and manifests clinically as so-called cretinism. Because neonatal hypothyroidism is easily detected and easily treated, neonatal screening for congenital hypothyroidism is widely applied.

- About 90% of cases are associated with thyroid dysgenesis (aplasia or hypoplasia), the result most commonly of maternal autoantibodies. Only about 2% have an inherited basis. Inherited thyroid dysgenesis may be caused by mutations in 1 of 3 transcription factors involved in thyroid formation—*TTF1, TTF-2,* and *PAX-8*.

- Around 10% are caused either by a defect in thyroid hormone biosynthesis or end-organ resistance, and most of these cases are inherited. In contrast to dysgenesis, defects in thyroid hormone biosynthesis are usually associated with a goiter. Thyroid hormone synthesis involves several steps, including iodine transport into the cell, synthesis of the protein thyroglobulin, and the joining (organification) of iodine to thyroglobulin. These defects are inherited as autosomal recessive traits. Thyroid peroxidase deficiency is perhaps the most common. Other defects include those within the iodine transport protein (reported in rare kindreds from Japan and in the Hutterites), defective sulfate transport (resulting in the Pendred syndrome), and mutations in the thyroglobulin gene. The Pendred syndrome is characterized by congenital hypothyroidism and sensorineural hearing loss. Multiple defects in the thyrotropin releasing hormone–TSH axis have also been described, some on the basis of G protein mutations.

- Thyroid hormone resistance (Refetoff syndrome) is also usually associated with goiter. Some patients are euthyroid, with the raised levels of thyroxine overcoming the end-organ resistance. Others are clinically hypothyroid, manifesting mental retardation and growth retardation. The disorder is inherited in an autosomal dominant fashion.

Autoimmune Thyroid Disease and Polyglandular Syndrome

- There are several categories of immune-mediated thyroid disease—Hashimoto thyroiditis, lymphocytic thyroiditis, granulomatous (deQuervain) thyroiditis, and Graves disease. Together, these disorders affect about 1% of the population, with a roughly 5-10:1 female to male ratio. Autoimmune thyroid diseases may occur in isolation or as part of a polyglandular autoimmune condition. In any case, these disorders tend to cluster within families, and the concordance rate among identical twins is about 80%.

- Hashimoto thyroiditis is characterized by circulating antimicrosomal and antithyroglobulin antibodies and histologic features including a lymphocytic infiltrate and Hürthle cell metaplasia. Lymphocytic thyroiditis is similar to Hashimoto thyroiditis but does not display Hürthle cell metaplasia. Studies point to a number of susceptibility loci, without a distinct monogenetic cause. In particular, there is strong

linkage to *HLA* gene loci (HLA-DR3, HLA-DR5), the *CTLA-4* (cytotoxic T lymphocyte antigen-4) gene on 2q33, and the *PTPN22* gene on 18q. Furthermore, Hashimoto thyroiditis occurs with increased frequency in Down syndrome.

- Graves disease is associated with circulating long-acting thyroid stimulating antibodies which are capable of acting on TSH receptors as agonists. Histologically, there may be a mild lymphocytic infiltrate, but the main feature (in untreated cases which are not seen much anymore in the histology laboratory) is papillary hyperplasia of follicular epithelium. Graves disease occurs with increased frequency in members of families that have not only Graves disease but also Hashimoto thyroiditis and type-1 diabetes mellitus. Like Hashimoto thyroiditis, the *CTLA4* gene appears to have strong influence on the development of Graves disease, and there is a relatively high incidence of HLA-DR3.

- Autoimmune polyglandular syndrome (APS) has 3 forms, types 1-3, characterized by differing combinations of autoimmune phenomena **T7.2**. Presentations may include hypothyroidism, Addison disease, and diabetes mellitus. Type 1 is also called the autoimmune polyendocrinopathy (candidiasis) ectodermal disease (APECED), and type 2 was previously called Schmidt syndrome.

T7.2
Autoimmune Polyglandular Syndromes

	Type 1	Type 2	Type 3
Common endocrine targets	Parathyroid Adrenal cortex (Addison disease) Ovary/testis Thyroid	Adrenal cortex (Addison disease) Thyroid Islets of Langerhans (diabetes mellitus)	Thyroid
Other features	Mucocutaneous candidiasis Vitiligo Autoimmune hepatitis Autoimmune enteropathy	Vitiligo	Vitiligo
Genetics	*AIRE* gene (21q) mutations	HLA-DR and DQ polymorphisms	Unknown

7: Endocrine Disorders and Disorders of Skeletal Growth

Diabetes Mellitus>Type-1 Diabetes Mellitus (DM; Insulin-Dependent DM); Type-2 Diabetes Mellitus;
Monogenetic Causes of DM

Diabetes Mellitus

Type-1 Diabetes Mellitus (DM; Insulin-Dependent DM)

- Type-1 DM is essentially an autoimmune condition in which the effect of genotype is best considered provocative or protective. Thus, inheritance is not strictly Mendelian. In fact, most cases lack a family history. However, first-degree relatives of affected persons have a higher-than-average risk of developing type-1 DM, siblings have a 5% to 10% chance of developing it, and identical twins have about 60% concordance.

- The greatest genetic impact on the acquisition of type-1 DM is exerted by the HLA class II genes on chromosome 6p21. Collectively, these loci are considered the IDDM1 locus in the context of type-1 diabetes genotypic discussions. Those with either the HLA-DR3 or HLA-DR4 alleles have a 2- to 3-fold increased risk of type-1 DM, while those homozygous for HLA-DR3 or HLA-DR4 or doubly heterozygous (HLA-DR3 and HLA-DR4) have an 10-fold risk. A less frequent anomaly, a point mutation in the HLA-DQβ_1, with the loss of Asp at position 57, confers a relative risk of more than 100. On the other hand, certain alleles at the HLA-DR locus confer relative protection against type-1 DM.

- Several additional loci appear to exert influences on the development of type-1 DM, including IDDM2 on chromosome 11p5.5 and IDDM12 on 2q33. IDDM2 is composed of a variable number of tandem repeats (VNTR), actually located adjacent to the insulin (*INS*) gene. A class I (short) allele, class II (intermediate) allele, or class III (long) allele may be found at the IDDM2 locus. Homozygosity for class I alleles is found in about 80% of those with type-1 DM (compared with around 50% of the general population). Class III alleles are believed to confer a degree of protection. Class II alleles are very rare. The IDDM12 locus is composed of several genes involved in T-cell activation.

Type-2 Diabetes Mellitus

- Genotype is 1 of many factors contributing to the development of type-2 DM. Type-2 DM is thus considered a multigenic (multifactorial) condition, and like type-1 DM, mendelian inheritance is not commonly seen.

- The effect of genotype is complex, with many genes having counterbalancing effects on glycemic control and insulin resistance. These genetic anomalies would be considered polymorphisms instead of disease-causing mutations. Among these are the glucose transporter 2 (*GLUT2*) gene, insulin gene, insulin receptor, adenosine triphosphate–sensitive transmembrane transporters, and others.

Monogenetic Causes of DM

- Pancreatic agenesis is extremely rare, thought to be the result of sporadic mutations in transcription factor genes. Agenesis causes absolute insulin deficiency, a form of type-1 DM.

- Mutations in the insulin gene or genes involved in insulin posttranslational modification can lead directly to insulin deficiency (type-1 DM).

- Mutations in the insulin receptor gene (particularly in association with inherited leprechaunism or Rabson-Mendenhall syndrome) can cause insulin resistance. Inherited leprechaunism is characterized by intrauterine growth retardation, postprandial hyperglycemia, and fasting hypoglycemia. Peripheral insulin resistance is marked, with profoundly elevated serum insulin levels. Rabson-Mendenhall syndrome is similar to inherited leprechaunism but with acanthosis nigricans and other anomalies.

- Cystic fibrosis (see chapter 8) leads to progressive pancreatic insufficiency, both exocrine and endocrine, with many who survive into the teenage years and nearly all those who survive into adulthood developing type-1 diabetes mellitus.

- Maturity-onset diabetes of the young (MODY)
  - The name derives from traditional systems of diabetes classification in which type-1 was generally classified as juvenile-onset diabetes and type-2 was usually classified as maturity-onset diabetes. It was recognized that a subset of children with diabetes had a clinical picture resembling maturity-onset diabetes, in that they were non–insulin dependent, and these cases were named MODY.
  - MODY is a form of non–insulin dependent (type-2) diabetes with autosomal dominant inheritance that usually develops in the young (often in childhood). It is responsible for about 5% of type-2 cases. Affected individuals are rarely obese.

□ There are in fact multiple genotypic forms of MODY. Accounting for the vast majority of cases are *GCK/MODY2* (glucokinase), *HNF4a/MODY1* (hepatocyte nuclear factor 4 alpha), *HNF1a/MODY3* (hepatocyte nuclear factor 1 alpha), *IPF1/MODY4* (insulin promoter factor 1), and *HNF1b/MODY5* (hepatocyte nuclear factor 1 beta).

References

Akintoye SO, Chebli C, Booher S, et al. Characterization of gsp-mediated growth hormone excess in the context of McCune-Albright syndrome. *J Clin Endocr Metab* 2002; 87: 5104-5112.

Albright F, Butler AM, Hampton AO, et al. Syndrome characterized by osteitis fibrosa disseminata, areas of pigmentation and endocrine dysfunction, with precocious puberty in females:report of five cases. *N Engl J Med* 1937; 216: 727-746.

Aldred MA, Aftimos S, Hall C, et al. Constitutional deletion of chromosome 20q in two patients affected with Albright hereditary osteodystrophy. *Am J Med Genet* 2002; 113: 167-172.

Boehmer AL, Brinkmann O, Bruggenwirth H, et al. Genotype versus phenotype in families with androgen insensitivity syndrome. *J Clin Endocrinol Metab* 2001; 86: 4151-4160.

Campbell R, Gosden CM, Bonthron DT. Parental origin of transcription from the human GNAS1 gene. *J Med Genet* 1994; 31: 607-614.

Candeliere GA, Glorieux FH, Prudhomme J, et al. Increased expression of the c-fos proto-oncogene in bone from patients with fibrous dysplasia. *N Engl J Med* 1995; 332: 1546-1551.

Collins MT, Sarlis NJ, Merino MJ, et al. Thyroid carcinoma in the McCune-Albright syndrome:contributory role of activating G(s)-alpha mutations. *J Clin Endocr Metab* 2003; 88: 4413-4417.

De Sanctis C, Lala R, Matarazzo P, et al. McCune-Albright syndrome:a longitudinal clinical study of 32 patients. *J Pediatr Endocr Metab* 1999; 12: 817-826.

Eisenbarth GS, Gottlieb PA. The immunoendocrinopathy syndromes. In:*Williams Textbook of Endocrinology*. 10th ed. Philadelphia, Pa: WB Saunders, 2003.

Farfel Z, Bourne HR, Iiri T. The expanding spectrum of G protein diseases. *N Engl J Med* 1999; 340: 1012-1020.

Forest MG. Prenatal diagnosis, treatment, and outcome in infants with congenital adrenal hyperplasia. *Curr Opin Endocrinol Diab* 1998; 4: 209-217.

References

Gottlieb B, Beitel LK, Wu JH, et al. The androgen receptor gene mutations database (ARDB): 2004 update. *Hum Mutat* 2004; 23: 527-533.

Hall JG. Genomic imprinting: review and relevance to human diseases. *Am J Hum Genet* 1990; 46: 857-873.

Haller MJ, Atkinson MA, Schatz D. Type 1 diabetes mellitus: etiology, presentation, and management. *Pediatr Clin North Am* 2005; 52: 1553-1578.

Happle R. The McCune-Albright syndrome: a lethal gene surviving by mosaicism. *Clin Genet* 1986; 29: 321-324.

Jääskeläinen J, Mongan NP, Harland S, et al. Five novel androgen receptor gene mutations associated with complete androgen insensitivity syndrome. *Hum Mutat* 2006; 27: 291.

Keegan CE, Killeen AA. An overview of molecular diagnosis of steroid 21-hydroxylase deficiency. *J Mol Diagnos* 2001; 3: 49-54.

Kirk JM, Brain CE, Carson DJ, et al. Cushing's syndrome caused by nodular adrenal hyperplasia in children with McCune-Albright syndrome. *J Pediatr* 1999; 134: 789-792.

Kovacs K, Giannini C, Scheithauer BW, et al. Pituitary changes in ataxia-telangiectasia syndrome: an immunocytochemical, in-situ hybridization, and DNA cytometric study of three cases. *Endocr Pathol* 1997; 8: 195-203.

LaFranchi S. Disorders of the thyroid gland. In: *Nelson Textbook of Pediatrics*. 17th ed. Philadelphia, Pa:WB Saunders, 2004.

Lee HH, Chang JG, Tsai CH, et al. Analysis of the chimeric CYP21P/CYP21 gene in steroid 21-hydroxylase deficiency. *Clin Chem* 2000; 46: 606-11.

Lumbroso S, Paris F, Sultan C. Activating Gs-alpha mutations: analysis of 113 patients with signs of McCune-Albright syndrome. *J Clin Endocr Metab* 2004; 89: 2107-2113.

McCarthy MI. Progress in defining the molecular basis of type 2 diabetes mellitus through susceptibility-gene identification. *Hum Mol Genet* 2004; 13 (review issue): R33-R41.

Mantovani G, Maghnie M, Weber G, et al. Growth hormone-releasing hormone resistance in pseudohypoparathyroidism type Ia: New evidence for imprinting of the Gs-alpha gene. *J Clin Endocr Metab* 2003; 88: 4070-4074.

Mantovani G, Romoli R, Weber G, et al. Mutational analysis of GNAS1 in patients with pseudohypoparathyroidism: Identification of two novel mutations. *J Clin Endocr Metab* 2000; 85: 4243-4248.

Mao R, Nelson L, Kates R, et al. Prenatal diagnosis of 21-hydroxylase deficiency caused by gene conversion and rearrangements: pitfalls and molecular diagnostic solutions. *Prenat Diagn* 2002; 22: 1171-1176.

Mercado AB, Wilson RC, Cheng KC, et al. Prenatal treatment and diagnosis of congenital adrenal hyperplasia owing to steroid 21-hydroxylase deficiency. *J Clin Endocrinol Metab* 1995; 80: 2014-2020.

Mullis PE. Genetics of growth hormone deficiency. *Endocrinol Metab Clin North Am* 2007; 36: 17-36.

Pang S. Congenital adrenal hyperplasia. *Endocrinol Metab Clin North Am* 1997; 26: 853-891.

Pang S, Shook MK. Current status of neonatal screening for congenital adrenal hyperplasia. *Curr Opin Pediatr* 1997; 9: 419-423.

Pugliese A. Genetics of type 1 diabetes. *Endocrinol Metab Clin N Am* 2004; 33: 1-16.

Rapaport R. Disorders of the gonads. In: *Nelson Textbook of Pediatrics*. 17th ed. Philadelphia, Pa: Saunders, 2004.

Reed MJ, Purohit A, Woo LWL, et al. Steroid sulfatase: molecular biology, regulation, and inhibition. *Endocr Rev* 2005; 26: 171-202.

Ruan QG, She J. Autoimmune polyglandular syndrome type 1 and the autoimmune regulator. *Clin Lab Med* 2004; 24: 305-317.

Speiser PW, White PC. Congenital adrenal hyperplasia. *N Engl J Med* 2003; 349: 776-788.

Spiegel AM, Weinstein LS. Inherited diseases involving G proteins and G protein–coupled receptors. *Annu Rev Med* 2004; 55: 27-39.

References

Taylor JC, Gough SC, Hunt PJ, et al. A genome-wide screen in 1119 relative pairs with autoimmune thyroid disease [published online ahead of print November 8, 2005]. *J Clin Endocrinol Metab* 2006; 91: 646-653.

Trajkovskia M, Mziauta H, Schwarz PE, et al. Genes of type 2 diabetes in β cells. *Endocrinol Metab Clin North Am* 2006; 35: 357-369.

Vaxillaire M, Froguel P. Genetic basis of maturity-onset diabetes of the young. *Endocrinol Metab Clin North Am* 2006; 35: 371-384.

Weinstein LS, Shenker A, Gejman PV, et al. Activating mutations of the stimulatory G protein in the McCune-Albright syndrome. *N Engl J Med* 1991; 325: 1688-1695.

White PC, Tusie-Luna MT, New MI, et al. Mutations in steroid 21-hydroxylase (CYP21). *Hum Mutat* 1994; 3: 373-378.

Chapter 8

Gastrointestinal, Hepatobiliary, and Pancreatic Diseases

Gastrointestinal Tract

Hirschsprung Disease

- The gastrointestinal (GI) tract normally has an extensive neural plexus, exerting its influence through synapses formed upon ganglion cells located within the intestinal wall. Throughout the length of colon, with the exception of the last 1 to 2 cm of rectum, clusters of ganglion cells can normally be found in the muscularis mucosa (Meissner submucosal plexus) and muscularis propria (Auerbach myenteric plexus).

- Hirschsprung disease is an example of a disease caused by abnormal migration of neural crest cells during fetal development (a neurocristopathy). Cells emerging from the neural crest migrate to the developing bowel and populate it with neurons, beginning proximally and proceeding distally. An interruption in this process, therefore, always involves the distalmost portions of colon and a variable length proximally.

- As Harald Hirschsprung described in the 19th century, untreated Hirschsprung disease results in death in infancy from toxic megacolon. Many years later it was recognized, based on histologic examination, that this disease is related to aganglionosis of a segment of the colon, a defect that always includes the distal rectum and a variable length proximal to and contiguous with the rectum.

- Hirschsprung disease is classified according to the length of colon involved with reference to the splenic flexure. Most cases are restricted to the rectum or rectosigmoid and considered short-segment Hirschsprung disease. Some cases involve only the very distal rectum and are considered ultra-short segment Hirschsprung disease. In about 15%, the aganglionosis extends proximal to the splenic flexure (long-segment Hirschsprung disease). Rare cases (<5%) involve the entire colon (total colonic aganglionosis).

- Short-segment disease is 4 times more common in males than in females; however, the numbers are essentially equal for long-segment Hirschsprung disease.

- Hirschsprung disease usually presents as failure to pass meconium (meconium ileus) in the first 48 hours of life. Those with very short affected segments may be capable of passing meconium, and will present somewhat later with constipation or other evidence of altered bowel motility. Of course, other common causes of meconium ileus must be considered,

including cystic fibrosis, intestinal atresia, and imperforate anus.

- The definitive diagnosis requires a biopsy specimen *taken more than 2 cm from* the dentate line (a specimen should not be taken from the normally aganglionic segment). Affected individuals show an absence of ganglion cells in association with axonal hypertrophy.

- A structural chromosomal abnormality is present in about 10% of cases, most commonly trisomy 21. Genes known to cause Hirschsprung disease are not found on 21, however, and include, among others, the *RET* gene (10q11.2), *GDNF* gene (5p), and *EDNRB* gene (13q). In addition, Hirschsprung disease is often a component of a larger syndrome, such as neurofibromatosis type 1 (NF1), multiple endocrine neoplasia type 2A (MEN2A), Waardenburg syndrome, congenital central hypoventilation (Haddad) syndrome, familial dysautonomia (Riley-Day) syndrome, and Smith-Lemli-Opitz syndrome.

- *RET* is a proto-oncogene in which germline (gain-of-function) mutations result in the MEN2A syndrome. *RET* mutations in a different exon lead to MEN2B which has no association with Hirschsprung disease. Loss-of-function *RET* mutations are found in Hirschsprung disease.

Esophageal Atresia

- The overall incidence of congenital structural anomalies of the esophagus is about 1 in 3000 live births, taking the form of esophageal atresia in most instances. Esophageal atresia may occur with or without a tracheoesophageal fistula (TEF) and with or without a larger syndrome, especially the VACTERL sequence (vertebral, anal, cardiac, tracheal, esophageal, renal, and limb). In fact, esophageal atresia occurs as an isolated anomaly in fewer than 10% of cases. There are several forms of TEF, the most common being the distal-type TEF (90% of cases) which communicates between the trachea and the distal end of the esophagus (distal to the stenosis). The second most common (5% of cases) is the so-called H type, in which a TEF is noted in association with a nonatretic esophagus.

- Esophageal atresia most often comes to clinical attention by producing polyhydramnios (amniotic fluid is normally swallowed by the fetus). Alternatively, it may present as difficulty with feeding. If the distal form of TEF is present, pneumonitis may develop

8: Gastrointestinal, Hepatobiliary, and Pancreatic Diseases

Gastrointestinal Tract>Esophageal Atresia; Pyloric Stenosis; Intestinal Atresia; Abdominal Wall Defects: Abdominal Wall Defects: Omphalocele and Gastroschisis

because of aspiration of gastric contents. The atresia is confirmed by failure to pass a nasogastric tube, and the presence of a distal TEF is confirmed by the radiographic presence of a gastric gas bubble (which would be absent without a distal TEF).

- Surgical management is occasionally straightforward but usually complex, particularly when the gap between the proximal and distal segments is long (>2 cm or >2 disc spaces). In such long-gap cases, multiple staged procedures are often necessary, with the application of tension to the free ends. Anastomotic leak, strictures, and recurrence of TEF are the main surgical complications, but swallowing problems may also be significant. All this occurs during a critical time for the learning of proper swallowing, which may subsequently be impaired.

Pyloric Stenosis

- Pyloric stenosis usually does not present immediately at birth. Instead, it presents in infants usually between 1 and 6 weeks of age, with projectile vomiting after meals. If not addressed, electrolyte abnormalities (metabolic alkalosis) and malnutrition can result. Anatomically, pyloric stenosis results from hypertrophy of the smooth muscle surrounding the pyloric channel.

- The pyloric valve may be palpable as mass (olive) in the epigastrium. The diagnosis can usually be confirmed by imaging. Dye studies reveal a classic string sign, and ultrasonography gives a classic double-track sign; however, these findings are not 100% specific (being potentially produced by pylorospasm); thus, strict quantitative ultrasonography criteria have been adopted. Surgical intervention (eg, pyloromyotomy) is highly successful.

- While a strict mendelian pattern of inheritance is not observed, familial clustering is, and concordance among identical twins is about 50%. Furthermore, pyloric stenosis is often present in association with Apert syndrome, Zellweger syndrome, trisomy 18, Smith-Lemli-Opitz syndrome, Cornelia de Lange syndrome, Turner syndrome, and Hirschsprung disease. The pathogenesis is presently considered multifactorial.

- Pyloric stenosis is most common in those of northern European descent. It is uncommon in blacks and rare in Asians. Males are affected approximately 4 times as often as females, firstborn infants are at highest risk,

and the incidence is increased in infants with type B and O blood groups. A child born to a mother with a history of pyloric stenosis is more likely to be affected than one born to a father who had pyloric stenosis. Pyloric stenosis is associated with other congenital defects, including tracheoesophageal fistula.

- The overall incidence is about 1 in 300 live births.

Intestinal Atresia

- Intestinal atresia is among the most common congenital defects of the GI tract, with an incidence of around 1 in 500 to 1 in 1000 live births. The term refers to a segment of stenotic intestine, thought to be the result of a failure of recanalization of the bowel which, at around 10 weeks, is present in the form of a solid cord. A vascular insult may underlie this failure. The most common location is the ileum, followed by jejunum and duodenum. Other congenital intestinal obstructions may be the result of an annular pancreas or a duodenal web (Ladd bands), both presenting as obstructions in the region of the ampulla of Vater.

- Most cases of intestinal atresia appear to represent sporadic events, however, about 30% of cases are associated with Down syndrome, and there are rare familial cases. Furthermore, a mutation of the fibroblast growth factor gene in mice has been shown to reproduce this phenotype. With regard to Mendelian disorders, atresia is seen frequently in Feingold syndrome, a rare autosomal-dominant disorder characterized by duodenal atresia, microcephaly, and limb malformations.

- Intestinal atresia may come to clinical attention as a result of polyhydramnios. After birth, it may present with bilious vomiting. A duodenal obstruction may be seen radiographically as a "double bubble" sign caused by a gastric gas bubble adjacent to the proximal duodenal gas bubble.

Abdominal Wall Defects: Omphalocele (Exomphalos) and Gastroschisis

- Omphalocele and gastroschisis are congenital abdominal wall defects that must be distinguished from one another, because their clinical implications are markedly different **T8.1**.

- The location of a gastroschisis is typically just to the right of the umbilicus. It is composed of loops of intestine without covering. In contrast an omphalocele is located in the midline, essentially in the umbilical

Gastrointestinal Tract>Abdominal Wall Defects: Omphalocele and Gastroschisis; Osler-Weber-Rendu Syndrome; Blue Rubber Bleb Nevus Syndrome; Microvillus Inclusion Disease

T8.1
Omphalocele vs Gastroschisis

	Omphalocele	**Gastroschisis**
Peritoneal covering	Yes	No
Contents	Often bowel, liver, and spleen	Often only bowel
Location	Umbilicus	Right of umbilicus
Associated anomalies	Common Gastrointestinal (35%) Cardiac (20%) Beckwith-Wiedemann (10%)	Uncommon, mainly gastrointestinal
Associated prematurity	10%	60%

cord. It is composed of multiple viscera, including intestine, liver, and spleen, and it is covered by a membrane composed of peritoneum and amnion.

- Abdominal wall defects occur sporadically, but gastroschisis is strongly associated with *decreased* maternal age. Importantly, the incidence of additional congenital anomalies is very high in association with omphalocele (60%) but relatively low in association with gastroschisis (10%). Furthermore, anomalies associated with gastroschisis are largely intestinal, whereas omphalocele is often associated with major cardiac defects, chromosomal anomalies (trisomy 21, trisomy 18, trisomy 13), or the Beckwith-Wiedemann syndrome.

- Abdominal wall defects can be diagnosed prenatally. Often there is an elevated maternal serum alpha fetoprotein (MSAFP) on routine prenatal screening, being much higher in gastroschisis than in omphalocele. Ultrasound easily detects the anatomic findings.

Osler-Weber-Rendu Syndrome (Hereditary Hemorrhagic Telangiectasia)

- This is a condition in which vascular walls are structurally abnormal, leading to recurrent episodes of bleeding, and it may initially be taken to represent a coagulation disorder.

- The initial manifestation in most patients, beginning in childhood, is epistaxis. In adolescence or young adulthood, skin lesions appear, taking the form of telangiectasias on the face, lips, ears, and chest. Similar lesions can be found on the oral mucosa.

In the 4th or 5th decade, GI bleeding arises, resulting from bleeding telangiectasias or arteriovenous malformations. Arteriovenous malformations may also form in the brain, lung, or liver.

- This is an autosomal dominant disorder with a frequency of about 1 in 5000. It can be caused by mutations in either the *ENG* gene or the *ACVRL1* gene. *ENG* is found at 9q34 and encodes endoglin. *ACVRL1* is found at 12q and encodes a serine/threonine protein kinase receptor. About 80% of all disease-causing mutations can be detected by direct sequence analysis, with another 10% detected by duplication/deletion analysis.

Blue Rubber Bleb Nevus Syndrome

- This rare autosomal recessive disorder somewhat resembles Osler-Weber-Rendu. It is characterized by the cutaneous hemangiomas and GI bleeding caused by vascular malformations, both manifestations presenting in infancy or early childhood.

- 3 types of cutaneous hemangiomas have been described. The first presents as soft compressible nodules (blue rubber blebs). The second is a blue-black punctate lesion, tender to palpation, found in great numbers on the trunk and extremities. The last type are large cavernous hemangiomas.

Microvillus Inclusion Disease (MID)

- MID is a cause of chronic malabsorptive malnutrition in infants. In fact, it is considered the most common cause of malabsorption to present in the neonatal period. It is inherited as an autosomal recessive trait.

- Characteristically, the wall of the small intestine is paper-thin. Small-bowel biopsy shows villus blunting, with overall mucosal atrophy and characteristic apical intracellular inclusions. Ultrastructurally, these consist of vesicles of invaginated brush border constituents, and traditionally, ultrastructural examination has been required for the diagnosis.

- There are several histochemical and immunohistochemical alternatives to electron microscopy. Periodic acid–Schiff (PAS) staining, polyclonal carcinoembryonic antigen, and CD10 normally highlight the brush border of intestinal epithelia in a linear apical pattern. All have also been shown to highlight the microvillus inclusions in MID by displaying cytoplasmic staining in a globular or grainy pattern.

Tufting Enteropathy (Intestinal Epithelial Dysplasia)

- Like MID, this has its onset in infancy and presents as a chronic malabsorptive state.

- Small-bowel biopsy shows widespread "tufts" of enterocytes.

- The enterocytes appear to express a paucity of the adhesion molecule E-cadherin.

Autoimmune Enteric Diseases: Celiac Sprue, Crohn Disease (CD), Ulcerative Colitis (UC), and Autoimmune Enteropathy

- Similar to most other well-studied autoimmune conditions, there appear to be inherited alleles that influence (but do not directly cause) the development of celiac sprue.

  - Celiac sprue is an autoimmune condition provoked by gluten. The disease may arise at any time after eating begins, and while many cases present in the pediatric age group, new diagnoses are frequently made in the elderly. Histologically, the duodenum is the site of greatest severity. In fully developed lesions, there is villous atrophy, but many of those affected have only an increase in intraepithelial lymphocytes without architectural changes. Furthermore, some cases present with histologic findings and no symptoms. Prolonged inflammation may lead to a risk of malnutrition (a common cause of idiopathic short stature and unexplained iron deficiency anemia) and of T-cell lymphoma (enteropathy-associated T cell

lymphoma). Extraintestinal manifestations include arthritis and dermatitis herpetiformis. Sprue is strongly associated with diabetes mellitus, IgA deficiency, and cystic fibrosis. Serologic markers in celiac sprue include antigliadin antibodies, antiendomyseal antibodies, and antitransglutaminase antibodies. Both biopsy findings and serologic findings abate with restriction of gluten.

  - The incidence of celiac sprue depends on how the disease is defined. Those with symptomatic disease represent only a small fraction of those with serologic or histologic findings consistent with celiac sprue. In the United States, the incidence of clinically significant celiac sprue is approximately 1 in 7000. However, the incidence based on serologic studies is as high as 1 in 1000. While the disease is present worldwide, it is relatively infrequent in sub-Saharan African, Chinese, and Japanese populations. Concordance for celiac sprue among identical twins is about 70%.

  - The HLA-DQ2 allele is present in about 95% of patients with celiac sprue (compared with around 30% of the general population). Alleles that encode DQ2 include DQA1*0501, DQA1*0505, and DQB1*0201/*0202. Nonetheless, only a minority of persons with HLA-DQ2 actually develop sprue. Clearly, other susceptibility genes and environmental influences are at work. HLA-DQ8 (allele DQB1*0302) is present in most of the remaining cases of celiac sprue. HLA typing may be useful in patients with equivocal biopsy and serologic findings. Those negative for DQ2 and DQ8 are extremely unlikely to have celiac sprue. Only about 1% of those with HLA DQ2 or DQ8 type have disease, however.

- Chronic inflammatory bowel disease (IBD) encompasses 2 distinct clinicopathologic syndromes: CD and UC. CD can affect any part of the intestine, and is characterized by discontinuous, transmural inflammatory lesions sometimes having a granulomatous component. UC affects the rectum and sometimes portions of the colon, always in a continuous fashion (at least initially), with inflammation that is superficial and not associated with granulomas.

  - Familial clustering has long been noted in cases of CD. The rate of concordant disease among siblings is about 15% to 30%. The relative risk among first-degree relatives is 15 times that of the

8: Gastrointestinal, Hepatobiliary, and Pancreatic Diseases

Gastrointestinal Tract>Autoimmune Enteric Diseases I Biliary>Caroli Disease, Congenital Hepatic Fibrosis and Related
Biliary Fibrocystic Diseases; Syndromic Paucity of Bile Ducts

general population, and the concordance among identical twins approaches 70%. Furthermore, Ashkenazi Jews have a relative risk of roughly 4-fold. Several susceptibility genes have been identified, including the *NOD2/CARD15* gene (IBD1 locus) on chromosome 16 and the *OCTN* gene (IBD5 locus) on 5q31. Interestingly, consistent associations with HLA polymorphisms have not been demonstrated in Crohn disease.

- ☐ Familial clustering is also evident in UC; however, the concordance rate for identical twins is only about 15% to 20% (much lower than CD). A sibling of an affected individual has a roughly 10% chance of being affected. Several susceptibility genes have been explored, including the IBD2 locus on chromosome 12.

- ☐ Interestingly, both UC and CD appear to be influenced by polymorphisms in the *MDR1* (multidrug resistance 1) gene. In particular, a C3435T polymorphism appears to be associated with both diseases.

- Genetic influences on isolated autoimmune enteropathy, a cause of gluten-independent bowel injury commonly found in children, have not been elucidated. However (like many autoimmune conditions), the disease is common in those with inherited immunodeficiency states.

Biliary

Caroli Disease, Congenital Hepatic Fibrosis (CHF), and Related Biliary Fibrocystic Diseases

- The conditions in this category are considered disorders of the ductal plate (ductal plate malformations). In fact, the classic histologic finding in congenital hepatic fibrosis—a sleevelike annular bile duct encircling a central core of connective tissue—is the normal appearance of the fetal liver at around 10 weeks. In the normal course of events, this ductal plate becomes reorganized into the portal triad as we normally envision it. This process is thought to be interrupted in ductal plate malformations.

- Both Caroli disease and CHF are strongly associated with autosomal recessive polycystic kidney disease (ARPKD) and nephronophthisis (see chapter 5). Like ARPKD, Caroli disease and CHF are caused by mutations in the *PKHD1* gene on 6p. This gene

encodes a protein called fibrocystin (polyductin) which is thought to be involved in the normal embryogenesis of the bile ducts and renal tubules.

- Caroli disease is characterized by segmental dilation of the intrahepatic bile ducts (and to a lesser extent, extrahepatic ducts), not related to obstruction. Dilation may be fusiform early, but in its mature form, is saccular. Stone formation and recurrent bouts of bacterial cholangitis typically complicate this syndrome. Caroli disease can be diagnosed with ultrasound or endoscopic retrograde cholangio pancreatography, showing the typical saccular or fusiform dilations in the intrahepatic bile ducts (without evidence of an obstruction). The liver biopsy may show features of ascending cholangitis. Strictly defined, Caroli disease is a term that refers to bile ductular ectasia without the other findings of CHF.

- CHF is characterized by enlargement of portal tracts by interstitial fibrosis within which are segmentally dilated and abnormally shaped (sleevelike) bile ducts. The result is biliary obstruction and portal hypertension. Because of the concomitant renal disease, palpable kidneys, progressive azotemia, and hypertension may be seen.

- Autosomal dominant polycystic kidney disease (ADPKD; see chapter 5) has associated hepatic cysts (and von Meyenburg complexes) in about half of patients. These differ from Caroli disease and CHF in that they are usually simple cysts, not in continuity with the ductal system. These are much more prominent in affected females.

- Other ductal plate malformation–related diseases include Joubert syndrome, Meckel-Gruber syndrome, and Bardet-Biedl syndrome.

Syndromic Paucity of Bile Ducts (Alagille Syndrome, Arteriohepatic Dysplasia)

- Alagille syndrome is an autosomal dominant disorder characterized by a set of dysmorphic features in association with a noninflammatory dearth of interlobular bile ducts.

- A paucity of interlobular bile ducts in infancy is frequently the result of causes other than Alagille syndrome, including congenital rubella syndrome and alpha-1 antitrypsin (AAT) deficiency.

- Mutations in the *JAG1* gene, responsible for encoding the protein Jagged1, have been identified in around 70% of cases. Jagged1 is a signaling protein involved in fetal development, serving as a ligand for Notch receptors. Genetic anomalies range from point mutations to entire gene deletion. A small percentage of patients with this syndrome have instead a mutation in the *NOTCH2* gene. Interestingly, *NOTCH1* mutations (translocations) are found in T-cell acute leukemias, and *NOTCH3* mutations cause cerebral autosomal dominant arteriopathy with subcortical infarcts and leukoencephalopathy (CADASIL). While the diagnosis of Alagille syndrome is based largely on clinical findings, mutations can be found in the *JAG1* gene in the vast majority of cases based on direct gene sequencing.

- Alagille syndrome usually presents with cholestasis, often in the neonatal period. Total bilirubin is elevated (ratio of conjugated-to-unconjugated bilirubin about 50:50), as is the alkaline phosphatase level. Additional features include facial dysmorphism (broad forehead, widely spaced eyes, small mandible, prominent ears), butterfly vertebrae, posterior embryotoxon of the eye, and congenital heart disease (especially peripheral pulmonic stenosis).

- At very early stages, the liver biopsy shows hepatitis resembling neonatal (giant cell) hepatitis. The number of bile ducts is normal at birth and progressively diminishes thereafter (hence the alternate designation of *the disappearing bile duct syndrome*). The characteristic paucity of bile ducts (duct-to–portal tract ratio less than 1:2) may not be apparent until after 6 months of age. Histologic examination shows no evidence of ductal inflammation and no injury to existing ducts. It is thought that the mechanism underlying bile duct paucity is the failure of ducts to continue to elongate after birth.

Gallstone Disease

- While a seemingly mundane aspect of the routine practice of pathology, heredity exerts a significant influence on the development of gallstones. These effects may be considered in 3 broad categories: (1) gender, (2) inherited diseases with metabolic by-products that enhance stone formation (eg, chronic hemolytic anemias) and (3) poorly understood but well-established familial and ethnic influences.

- Females are roughly twice as likely to develop stones than males. First-degree relatives of patients with gallstones have a roughly 5-fold increased risk of having gallstones. Furthermore, certain ethnic groups—eg, Native Americans, especially the Pima

Indians, with a 70% lifetime risk, and Scandinavians with a 50% risk—have increased risk of developing gallstones.

- With regard to inherited disease, the risk relates to the type of stone. Cholesterol (yellow) stones are promoted by conditions associated with enhanced cholesterol excretion; eg, increased activity of HMG CoA reductase. Black pigment stones are promoted by inherited chronic hemolytic conditions.

Extrahepatic Biliary Atresia (EHBA)

- The influence of genetics in EHBA is unclear. At this time, it appears that certain inherited factors influence disease susceptibility. In further defining the pathogenesis of EHBA, it is helpful to understand that there are 2 somewhat distinct types. 1 is the more common neonatal form that presents with jaundice when the infant is several weeks old. This type of EHBA tends to occur in isolation, and pathogenesis appears to be related to perinatal injury perhaps related to a virus. In this regard, a seasonality has been demonstrated in its incidence. The second, less common, type may be thought of as a true congenital anomaly, developing in fetal life, in which there are often associated extrahepatic anomalies, particularly splenic (polysplenia syndrome) and defects of laterality (situs inversus). Some have advocated the term *biliary atresia splenic malformation* (BASM) syndrome for this association.

- From a practical point of view, the challenge lies in recognizing EHBA because there are numerous causes of neonatal jaundice, and the benefit of surgical intervention is exquisitely time-sensitive. The surgical approach to EHBA, the creation of a portoenterostomy as described by Morio Kasai in 1959, can potentially cure a once uniformly fatal disease. However, outcome is most favorable if this surgery is undertaken before 6 weeks of age and drops off precipitously after 8 weeks. The alternative to the Kasai procedure is liver transplantation.

- Jaundice that results from conjugated (direct) hyperbilirubinemia is the most common presenting symptom. In classic cases, infants have clay- or gray-colored acholic stool. The differential diagnosis is long, but early consideration should be given to liver biopsy and radiographic imaging of the biliary system. In addition to other findings, the absence of rapid emptying of dye into the duodenum and the inability to visualize a gallbladder support a diagnosis of EHBA. Liver

8: Gastrointestinal, Hepatobiliary, and Pancreatic Diseases

Biliary>Extrahepatic Biliary Atresia I Hepatic>Medium-Chain Acyl-Coenzyme A Dehydrogenase Deficiency; Hereditary Hemochromatosis

biopsy showing evidence of extrahepatic obstruction (portal neutrophilic inflammation and profound bile ductular proliferation) further supports the diagnosis. Liver biopsy interpretation in this setting is often not straightforward, however, because of the overlap with neonatal (giant cell) hepatitis. Essentially, the liver biopsy should be viewed as a means to exclude other causes of neonatal jaundice and to identify histologic changes consistent with EHBA. Pathologists may also be called on intraoperatively; frozen section evaluation can aid in determining the suitability of a particular site for transection of the porta hepatis.

- As stated before, a genetic influence on EHBA is most likely in the true congenital type. There is more-than-chance concordance of EHBA in identical twins and a small number of reports of familial EHBA. Nonetheless, the pattern is far from mendelian, and the disease is currently considered multifactorial.

Hepatic

Medium-Chain Acyl-Coenzyme A Dehydrogenase (MCAD) Deficiency

- When a child presents with hepatic failure and is found on biopsy (or autopsy) to have widespread microvesicular steatosis, the diagnosis of idiopathic Reye syndrome is suggested. However, cases previously classified as Reye syndrome are increasingly found to be the result of underlying metabolic defects, including respiratory chain disorders, disorders of fatty acid oxidation (the most common being MCAD deficiency), and carnitine transport disorders.

- See chapter 10

Hereditary Hemochromatosis (HH)

- HH is the most common inherited disease in persons of northern European ancestry. The prevalence in the United States is approximately 1 in 300. The prevalence is lower among American Hispanics (1 in 3000), American blacks (1 in 10,000), and Asian Americans (1 in 1 million).

- HH is inherited as an autosomal recessive disease. The vast majority of cases are caused by 1 of 2 point mutations **T8.2** of the *HFE* gene on chromosome 6p21.3, within the HLA locus (previously called HLA-H). Most affected individuals (60%-90%) are homozygous for the C282Y (845A) mutation, and the remaining cases are caused by compound heterozygosity for C282Y and the H63D (187G) mutation. The C282Y mutation is caused by a G to A substitution at nucleotide 845 that results in a tyrosine-for-cysteine substitution at amino acid 282 (nucleotide 845). This disrupts a disulphide bond, the effect of which is impaired association of the HFE protein with β2-microglobulin and thereby decreased expression of HFE on the cell surface. The H63D mutation (or polymorphism) is quite common in Caucasians, being present in 25% of the population. It only causes disease when coinherited with a C282Y mutation (compound heterozygote). However, the compound heterozygotes represent about 2% of the population, and only a small minority of them will develop clinical disease.

- There is a less common group of non-*HFE*-related cases. Juvenile hereditary hemochromatosis (sometimes called type 2 HHC) has an earlier age at onset and more severe manifestations than usual type HHC. Juvenile HHC is caused by mutations in either the *HJV* (hemojuvelin) gene or the *HAMP* gene.

T8.2
Hereditary Hemochromatosis-Associated Genes

Gene	Location	Disease
HFE (most common variants: C282Y, H63D, S65C)	6p21.3	Hereditary hemochromatosis
HFE2 (hemojuvlin)	1q21	Juvenile hemochromatosis A
HAMP (hepcidin)	19q13	Juvenile hemochromatosis B
TFR2 (transferrin receptor)	7q22	Hemochromatosis type 3
FTH1 (ferritin heavy chain)	11q13	Familial iron overload

- Hemochromatosis displays a low rate of penetrance. Disease is most likely to develop in those homozygous for C282Y, but even in these cases clinically significant hemochromatosis arises at a low rate. Slightly less severe but still capable of fully manifesting hemochromatosis are compound heterozygotes for C282Y/H63D. Homozygotes for H63D are clinically well. Simple heterozygotes for either C282Y or H63D are generally healthy, with the following caveats: many have abnormal serum iron studies reflecting some degree of iron overload, and there is a greater likelihood of progression in other forms of hepatic injury, such as steatohepatitis.

- The basic defect in HH is enhanced intestinal iron absorption. The normal adult absorbs only a small percentage of ingested iron, amounting to about 1 to 2 mg per day. Absorption is regulated by the demand for iron, through a feedback loop which is interrupted in HH. The mechanisms for this have not been fully elucidated, but a protein hormone called hepcidin appears to be involved. Hepcidin is synthesized in the liver at a rate influenced by iron stores (it is also an acute phase reactant), and it exerts an inhibitory effect on iron absorption. In HH, hepcidin levels are low. Iron absorption in excess of what can be used by the reticuloendothelial system results in iron deposition in hepatocytes, pancreas, pituitary, synovium, heart, and skin. This causes damage to the liver (usually pauci-inflammatory fibrosis progressing to cirrhosis), pancreas (fibrosis with impairment of islet cell function leading to diabetes), pituitary gland (hypogonadotrophic hypogonadism leading to infertility—not much direct impact on the gonads), joints (osteoarthritis), heart (dilated or restrictive cardiomyopathy), and skin (bronzing secondary to increased melanin). It has been suggested that increased iron may lead to oxidative damage to DNA and the increased risk of hepatocellular (and other) carcinomas. Regardless of genotype, women are half as likely as men to develop complications of hemochromatosis.

- Screening involves serum iron studies, especially percentage of transferrin saturation and ferritin (both elevated in HH). A transferrin saturation of at least 45% has a sensitivity of more than 95%, and this is the most widely recommended single screening assay (suggested cut-offs vary from 45%-60%, and an elevated value should lead to repeat testing). However, specificity is hampered by a number of causes of secondary siderosis **T8.3**, including steatohepatitis, chronic hemolytic anemia, dietary iron overload (eg, excessive iron supplementation, Bantu siderosis), chronic transfusions, sideroblastic anemia, and porphyria cutanea tarda.

- The traditional confirmatory test has been liver biopsy with either qualitative or quantitative iron assessment. The liver biopsy displays increased hepatocellular iron, particularly when stained with Prussian blue, with the greatest deposition in periportal (zone 1) hepatocytes. Semiquantitative iron grading (0-4+ scale) correlates extremely well with hepatic iron quantitation, especially at the extremes (0-1+ and 4+). Hepatic iron can be measured quantitatively by means of atomic absorption spectrophotometry, and expressed either as the hepatic iron concentration (micromoles of iron per gram of dry liver weight) or as the hepatic iron index (hepatic iron concentration divided by age in years). A normal hepatic iron index is lower than 1.1, and a value higher than 1.9 is considered diagnostic of HH. Once cirrhosis is established, the value of the hepatic iron index is lower.

- Confirmation by molecular methods may substitute for liver biopsy in appropriate settings. The molecular diagnosis of HH is an excellent example of the application of targeted mutation analysis. Because nearly all affected persons have either C282Y or H63D, it is cost-effective to look for only these 2 alleles. The most common methods for detecting these alleles are PCR-ASO (dot-blot) and restriction fragment length polymorphism (RFLP) after polymerase chain reaction (PCR) amplification (PCR-RFLP) in which the diagnostic restriction fragments are detected by gel electrophoresis.

T8.3
Causes of Hemochromatosis/Hemosiderosis

Hereditary	Acquired
Hereditary hemochromatosis	Chronic transfusion
Porphyria cutanea tarda	Chronic hemolytis
Atransferrinemia	Chronic liver disease (steatohepatitis, hepatitis C)
	Dietary iron overload (eg, Bantu siderosis)

Wilson Disease (Hepatolenticular Degeneration)

- Wilson disease is an autosomal recessive disorder that occurs with a frequency of about 1 in 30,000. It is caused by mutations in the *ATP7B* gene on chromosome 13. This gene encodes an adenosine triphosphatase (ATPase) involved in binding copper to ceruloplasmin.

- Wilson disease may present in 1 of 3 ways—liver disease, neuropsychiatric disease, or hemolysis—usually in childhood or adolescence **T8.4**. Hepatitis caused by Wilson disease often presents acutely with jaundice and abdominal pain, but it may present with chronic hepatitis. Sometimes this is discovered only incidentally through abnormal liver function tests. Often coincident with hepatitis is a nonimmune hemolytic anemia. Kayser-Fleischer rings often develop in association with neurologic disease. The neurologic manifestations were the basis for the first description of Wilson disease by Samuel Alexander Kinnier Wilson in 1912. The neurologic manifestations are protean and may include movement disorders (dysarthria, tremors, rigidity, bradykinesia, and abnormal gait) and psychosis.

- It is important to think of the possibility of Wilson disease when examining a liver biopsy specimen from a young adult with hepatitis. The liver biopsy shows glycogenated nuclei, steatosis, and inflammation that may mimic the pattern of chronic viral hepatitis. Fibrosis ultimately leads to cirrhosis. Unlike liver iron stains, hepatic copper stains are unreliable in

comparison with formal hepatic copper quantitation (which is considered the gold standard). Furthermore, the finding of stainable copper is highly nonspecific and may be seen in steatohepatitis and cholestasis. In secondary forms of copper accumulation (eg, cholestasis), the quantitative hepatic copper is in the range of 0.55 to 1.26 µmol/g, whereas in Wilson disease it is often greater than 4 µmol/g.

- The plasma ceruloplasmin may serve as a screening test. Low levels are found in Wilson disease, but there are several causes of falsely elevated and falsely depressed levels. In fully established Wilson disease, the serum copper is elevated; however, at various stages, the copper may be low, normal, or high. The urinary copper excretion is usually elevated. There are too many disease-causing mutations in *ATP7B* for molecular diagnosis to be practical at this time.

Alpha-1 Antitrypsin (AAT) Deficiency

- The *SERPINA1* (*PI*) gene on chromosome 14q31-32.3 is the site of moderate polymorphism. The normal (wild-type) genotype consists of homozygosity for the M allele (denoted PI-MM). About 10% of the normal Caucasian population is heterozygous for M and some other allele, of which there are about 75. The alleles are named according to the electrophoretic mobility of the encoded protein; fastest variants are A, slowest Z.

- Aside from rare examples, nearly all clinically relevant AAT deficiency is associated with at least 1 copy of the Z allele (Glu342Lys). The vast majority of affected patients have either PI-ZZ or PI-SZ. The S allele (Glu264Val) is by itself incapable of causing clinical disease, but homozygosity for S leads to modest reductions in plasma AAT **T8.5**.

- The Z allele has a frequency in the US population of about 1% to 2%. In Europe, the allele frequency is highest in the North (5% in Scandinavians) and lowest in the South (1% of Italians). The S allele has the opposite distribution: 10% in Southern Europe, 5% in the north.

- AAT deficiency is thus inherited as an autosomal recessive trait. It presents **T8.6** as neonatal hepatitis in a significant portion of patients. Others are spared as neonates and may present instead with early-onset emphysema, cirrhosis, hepatocellular carcinoma, or panniculitis. There appears to be an increased incidence of Wegener granulomatosis and other vasculitides. In contrast to usual-type emphysema

T8.4
Clinical Presentations of Wilson Disease

Elevated liver function tests

Acute hepatitis

Chronic hepatitis

Cirrhosis

Kayser-Fleischer rings

Neurologic disease (dysarthria, tremor, bradykinesia, abnormal gait, choreiform movement disorder, psychosis)

Renal insufficiency

Arthropathy (osteochondritis dissecans)

Hemolysis

8: Gastrointestinal, Hepatobiliary, and Pancreatic Diseases

Hepatic>Alpha-1 Antitrypsin Deficiency; Disorders of Bilirubin Conjugation: Gilbert Syndrome and Crigler-Najjar Syndromes

T8.5

Alpha-1 Antitrypsin Deficiency–Associated Alleles

Genotype	Prevalence (%)	Approximate AAT (mg/dL)
MM	90	150-350
MS	6	125-300
MZ	5	100-200
SS	<1	100-200
SZ	<1	75-120
ZZ	<1	20-50

which is centro-acinar and upper lobe–predominant, AAT-associated emphysema has panacinar histopathology and basilar predominance.

- AAT is a member of the serpin family of protease inhibitors, related to C1 esterase inhibitor and antithrombin. The serpins exert their effects through a unique mechanism involving a profound change in conformation on binding the target protease. This reliance on conformation makes them exquisitely sensitive to specific amino acid substitutions in the "hinge" regions. Interestingly, the hepatic effects of AAT deficiency are not related to any decrement in protease inhibition. The conformational effects of disease-causing mutations lead to polymerization of AAT in hepatocytes. Polymerization prevents effective secretion of AAT into the blood and leads to the accumulation of AAT in the hepatocyte endoplasmic reticulum (visible as PAS-positive droplets). This mechanism of organ damage caused by conformation-driven intracellular accumulation has been termed "conformational disease" and is a mechanism shared with Alzheimer and Pick diseases (see chapter 11).

Disorders of Bilirubin Conjugation: Gilbert Syndrome and Crigler-Najjar Syndromes

- Gilbert syndrome is a relatively common (around 5% of the population) benign condition that presents as episodic mild hyperbilirubinemia **T8.7**, brought on by fasting, infection, or other physiologic stress. It results from defective bilirubin glucuronidation caused by a mild to moderate deficiency in bilirubin glucuronosyl transferase. Thus, jaundice in Gilbert syndrome is related to elevated unconjugated bilirubin. Bilirubin glucoronosyl transferase is encoded by the *UGT1A1* gene on chromosome 2. As with most genes, this contains a noncoding 5' promoter sequence, a component of which is the TATAA box. The patient with Gilbert syndrome has a normal coding *UGT1A1* nucleotide sequence; the abnormality lies in the 5' TATAA box which contains an abnormal extra TA. The longer-than-usual TATAA results in reduced gene expression. 2 abnormal gene promoters must be inherited to cause enzyme activity low enough to be clinically apparent; thus Gilbert syndrome is considered an autosomal recessive condition.

T8.6

Clinical Presentations of Alpha-1-Antitrypsin Deficiency

Neonates, infants, young children	Older children, adults
Neonatal hepatitis	Chronic hepatitis
Neonatal cholestasis	Cirrhosis
	Hepatocellular carcinoma
	Chronic obstructive pulmonary disease

8: Gastrointestinal, Hepatobiliary, and Pancreatic Diseases

Hepatic>Disorders of Bilirubin Conjugation: Gilbert Syndrome and Crigler-Najjar Syndromes; Disorders of Bilirubin Canalicular Secretion: DJS and Rotor Syndrome; Autoimmune Liver Disease: Autoimmune Hepatitis, AC and PBC

T8.7
Hereditary Hyperbilirubinemia

Syndrome	Bilirubin type	Inheritance	Defect	Comment
Crigler-Najjar I	Unconjugated	Autosomal recessive	Absent UDP-glucoronosyl tranferase	Fatal
Crigler-Najjar II	Unconjugated	Autosomal dominant	Decreased UDP-glucoronosyl transferase	Benign, occasional kernicterus
Gilbert	Unconjugated	Autosomal dominant	Decreased UDP-glucoronosyl transferase	Benign, present in about 5% of population
Dubin-Johnson	Conjugated	Autosomal recessive	Decreased secretion	Benign, liver is pigmented
Rotor	Conjugated	Autosomal recessive	Decreased secretion	Benign, liver not pigmented

- Crigler-Najjar syndromes, on the other hand, are caused by mutations in the *UGT1A1* coding sequence. Both types of Crigler-Najjar syndrome cause more severe unconjugated hyperbilirubinemia than does Gilbert syndrome. In type I Crigler-Najjar syndrome, there is no detectable glucuronosyl transferase activity, leading to severe jaundice beginning in the neonatal period, often complicated by kernicterus. In type II Crigler-Najjar syndrome (also called *Arias syndrome*), there is some glucuronosyl transferase activity, usually less than 10% of normal, and jaundice presents somewhat later.

Disorders of Bilirubin Canalicular Secretion: Dubin-Johnson Syndrome and Rotor Syndrome

- Following bilirubin conjugation, it must be secreted into the canalicular system. A failure in this step typifies these fairly benign clinical disorders and is associated with conjugated hyperbilirubinemia.

- Dubin-Johnson syndrome is an autosomal recessive disorder that is caused by a mutation in the *MRP2* (multidrug resistance protein 2) gene on 10q, which encodes a protein (MRP2) that is also known as the canalicular multispecific organic anion transporter (cMOAT). It is responsible for escorting multiple organic anions across the cell membrane and into the canalicular system. Several different mutations in the *MRP2* gene have been identified in patients with Dubin-Johnson. The hepatic parenchyma is heavily pigmented, on both gross and microscopic examination, in Dubin-Johnson syndrome. However, there is no associated evidence of hepatic injury.

- While bilirubin secretion appears to be the underlying defect in Rotor syndrome as well, there is no hepatic pigment accumulation in this disease. Furthermore, the genetic defect in Rotor syndrome has not been elucidated.

Autoimmune Liver Disease: Autoimmune Hepatitis, Autoimmune Cholangitis, and Primary Biliary Cirrhosis

- Autoimmune hepatitis (AIH)

  □ Laboratory findings include hypergammaglobulinemia (predominantly increased polyclonal IgG) and a specific set of autoantibodies: antinuclear antibody, anti–smooth muscle antibody (SMA), anti–liver kidney microsome antibody (LKM1, an antibody against CYP 2D6), and in some cases anti–soluble liver antigen/liver pancreas (SLA/LP) antibody. Anti-SMA and Anti-LKM do not occur in the same patient together; the particular antibody present determines whether the patient has type 1 (anti-SMA) or type 2 (anti-LKM) AIH. Type 2 is the more rapidly progressive of the 2, but both appear to progress to cirrhosis with great regularity.

  □ Histologically, there is chronic hepatitis with a lymphoplasmacytic portal infiltrate and characteristically brisk limiting plate necrosis. Bile ducts are largely spared.

  □ In many cases, AIH is associated with extrahepatic autoimmune disease. Type 1 AIH is associated with UC, arthritis, immune thrombocytopenic purpura (ITP), and autoimmune hemolytic anemia (AIHA); type 2 is associated with type 1 diabetes mellitus, thyroiditis, autoimmune enteropathy, and autoimmune polyglandular syndrome type 1 (see chapter 7).

8: Gastrointestinal, Hepatobiliary, and Pancreatic Diseases

Hepatic>Autoimmune Liver Disease: Autoimmune Hepatitis, Autoimmune Cholangitis, and Primary Biliary Cirrhosis |
Pancreas>Hereditary Pancreatitis

☐ As is typical of autoimmune conditions, AIH tends to occur in families with a general predisposition for autoimmunity. Polymorphisms in the *CTLA-4* gene appear to influence the likelihood of AIH. The *AIRE* (autoimmune regulator) gene that has been implicated in autoimmune polyglandular syndrome type 1 (APECED) also appears to influence the likelihood of AIH type 2. In fact, AIH is a feature of about 1 in 4 cases of the APECED. Susceptibility to AIH is also associated with particular HLA-DRB1 alleles (DRB1*1301 for type 1 and DRB1*0201 for type 2).

■ Primary biliary cirrhosis (PBC)

☐ Presents histopathologically as a lymphoplasmacytic infiltrate with direct infiltration of interlobular bile ducts and progressive bile duct destruction (chronic nonsuppurative destructive cholangitis). Anti–mitochondrial antibodies are present in more than 95% of cases.

☐ PBC occurs with increased incidence in relatives of affected persons. The most common HLA association is with HLA-DR8. Class 3 (complement) HLA components have also shown an association, especially C4A*Q0.

Pancreas

Hereditary Pancreatitis

■ Hereditary pancreatitis is characterized by recurrent episodes of pancreatitis beginning in childhood. Several heritable forms of pancreatitis have been described that may be placed into 4 categories. The first and most common form is that related to cystic fibrosis (CF; see following subsection on CF). Second, because pancreatitis can be caused by metabolic derangements, notably hypercalcemia and hyperlipidemia, inherited forms of hypercalcemia and hyperlipidemia (especially type IV with hypertriglyceridemia) can be associated with chronic pancreatitis (see chapter 10). Third, several single-gene defects cause principally pancreatitis, without a wide range of extrapancreatic disease (see following subsection), including mutations of cationic trypsinogen (*PRSS1*) and pancreatic secretory trypsin inhibitor (*SPINK1*). Lastly, pancreatitis is a cardinal feature of several distinct inherited syndromes, including Pearson syndrome.

■ Cystic fibrosis

☐ The *CFTR* gene encodes the CF transmembrane regulator (CFTR), an epithelial transmembrane protein that serves as a regulated chloride channel. CFTR is expressed largely on the surface of epithelial cells of airways, the GI tract, pancreaticobiliary system, sweat glands, and genitourinary system. The *CFTR* gene is very large, composed of 27 exons, and a wide range of mutations are possible. When loss-of-function mutations occur, the ion channel abnormality results in multisystem disease affecting the upper and lower aerodigestive tract, hepatobiliary system, GI tract, pancreas, and male reproductive tract.

☐ CF is an autosomal recessive disease that affects about 1 in 2000 live births in Caucasians. The gene frequency in Caucasians is about 1 in 20. Among other groups of Americans, the incidence is lower—about 1 in 10,000 Hispanic births, 1 in 15,000 African American births, and 1 in 30,000 Asian American births.

☐ CF is capable of causing chronic pancreatitis resulting in eventual exocrine and endocrine deficiency. Mutations impair ion transport and thus water transport, leading to dehydrated, viscous secretions. These cause obstruction of pancreatic ducts, leading to pancreatitis.

☐ The manifestations are, of course, not limited to the pancreas **T8.8**. The earliest manifestation of CF is sometimes a meconium ileus. Liver disease can result from biliary obstruction. CF is also a cause of chronic lung disease, again related to viscous secretions, leading to bronchiectasis and eventual pulmonary insufficiency. Chronic recalcitrant infections take root in these tenacious secretions. Childhood pulmonary infections caused by *Staphylococcus aureus, Burkholderia cepacia,* or *Pseudomonas aeruginosa* is strong presumptive evidence of CF. In particular, mucoid forms of *Pseudomonas* are considered strongly suggestive of CF. CF is responsible for many cases of sinusitis and nasal polyps, particularly in children. Lastly, as a direct consequence of the ion channel disorder, CF can lead to severe salt loss and hyponatremia.

☐ The aforementioned generalities notwithstanding, in any given case, certain organs may be relatively spared; conversely, there are cases in which manifestations are restricted to a single organ. For example, some cases of CF present only as

Pancreas>Hereditary Pancreatitis

T8.8
Most Common Presentations of Cystic Fibrosis (in order of Decreasing Frequency)

Recurrent pneumonia and/or bronchiectasis

Unexplained malnutrition or failure to thrive

Meconium ileus

Hyponatremia, especially with hypochloremia and metabolic alkalosis

Rectal prolapse

Unexplained chronic diarrhea

Refractory sinusitis or asthma

Nasal polyps in childhood

Chronic, recurrent, pancreatitis

Hepatic disease (focal biliary obstruction, unexplained jaundice)

Male infertility

idiopathic pancreatitis. In some males, only the function of the vas deferens is affected; congenital bilateral absence of vas deferens (CBAVD) occurs frequently in isolation, without multisystem disease. These variations are thought to be the result of other inherited (modifier genes) or environmental influences. The severity of lung disease, for example, varies tremendously, even among those with identical CFTR genotype. The myeloperoxidase (MPO) activity within circulating neutrophils is known to vary among individuals, and the MPO activity has been shown to correlate with the FEV1/FVC in patients with CF. Another example is a locus on chromosome 19 that appears to be strongly associated with meconium ileus. The degree of both pulmonary and hepatic involvement appears to vary with the AAT genotype. Interestingly, it has been found that among alcoholics who develop chronic calcifying pancreatitis, CFTR mutations are quite common.

☐ The diagnosis of CF can be established, in a patient with suggestive clinical features, with 1 of the following: molecular testing, 2 consecutive abnormal pilocarpine iontophoresis sweat chloride tests, or an abnormal transepithelial nasal potential difference measurement. Many states have implemented newborn screening for CF. The method commonly used for this is an immunoreactive trypsinogen (IRT) assay,

performed on blood spots. IRT levels are elevated in CF until the age of about 2 months. This finding must be confirmed by another modality and should not be used after about 2 months of age. The sweat test is difficult to perform reproducibly. Positive results should be confirmed with a repeat test, and if the results are negative, the test should be repeated if suspicion is high. False-positive and false-negative results are common. Increased potential (voltage) differences across nasal epithelium have been used to confirm the diagnosis in patients with borderline sweat tests. Heterozygotes are asymptomatic and, to date, there is no test capable of detecting them aside from DNA studies.

☐ Mutations in the *CFTR* gene, on 7q31.2, are the cause of CF. Over 1000 such mutations have been described T8.9. Several multiple-mutation targeted mutation analysis panels are clinically available, generally probing for 20 to 25 common mutations. Such panels are capable of detecting about 90% of cases overall; however, because of population differences, the detection rate is lower in Hispanics and African Americans. Direct sequence analysis is capable of detecting more than 98% of mutations, but because of the size of this gene, are labor-intensive and expensive.

☐ The most common disease-causing mutation is ΔF508 (present in approximately 70% of affected individuals). The ΔF508 mutation is a 3-nucleotide deletion of codon 508, encoding a CFTR protein that lacks a phenylalanine (F) residue at position 508. The mutation results in a protein that, though functional, is rapidly degraded.

T8.9
Most Common *CFTR* Gene Mutations

Mutation	Frequency in Affected Persons (%)
ΔF508	66.0
G542X	2.4
G551D	1.6
N1303K	1.3
W1282X	1.2
R553X	0.7

8: Gastrointestinal, Hepatobiliary, and Pancreatic Diseases

Pancreas>Hereditary Pancreatitis; Pancreatic Lipomatosis Syndromes: Shwachman-Diamond Syndrome
and Johanson-Blizzard Syndrome

- About 5% to 10% of *CFTR* mutations are caused by premature truncation, and these are particularly common in Ashkenazi Jews. The W1282X mutation, a truncating mutation, occurs in 60% of the Ashkenazi Jews with CF.

- Other kinds of *CFTR* mutations, and in fact some non-*CFTR* mutations can rarely give rise to CF-like disease. Such cases often result in a phenotype with limited or late-onset manifestations (so-called *variant cystic fibrosis*).

- The cationic trypsinogen (*PRSS1*) gene is found on chromosome 7q35. The pancreatitis-associated cationic trypsinogen (*PRSS1*) mutations, most commonly an arginine-to-histidine (R122H) substitution, result in a type of trypsinogen that is capable of activation (to trypsin) but resistant to deactivation. This causes an autosomal dominant form of inherited pancreatitis, in which patients appear to also be at increased risk for pancreatic adenocarcinoma. Trypsinogen exists as 2 main types: cationic (about 2/3 of all enzyme) and anionic (encoded by *PRSS2*). A small fraction is mesotrypsinogen, encoded by *PRSS3*. Proteolytic cleavage by enterokinase or trypsin itself results in the active form, trypsin. Trypsin is then rapidly degraded. In addition to the arginine substitution (R122H), several PRSS1 mutations have been described that lead to resistance to degradation or gain of function. The second most common such mutation is an asparagine-to-isoleucine substitution, N29I.

- Pancreatic trypsin inhibitor (PSTI), also known as SPINK1 or serine protease inhibitor, Kazal type 1, normally acts to protect the pancreas from autodigestion. Pancreatic secretory trypsin inhibitor (*SPINK1*) gene mutations, especially the N34S substituation, result in a similar clinical phenotype.

- Pearson syndrome is an extremely rare cause of chronic pancreatitis showing autosomal dominant inheritance and an association with marrow failure. Despite its rarity, the disease is fascinating because it is a chromosomal breakage syndrome affecting the mitochondrial DNA. The marrow shows sideroblastic anemia with vacuolization of precursors, and the pancreas shows fibrosis typical of chronic pancreatitis. The molecular defect is a microdeletion in the mitochondrial DNA.

- Tropical pancreatitis is a form of early-onset chronic pancreatitis found in tropical regions that tends to cluster within families. However, it does not appear to have a Mendelian pattern of inheritance, and the pathogenesis of this syndrome is not clear.

Pancreatic Lipomatosis Syndromes: Shwachman-Diamond Syndrome and Johanson-Blizzard Syndrome

- Generally thought of as a bone marrow failure syndrome, nearly all patients with Shwachman-Diamond syndrome also have exocrine pancreatic insufficiency. Note that this syndrome is distinct from Blackfann-Diamond syndrome (pure red cell aplasia, no pancreatic disease). Also note that this syndrome is not a cause of pancreatitis. The hematologic findings include cyclic neutropenia, eventually leading to aplastic anemia, myelodysplasia, and possibly acute leukemia. Neutropenia leads to recurrent infections, particularly skin infections, osteomyelitis, otitis media, and sinusitis. Pancreatic insufficiency may manifest itself in infancy as steatorrhea, malabsorption, and malnutrition. The histologic features are similar to those seen in Johanson-Blizzard syndrome: the acini are devoid of exocrine cells and replaced with adipose tissue. The islets are preserved and disposed in a background of adipose tissue (pancreatic lipomatosis). Unlike chronic pancreatitis, there is no fibrosis. Interestingly, over time some patients begin to develop some exocrine pancreatic function, and their symptoms improve. The syndrome is caused by mutations in a gene known as *SBDS* (Shwachman-Bodian-Diamond syndrome). While the function of the gene is unknown, mutations in it appear to arise as a result of exchange of genetic material with a nearby pseudogene (*SBDSP*) in a manner similar to the mechanism of mutation in congenital adrenal hyperplasia (gene conversion).

- Johanson-Blizzard syndrome is characterized by hypoplasia of the nasal alae, pancreatic exocrine insufficiency, hypothyroidism, and deafness. Like Shwachman-Diamond syndrome, there is lipomatous change in the pancreas (replacement of acinin with adipocytes), with preservation of the pancreatic ducts and islets. Johanson-Blizzard syndrome is caused by mutations in the UBR1 gene.

References

Adams PC, Deugnier Y, Moirand R, et al. The relationship between iron overload, clinical symptoms, and age in 410 patients with genetic hemochromatosis. *Hepatology* 1997; 25: 162-166.

Albers S, Levy HL, Irons M, et al. Compound heterozygosity in four asymptomatic siblings with medium-chain acyl-CoA dehydrogenase deficiency. *J Inherit Metab Dis* 2001; 24: 417-418.

Angrist M, Bolk S, Halushka M, et al. Germline mutations in glial cell line-derived neurotrophic factor (GDNF) and RET in a Hirschsprung disease patient. *Nat Genet* 1996; 14: 341-344.

Angrist M, Bolk S, Thiel B, et al. Mutation analysis of the RET receptor tyrosine kinase in Hirschsprung disease. *Hum Mol Genet* 1995; 4: 821-830.

Aono S, Adachi Y, Uyama E, et al Analysis of genes for bilirubin UDP-glucuronosyltransferase in Gilbert's syndrome. *Lancet* 1995; 345(8955): 958-959.

Bacon BR, Powell LW, Adams PC, et al. Molecular medicine and hemochromatosis: at the crossroads. *Gastroenterology* 1999; 116: 193-207.

Bagolan P, Iacobelli BB, De Angelis P, et al. Long gap esophageal atresia and esophageal replacement: moving toward a separation? *J Pediatr Surg* 2004; 39: 1084-1090.

Bahuau M, Pelet A, Vidaud D, et al. GDNF as a candidate modifier in a type 1 neurofibromatosis (NF1) enteric phenotype. *J Med Genet* 2001; 38: 638-643.

Barman KK, Premalatha G, Mohan V. Tropical chronic pancreatitis. *Postgrad Med J* 2003; 79(937): 606-615.

Bates MD, Balistreri WF. The liver and biliary system. In: *Nelson Textbook of Pediatrics*. 17th ed. Philadelphia, Pa: WB Saunders, 2004.

Bennett MJ, Rinaldo P, Millington DS, et al. Medium-chain acyl-CoA dehydrogenase deficiency: postmortem diagnosis in a case of sudden infant death and neonatal diagnosis of an affect sibling. *Pediatr Pathol* 1991; 11: 889-895.

Beutler E, Felitti VJ, Koziol JA, et al. Penetrance of 845G→A (C282Y) HFE hereditary haemochromatosis mutation in the USA. *Lancet* 2002; 359: 211-218.

Bhatia E, Durie P, Zielenski J, et al. Mutations in the cystic fibrosis transmembrane regulator gene in patients with tropical calcific pancreatitis. *Am J Gastroenterol* 2000; 95: 3658-3659.

Boles RG, Buck EA, Blitzer MG, et al. Retrospective biochemical screening of fatty acid oxidation disorders in postmortem livers of 418 cases of sudden death in the first year of life. *J Pediatr* 1998; 132: 924-933.

Boocock GR, Morrison JA, Popovic M, et al. Mutations in SBDS are associated with Shwachman-Diamond syndrome. *Nat Genet* 2003; 33: 97-101.

Bosma PJ, Chowdhury JR, Bakker C, et al. The genetic basis of the reduced expression of bilirubin UDP- glucuronosyl-transferase 1 in Gilbert's syndrome. *N Engl J Med* 1995; 333(18): 1171-1175.

Branski D, Fasano A, Troncone R. Latest developments in the pathogenesis and treatment of celiac disease. *J Pediatr* 2006; 149: 295-300.

Bulaj ZJ, Griffen LM, Jorde LB, et al. Clinical and biochemical abnormalities in people heterozygous for hemochromatosis. *N Engl J Med* 1996; 335: 1799-1805.

Burdick JS, Tompson ML. Anatomy, histology, embryology, and developmental anomalies of the pancreas. In: *Sleisenger & Fordtran's Gastrointestinal and Liver Disease*. 8th ed. Philadelphia, Pa: Elsevier Saunders, 2006.

Burt MJ, George PM, Upton JD, et al. The significance of haemochromatosis gene mutations in the general population: implications for screening. Gut *1998*; 43: 830-836.

Carrell RW, Lomas DA. Conformational disease. *Lancet* 1997; 350:134-138.

Carrell RW, Lomas DA. Alpha 1-antitrypsin deficiency: a model for conformational diseases. *N Engl J Med* 2002; 346: 45-53.

Celli J, van Bokhoven H, Brunner HG. Feingold syndrome: clinical review and genetic mapping. *Am J Med Genet* 2003; 122: 294-300.

References

Cuthbert AP, Fisher SA, Mirza MM, et al. The contribution of NOD2 gene mutations to the risk and site of disease in inflammatory bowel disease. *Gastroenterology* 2002; 122: 867-874.

Davenport M, Tizzard SA, Underhill J, et al. The biliary atresia splenic malformation syndrome: a 28-year single-center retrospective study. *J Pediatr* 2006; 149: 393-400.

De Gobbi M, Roetto A, Piperno A, et al. Natural history of juvenile haemochromatosis. *Br J Haematol* 2002; 117: 973-979.

Drumm ML, Konstan MW, Schluchter MD, et al. Genetic modifiers of lung disease in cystic fibrosis. *N Engl J Med* 2005; 353: 1443-1453.

Ellis I. Genetic counseling for hereditary pancreatitis: the role of molecular genetics testing for the cationic trypsinogen gene, cystic fibrosis and serine protease inhibitor Kazal type 1. *Gastroenterol Clin North Am* 2004; 33: 839-854.

Eng C, Mulligan LM. Mutations of the RET proto-oncogene in the multiple endocrine neoplasia type 2 syndromes, related sporadic tumours, and hirschsprung disease. *Hum Mutat* 1997; 9: 97-109.

Favareto F, Caprino D, Micalizzi C, et al. New clinical aspects of Pearson's syndrome: report of three cases. *Haematologica* 1989; 74: 591-594.

Fitze G, Appelt H, Konig IR, et al. Functional haplotypes of the RET proto-oncogene promoter are associated with Hirschsprung disease (HSCR). *Hum Mol Genet* 2003; 12: 3207-3214.

Forsmark CE. Chronic pancreatitis. In: *Sleisenger & Fordtran's Gastrointestinal and Liver Disease.* 8th ed. Philadelphia, Pa: Elsevier Saunders, 2006.

Franchini M, Veneri D. Recent advances in hereditary hemochromatosis. *Ann Hematol* 2005; 84: 347-352.

Gaffney D, Fell GS, O'Reilly D. Wilson's disease: acute and presymptomatic laboratory diagnosis and monitoring. *J Clin Pathol* 2000; 53: 807-812.

Ganz T. Hepcidin, a key regulator of iron metabolism and mediator of anemia of inflammation. *Blood* 2003; 102: 783-788.

Garcia-Barcelo M, Sham M, Lee W, et al. Highly recurrent RET mutations and novel mutations in genes of the receptor tyrosine kinase and endothelin receptor B pathways in Chinese patients with sporadic Hirschsprung disease. *Clin Chem* 2004; 50: 93-100.

Gariepy E. Developmental disorders of the enteric nervous system: genetic and molecular bases. *J Pediatr Gastroenterol Nutr* 2004; 39: 5-11.

Garner HP, Phillips JR, Herron JG, et al. Peroxidase activity within circulating neutrophils correlates with pulmonary phenotype in cystic fibrosis. *J Lab Clin Med* 2004; 144: 127-133.

Gath R, Goessling A, Keller KM, et al. Analysis of the RET, GDNF, EDN3, and EDNRB genes in patients with intestinal neuronal dysplasia and Hirschsprung disease. *Gut* 2001; 48: 671-675.

Gershoni-Baruch R, Lerner A, Braun J, et al. Johanson-Blizzard syndrome: clinical spectrum and further delineation of the syndrome. *Am J Med Genet* 1990; 35: 546-551.

Grody WW. Cystic fibrosis: molecular diagnosis, population screening, and public policy. *Arch Pathol Lab Med* 1999; 123: 1041-1046.

Groisman GM, Amar M, Livne E. CD10: a valuable tool for the light microscopic diagnosis of microvillous inclusion disease (familial microvillous atrophy). *Am J Surg Pathol* 2002; 26: 902-907.

Hampe J, Frenzel H, Mirza MM, et al. Evidence for a NOD2-independent susceptibility locus for inflammatory bowel disease on chromosome 16p. *Proc Natl Acad Sci* 2002; 99: 321-326.

Hampe J, Grebe J, Nikolaus S, et al. Association of NOD2 (CARD 15) genotype with clinical course of Crohn's disease: a cohort study. *Lancet* 2002; 359: 1661-1665.

Huntington JA, Read RJ, Carrell RW. Structure of a serpin-protease complex shows inhibition by deformation. *Nature* 2000; 407: 923-926.

Hwang PJ, Kousseff BG. Omphalocele and gastroschisis: an 18-year review study. *Genet Med* 2004; 6: 232-236.

References

Inoue K, Shimotake T, Iwai N. Mutational analysis of RET/GDNF/NTN genes in children with total colonic aganglionosis with small bowel involvement. *Am J Med Genet* 2000; 93: 278-284.

Johnson CA, Gissen P, Sergi C. Molecular pathology and genetics of congenital hepatorenal fibrocystic syndromes. *J Med Genet* 2003; 40: 311-319.

Jones NL, Hofley PM, Durie PR. Pathophysiology of the pancreatic defect in Johanson-Blizzard syndrome: a disorder of acinar development. *J Pediatr* 1994; 125: 406-408.

Kamath BM, Piccoli DA. Heritable disorders of the bile ducts. *Gastroenterol Clin North Am* 2003; 32: 857-875.

Kanard RC, Fairbanks TJ, De Langhe SP. Fibroblast growth factor-10 serves a regulatory role in duodenal development. *J Pediatr Surg* 2005; 40: 313-316.

Kimble RM, Harding J, Kolbe A. Additional congenital anomalies in babies with gut atresia or stenosis: when to investigate, and which investigation. *Pediatr Surg Int* 1997; 12: 565-570.

Kimura K, Nishijima E, Tsugawa C, et al. Multistaged extrathoracic esophageal elongation procedure for long gap esophageal atresia: experience with 12 patients. *J Pediatr Surg* 2001; 36: 1725-1727.

Lachaux A, Descos B, Plauchu H, et al. Familial extrahepatic biliary atresia. *J Pediatr Gastroenterol Nutr* 1988; 7: 280-283.

Lankisch TO, Strassburg CP, Debray D, et al. Detection of autoimmune regulator gene mutations in children with type 2 autoimmune hepatitis and extrahepatic immune-mediated diseases. *J Pediatr* 2005; 146: 839-842.

Alvarez F. Autoimmune hepatitis and primary sclerosing cholangitis. *Clin Liver Dis* 2006; 10: 89-107.

Lantermann A, Hampe J, Kim WH, et al. Investigation of HLA-DPA1 genotypes as predictors of inflammatory bowel disease in the German, South African, and South Korean populations. *Int J Colorectal Dis* 2002; 17: 238-244.

Ledbetter DJ. Gastroschisis and omphalocele. *Surg Clin North Am* 2006; 86: 249-260.

Lopes MF, Reis A, Coutinho S, Pires A. Very long gap esophageal atresia successfully treated by esophageal lengthening using external traction sutures. *J Pediatr Surg* 2004; 39: 1286-1287.

Lovicu M, Dessi V, Zappu A, et al. Efficient strategy for molecular diagnosis of Wilson disease in the Sardinian population. *Clin Chem* 2003; 49: 496-498.

McCandless SE, Millington DS, Andresen BS, et al. Clinical findings in MCAD patients heterozygous for the common mutation identified by MS/MS newborn screening. *Am J Hum Genet* 2002; 71(suppl): 419.

Mack DR, Forstner GG, Wilschanski M, et al. Shwachman syndrome: exocrine pancreatic dysfunction and variable phenotypic expression. *Gastroenterology* 1996; 111: 1593-1602.

Mak V, Zielenski J, Tsui LC, et al. Cystic fibrosis gene mutations and infertile men with primary testicular failure. *Hum Reprod* 2000; 15: 436-439.

Mathew CG, Lewis CM. Genetics of inflammatory bowel disease: progress and prospects. *Hum Mol Genet* 2004; 13: R161-R168.

Mattman A, Huntsman D, Lockitch G, et al. Transferrin receptor 2 (TfR2) and HFE mutational analysis in non-C282Y iron overload: Identification of a novel TfR2 mutation. *Blood* 2002; 100: 1075-1077.

Mohan V, Premalatha G, Pitchumoni CS. Tropical chronic pancreatitis: an update. *J Clin Gastroenterol* 2003; 36: 337-346.

Moirand R, Adams PC, Bicheler V, et al. Clinical features of genetic hemochromatosis in women compared with men. *Ann Intern Med* 1997; 127: 105-110.

Mura C, Raguenes O, Ferec C. HFE mutation analysis in 711 hemochromatosis probands: evidence for S65C implication in mild form of hemochromatosis. *Blood* 1999; 93: 2502-2505.

Nichols L, Dickson G, Phan PG, et al. Iron binding saturation and genotypic testing for hereditary hemochromatosis in patients with liver disease. *Am J Clin Pathol* 2006; 125: 236-240.

References

Nielsen P, Carpinteiro S, Fischer R, et al. Prevalence of the C282Y and H63D mutations in the HFE gene in patients with hereditary haemochromatosis and in control subjects from Northern Germany. *Br J Haematol* 1998; 103: 842-845.

Oda T, Elkahloun AG, Pike BL, et al. Mutations in the human Jagged1 gene are responsible for Alagille syndrome. *Nat Genet* 1997; 16: 235-242.

Parisi MA, Kapur RP. Genetics of Hirschsprung disease. *Curr Opin Pediatr* 2000; 12: 610-617.

Parkes M, Barmada MM, Satsangi J, et al. The IBD2 locus shows linkage heterogeneity between ulcerative colitis and Crohn disease. *Am J Hum Genet* 2000; 67: 1605-1610.

Perlmutter DH, Shepherd RW. Extrahepatic biliary atresia: a disease or a phenotype? *Hepatology* 2002; 35: 1297-1304.

Phatak PD, Sham RL, Raubertas RF, et al. Prevalence of hereditary hemochromatosis in 16031 primary care patients. *Ann Intern Med* 1998; 129: 954-961.

Phillips AD, Schmitz J. Familial villous atrophy: a clinicopathological survey of 23 cases. *J Pediatr Gastroenterol Nutr* 1992; 14:380.

Pietrangelo A. Hereditary hemochromatosis: a new look at an old disease. *N Engl J Med* 2004; 350(23): 2383-2397.

Poki HO, Holland AJ, Pitkin J. Double bubble, double trouble. *Pediatr Surg Int* 2005; 21: 428-431.

Press RD. Hereditary hemochromatosis: impact of molecular and iron-based testing on the diagnosis, treatment, and prevention of a common, chronic disease. *Arch Pathol Lab Med* 1999; 123: 1053-1059.

Qian Q, Li A, King BF, Kamath PS, et al. Clinical profile of autosomal dominant polycystic liver disease. *Hepatology* 2003; 37: 164-171.

Rinaldo P, Matern D, Bennett MJ. Fatty acid oxidation disorders. *Annu Rev Physiol* 2002; 64: 477-502.

Rinaldo P, Yoon HR, Yu C, et al. Sudden and unexpected neonatal death: a protocol for the postmortem diagnosis of fatty acid oxidation disorders. *Semin Perinatol* 1999; 23: 204-210.

Rossi E, Olynyk JK, Cullen DJ, et al. Compound heterozygous hemochromatosis: Genotype predicts increased iron and erythrocyte indices in women. *Clin Chem* 2000; 46: 162-166.

Rowe SM, Miller S, Sorscher EJ. Cystic fibrosis. *N Engl J Med* 2005; 352:1992-2001.

Sancandi M, Griseri P, Pesce B, et al. Single nucleotide polymorphic alleles in the 5' region of the RET proto-oncogene define a risk haplotype in Hirschsprung's disease. *J Med Genet* 2003; 40: 714-718.

Schreiber S, Rosenstiel P, Hampe J, et al. Activation of signal transducer and activator of transcription (STAT) 1 in human chronic inflammatory bowel disease. *Gut* 2002; 51: 379-385.

Schuppan D. Current concepts of celiac disease pathogenesis. *Gastroenterology* 2000; 119: 234-242.

Schwab M, Schaeffeler E, Marx C, et al. Association between the C3435T MDR1 gene polymorphism and susceptibility for ulcerative colitis. *Gastroenterology* 2003; 124(1): 26-33.

Sharer N, Schwarz M, Malone G, et al. Mutations of the cystic fibrosis gene in patients with chronic pancreatitis. *N Engl J Med* 1998; 339: 645-652.

Skandalakis JE, Ellis H. Embryologic and anatomic basis of esophageal surgery. *Surg Clin North Am* 2000; 80: 85.

Smith VV, Eng C, Milla PJ. Intestinal ganglioneuromatosis and multiple endocrine neoplasia type 2B: implications for treatment. *Gut* 1999; 45: 143-146.

Spitz L, Kiely EM, Morecroft JA, et al. Oesophageal atresia: at-risk groups for the 1990s. *J Pediatr Surg* 1994; 29: 723-725.

Stewart DR, Von Allmen D. The genetics of Hirschsprung disease. *Gastroenterol Clin North Am* 2003; 32: 819-837.

Tavill AS. Diagnosis and management of hemochromatosis. *Hepatology* 2001; 33: 1321-1328.

Tortorelli S, Tokunaga C, Strauss AW, et al. Correlation of genotype and biochemical phenotype in 106 patients with MCAD deficiency. *J Inherit Metab Dis* 2004; 27(suppl 1): 102.

References

Uphoff TS, Highsmith WE. Introduction to molecular cystic fibrosis testing. *Clin Lab Sci* 2006; 19: 24-31.

Warner BW. Pediatric surgery. In: *Sabiston Textbook of Surgery.* 17th Ed. Philadelphia, Pa: Elsevier Saunders, 2004.

Weiss FU, Simon P, Mayerle J, et al. Germline mutations and gene polymorphism associated with human pancreatitis *Endocrinol Metab Clin North Am* 2006; 35: 289-302.

Wilson PD. Polycystic kidney disease. *N Engl J Med* 2004; 350: 151-164.

Yen AW, Fancher TL, Bowlus CL. Revisiting hereditary hemochromatosis: current concepts and progress. *Am J Med* 2006; 119: 391-399.

Zenker M, Mayerle J, Reis A, et al. Genetic basis and pancreatic biology of Johanson-Blizzard syndrome. *Endocrinol Metab Clin North Am* 2006; 35: 243-243.

Zenker M, Mayerle J, Lerch MM, et al. Deficiency of UBR1, a ubiquitin ligase of the N-end rule pathway, causes pancreatic dysfunction, malformations and mental retardation (Johanson-Blizzard syndrome). *Nat Genet* 2005; 37: 1345-1350.

Zielenski J. Genotype and phenotype in cystic fibrosis. *Respiration* 2000; 67: 117-133.

Zielenski J, Corey M, Rozmahel R. Detection of a cystic fibrosis modifier locus for meconium ileus on human chromosome 19q13. *Nat Genet* 1999; 22: 128-129.

Zschocke J, Schulze A, Lindner M, et al. Molecular and functional characterisation of mild MCAD deficiency. *Hum Genet* 2001; 108: 404-408.

Zytkovicz TH, Fitzgerald EF, Marsden D, et al. Tandem mass spectrometric analysis for amino, organic, and fatty acid disorders in newborn dried blood spots: a two-year summary from the New England newborn screening program. *Clin Chem* 2001; 47: 1945-1955.

Chapter 9

Immunologic Disorders, Immunodeficiency, and Autoimmunity

B-Cell and Immunoglobulin Defects

Bruton (X-Linked) Agammaglobulinemia

- Defective B-cell function generally results in recurrent bacterial infections, especially sinopulmonary infections, and recalcitrant intestinal infection with nonbacterial organisms such as Enteroviruses and *Giardia lamblia*. Enhanced susceptibility is particular to encapsulated bacteria (especially staphylococci, streptococci, and hemophilus) and certain viruses (especially polio, hepatitis, and Enteroviruses). Opportunistic fungal and viral infections are not a major feature of B-cell defects. The manifestations begin at or after 6 months of age, when transplacentally acquired maternal antibodies wane. Such a presentation should provoke evaluation for other conditions as well, especially cystic fibrosis (See Chapter 8). Besides infection, like most immunodeficiency conditions, Bruton agammaglobulinemia is associated with a predisposition to both autoimmunity and malignancy.

- Bruton agammaglobulinemia is an X-linked disorder in which affected males commonly present with chronic diarrhea. When reviewing a duodenal biopsy, particularly in a child or young adult, one must ensure that plasma cells are present in the lamina propria. The absence of plasma cells in the intestinal mucosa is distinctly abnormal and should prompt evaluation for a B-cell defect.

- Bruton agammaglobulinemia results from an arrest in B-cell development, such that neither mature B cells nor plasma cells can be found in the tissues. Serum IgG levels are markedly reduced (<200 mg/dL) as are circulating B cells (<1% of circulating lymphocytes by flow cytometry). Pre-B cells are found in lymph nodes and bone marrow. Lymph nodes lack germinal centers and plasma cells. Tonsils are rudimentary.

- Transient hypogammaglobulinemia of infancy

  □ Bruton agammaglobulinemia must be distinguished from transient hypogammaglobulinemia. Though fleeting, this condition is not entirely benign and may result in serious life-threatening infection.

  □ Most of the immunoglobulin found in the serum of neonates is transplacentally acquired maternal antibodies. These persist for about 3 to 6 months, coinciding with the onset of autonomous antibody production, which is usually fully in order by 6 months of age. Transient hypogammaglobulinemia of infancy is caused by a delay in endogenous antibody production, resulting in a window of vulnerability.

  □ This disorder does not have a specific inherited basis, and it is most commonly seen in premature infants. Temporary intravenous immunoglobulin administration can help prevent infection until antibody production emerges, usually by 12 months of age

- The Bruton tyrosine kinase (*BTK*) gene, sometimes called *agammaglobulinemia tyrosine kinase* (ATK), is on the X chromosome. It encodes the BTK tyrosine kinase protein and is normally expressed on the surface of B cells. Several different mutations cause a Bruton phenotype with differing levels of severity.

Common Variable Immunodeficiency (CVI)

- CVI is common in comparison with other forms of inherited (primary) immunodeficiency. While its principal feature is low serum immunoglobulin (IgG, IgM, and IgA), many cases also have a component of T-cell deficiency.

- CVI is variable with regard to clinical severity and age at onset; nonetheless, most cases present before the age of 30 years. Affected patients present with recurrent upper and lower respiratory tract infections (*Streptococcus pneumoniae, Haemophilus influenzae,* and *Mycoplasma pneumoniae*), intestinal bacterial overgrowth, and/or intestinal *G lamblia* infection. The development of bronchiectasis is extremely common.

- Autoimmune disorders are frequent, and there is a manyfold increase in the incidence of malignancy. For example, there is a nearly 50-fold increase in risk for gastric adenocarcinoma, and a 30-fold increase in risk for lymphoma.

- While not strictly Mendelian in its inheritance, patients with CVI tend to come from families with a history of immune dysregulation. First-degree relatives may manifest a similar CVI phenotype, but often they instead have selective IgA deficiency and/or autoimmunity.

- The B cells lack the capacity to differentiate into plasma cells. The number of B cells found in blood and tissue is normal, but the number of plasma cells is low, and the serum immunoglobulin level is low. Germinal centers are hyperplastic; the typical small bowel morphology includes pronounced reactive follicular lymphoid hyperplasia in the face of a distinctly low number of plasma cells.

Selective IgA Deficiency

- Like CVI, this is a common inherited immunodeficiency, affecting around 1 in 700 people in North America and Europe. The incidence is much lower in the East.

- These patients suffer from recurrent respiratory and gastrointestinal bacterial infections, a high incidence of autoimmunity (especially rheumatoid arthritis and systemic lupus erythematosis [SLE]), and allergy (especially allergic rhinitis, eczema, asthma, and a risk for anaphylaxis resulting from transfusion of IgA-containing blood products).

- The serum IgA concentration is below 5 mg/dL.

- Inheritance is variable, and IgA deficiency may represent a common final pathway for a number of inherited and acquired defects. Many cases are familial with autosomal recessive inheritance, others autosomal dominant, and still others apparently sporadic. Furthermore, IgA deficiency can be transient in childhood, and in some cases, patients who are thoroughly studied turn out to be best classified as having CVI or ataxia-telangiectasia.

Job (Hyper-IgE) Syndrome

- While not necessarily a B-cell defect, a highly characteristic feature of Job syndrome (named in reminiscence of the Biblical Job), is a very high serum IgE level. In particular, there is a high selective IgE anti-staphylococcal antibody. The IgE level appears to be an effect, however, of exquisite susceptibility to staphylococcal infection that is caused by a neutrophil chemotactic defect. Recurrent staphylococcal skin infections (furuncles, carbuncles) are the reason for the allusion to Job (covered in boils).

- Additional manifestations include staphylococcal visceral infections, staphylococcal osteomyelitis, fungal infections of the lung, chronic mucocutaneous candidiasis, and dental abnormalities (delayed shedding of primary teeth).

- The serum IgE level exceeds 2500 IU/mL, and peripheral eosinophilia is usually noted.

- Job syndrome is believed to be transmitted by autosomal dominant inheritance. At this time, the molecular defect and pathophysiology are not well understood.

Hyperimmunoglobulin M (Hyper-IgM) Syndrome

- This is another condition in which the noted anomaly (high IgM) appears to be the result of a defect in another immune system component, in this case T cells. Isotype switching is a process in which IgM-producing B cells are provoked, by T-cell–secreted cytokines, to switch to production of other isotypes (IgG, IgA, IgE). This switch usually takes place on repeated exposure to foreign antigen. The hyper-IgM syndrome is thought to be the result of a fundamental defect in the T-cell contribution to this process. The disorder presents with recurrent infections, increased serum IgM, and low levels of other immunoglobulin isotypes.

- In addition to high IgM, serum IgD may sometimes be elevated. Peripheral blood B cells are present in normal numbers. T cells lack expression of either CD40 or the ligand for CD40 (CD40L).

- There are several types of hyper-IgM. The most common type is X-linked recessive and is caused by mutations in the gene for CD40L, located on Xq26. Some cases are caused by mutations in CD40 itself, and these display autosomal recessive patterns of inheritance.

T-Cell and Combined Defects

DiGeorge Syndrome/Velocardiofacial Syndrome

- Among the many features of DiGeorge syndrome is failure of the third and fourth pharyngeal pouches to develop. Inherent in this maldevelopment is a hypoplastic thymus (T-cell defect), hypoplastic parathyroids (hypocalcemia, neonatal tetany), and anomalies of the great vessels (aortic arch). There is a typical facial dysmorphism (hypertelorism, low set ears, prominent nose, mandibular hypoplasia, retrognathia), bifid uvula, and a higher than usual incidence of esophageal atresia.

- The immunodeficiency manifests in typical T-cell defect fashion: opportunistic pathogens such as fungi, viruses, and *Pneumocystis carinii* are commonly encountered. The risk of transfusion-associated graft-versus-host disease is also increased. Note that, because of the central role of T cells in orchestrating the immune response, T-cell disorders often engender a certain degree of B-cell deficiency.

- Examined lymph nodes have depleted paracortical areas, and the spleen has poorly developed periarteriolar lymphatic sheaths (PALS).

- DiGeorge syndrome results from deletion (so-called microdeletion) of band 22q11.2, affecting a series of genes simultaneously (a contiguous gene syndrome). Depending on the nature and extent of the deletion, which is variable, the result may be DiGeorge syndrome, the very similar (if not identical) velocardiofacial syndrome, Shprintzen syndrome, or, occasionally, isolated conotruncal cardiac defects. Deletions on 10p13p14 (DiGeorge syndrome II locus) have also been associated with the phenotypic features of DiGeorge syndrome (DiGeorge syndrome II).

- A dual-probe fluorescence in situ hybridization assay is available for assessing these loci, with a sensitivity of about 95%. Most will demonstrate a deletion of 22q11.2, with the deletion of 10p13p14 being rare.

- DiGeorge syndrome occurs in up to 1 in 4000 births. It does not display Mendelian inheritance and instead occurs sporadically. Some cases have been associated with in utero exposure to accutane.

Severe Combined Immunodeficiency (SCID)

- SCID is a group of disorders characterized by decreased or absent T-cell function; often this is of sufficient severity to result also in low to undetectable immunoglobulin levels, B-cell numbers, and natural killer (NK) cell numbers. These defects result in severe, life-threatening, immunodeficiency that is usually only treatable by bone marrow transplantation.

- SCID affects about 1 in 50,000 births. Most affect patients are male (about 4: 1). About 1 in 3 cases is inherited, while the remainder appear to be the result of a sporadic molecular defect.

- The unifying feature of SCID is the paucity of mature T cells; SCID is further classified according to the affected NK and B lymphocyte subsets. There is good correlation between the subset patterns and the genetic basis. Thus, lymphocyte subset analysis (by flow cytometry) can be used to screen for the disease and to guide additional genetic testing.

- SCID is caused by a great variety of genetic defects **T9.1**. The most common form (50% of cases) is X-linked recessive and occurs because of a defect in the *interleukin (IL) receptor family*, especially IL-2, IL-7,

and others. The most common underlying mutation is found in the gene that encodes the common γ chain (CγC) of the IL receptor, located at Xq13.1. In such cases, peripheral blood flow cytometry shows a paucity of mature T- and NK-cells. The number of circulating B cells is normal.

- Many of the remaining cases are autosomal recessive. The most common AR form of SCID (15% of cases) is a deficiency in the enzyme *adenosine deaminase* (ADA). ADA is a key enzyme in the purine salvage pathway, and developing lymphoid cells appear to be exquisitely sensitive to its deficiency. Another autosomal recessive form of SCID is called *reticular dysgenesis*. It is because of a defect at the stem cell level that results in severe deficiency of neutrophils, B cells, NK cells, and T cells. It may go so far as to affect red cells and platelets. The thymus and lymph nodes are severely hypoplastic. Other recessive forms of SCID include CD45 deficiency, JAK3 deficiency, purine nucleoside phosphorylase (PNP) deficiency, CD3 deficiency, and RAG1/RAG2 deficiency.

T9.1
Forms of Severe Combined Immunodeficiency

Cause	Affected Lymphocyte Subsets	Inheritance
Common γ chain (CγC) deficiency	T, NK	XLR
Adenosine deaminase (ADA) deficiency	T, NK, B	AR
Reticular dysgenesis	T, NK, B	AR
RAG1/RAG2 deficiency	T, B	AR
Omenn syndrome	T, B	AR
JAK3 deficiency	T, NK	AR

Nezelof Syndrome (Isolated Thymic Aplasia)

- Nezelof syndrome is characterized by T-cell deficiency, thymic aplasia, and normal immunoglobulin levels. The lack of associated anatomic anomalies distinguishes this from DiGeorge syndrome; the lack of associated immune system defects distinguishes it from SCID.

- Affected children have recurrent bronchopulmonary infection and mucocutaneous candidiasis.

- The genetic basis has not been elucidated.

Wiskott-Aldrich Syndrome (WAS)

- WAS is an X-linked disease characterized by the triad of eczema, thrombocytopenia, and immunodeficiency. Peripheral blood platelets are small and uniform. There is loss of the CD43 antigen on circulating leukocytes and platelets. The immunodeficiency is caused by defects in both the T-cell and B-cell arms of the immune system.

- WAS initially manifests with bleeding—mucocutaneous petechiae and/or severe bleeding from the gastrointenstinal (GI) tract or nose—caused by severe thrombocytopenia that is present at birth. Later, eczema appears in typical eczema locations (antecubital and popliteal fossae). Bacterial infections take the form of otitis media, sinusitis, and pneumonia. The immune deficiency causes particular susceptibility to pneumococci and other encapsulated bacteria, *P. carinii,* and herpes viruses (HSV, VZV). Lastly, there is an increased risk for autoimmune disease, and a high incidence of malignancies.

- The most common causes of death, in decreasing frequency, are infection, bleeding, and malignancy.

- The responsible *WAS* gene is located on the X chromosome and has been associated with other forms of disease as well, including X-linked thrombocytopenia and X-linked congenital neutropenia. WAS protein (WASP) refers to the product of the *WAS* gene. WASP is found mainly in hematopoietic cells and appears to be responsible for the cytoskeletal malleability that is necessary for physiologic activities (eg, the dissolution of megakaryocytes to form mature platelets).

Syndromes Culminating in Fulminant Hemophagocytic Syndrome: Chediak-Higashi Syndrome, Griscelli Syndrome, Duncan Disease, and Familial Hemophagocytic Lymphohistiocytosis (FHL)

- Chediak-Higashi syndrome

  □ An autosomal recessive condition that presents as neutropenia, recurrent infection, thrombocytopenia, and oculocutaneous albinism. In late stages, an accelerated phase may develop, characterized by a fulminant hemophagocytic syndrome (HPS). As in sporadic cases of HPS, this appears to be triggered by viral infection, especially Epstein-Barr virus.

  □ Granulocytes, lymphocytes, and monocytes show giant cytoplasmic granules, representing abnormally fused lysosomes. In fact, abnormal granules can be found in all granule-forming cells, including melanocytes. Microscopic examination of hair shafts reveals giant melanosome granules in them (the hair color is abnormally light and "ashen" in affected individuals).

  □ The basic abnormality is defective degranulation, caused by mutations in the *LYST* (*CHS1*) gene, thought to be involved in lysosome trafficking.

- Griscelli syndrome is caused by mutations in the *RAB27A* gene, which encodes a GTPase involved in intracellular lysosome trafficking. Its manifestations are apparently similar to Chediak-Higashi syndrome.

- Duncan disease (X-linked lymphoproliferative disease)

  □ Duncan disease typically presents as a fulminant and often fatal immune response to Epstein-Barr virus (EBV) infection. EBV infection induces a fulminant hemophagocytic syndrome, the development of a neoplastic B cell proliferation, and/or fulminant hepatic failure, concomitant with an inverted CD4: CD8 ratio in the peripheral blood.

  □ Even before EBV infection occurs, affected individuals often have a CVI-like immune system defect, especially manifesting hypogammaglobulinemia with or without decreased B-, T-, or NK subsets.

  □ The median life-span is about 10 years.

  □ The *SH2D1A* gene, found at Xq25, has been implicated in this disease.

141

9: Immunologic Disorders, Immunodeficiency, and Autoimmunity

T-Cell and Combined Defects>Syndromes Culminating in Fulminant Hemophagocytic Syndrome; Chronic Mucocutaneous Candidiasis; CHH Syndrome; IPEX Syndrome | Granulocyte Defects>Inherited Neutropenias

- FHL is caused by a perforin deficiency and is characterized by the occurance of HPS at a very young age. The defect is manifested in T cells and NK cells, in which perforin is a critical component of cytotoxic granules.

Chronic Mucocutaneous Candidiasis

- Chronic, recalcitrant candidal infection is a problem common to T-cell defects. A disorder in which this is a predominant or isolated feature has been called chronic mucocutaneous candidiasis, thought to be the result of a highly selective defect in T-cell immunity to candida.

- Chronic mucocutaneous candidiasis often coexists with autoimmune endocrinopathies. In fact, type 1 autoimmune polyendocrinopathy or APECED (see chapter 7) overlaps with this syndrome.

- A syndrome resembling chronic mucocutaneous candidiasis may also be a presentation of thymoma.

Cartilage-Hair Hypoplasia (CHH) Syndrome

- CHH syndrome is an autosomal recessive disorder characterized by immunodeficiency (T-cell defects and neutropenia), short stature (because of metaphyseal chondrodysplasia), and sparse hair. While rare overall, the disease is relatively common among the Amish and in parts of Finland.

- T cells are decreased in number, IgA and IgG are decreased, and neutrophils are reduced in number. There is usually also anemia and reticulocytopenia.

- CHH is caused by mutations in *RMRP*, a gene that encodes an untranslated mRNA.

Immune Dysregulation, Polyendocrinopathy, Enteropathy, and X-Linked Inheritance (IPEX) Syndrome

- IPEX is caused by mutations in a gene located on the X chromosome that encodes the protein FoxP3. This protein is expressed in a group of CD4-positive, CD25-positive T cells involved in orchestration, especially suppression, of the immune response.

- The endocrinopathy most often takes the form of diabetes mellitus or hypothyroidism, manifestations that are thought to have an autoimmune basis. In fact, the thyroid histology resembles Hashimoto thyroiditis.

- The enteropathy, likewise, resembles inflammatory bowel disease.

Granulocyte Defects

Inherited Neutropenias: Congenital Neutropenia (Kostmann Syndrome) and Cyclic Neutropenia T9.2

- These diseases present with recurrent fever, cervical lymphadenopathy, oral ulcers, gingivitis, sinusitis, and pharyngitis. The more severe form of the disease (congenital neutropenia or Kostmann syndrome) may present in the neonatal period with omphalitis, followed in infancy by infectious complications such as pneumonia, intractable diarrhea, and abscesses. The later development of acute myelogenous leukemia afflicts a significant minority.

- The milder form (cyclic neutropenia) has intervals of fever, often accompanied by 1 or more foci of inflammation—such as oral ulcers, pharyngitis, sinusitis, perianal ulceration, or colonic ulceration—during which neutropenia can be found. The neutrophil count varies from normal to essentially none in a roughly 21-day cycle; the period of neutropenia lasts several days during which the patient is at risk for severe infections.

T9.2
Inherited Disorders with Neutropenia as a Component

Kostmann syndrome
Cyclic neutropenia
Myelokathexis (WHIM syndrome)
Chediak-Higashi syndrome
Reticular dysgenesis
Hermansky-Pudlak syndrome (with defect in platelets and albinism)
Glycogen storage disease type 1b
Barth syndrome
Shwachman-Diamond syndrome (pancytopenia)
Dyskeratosis congenita (anemia, thrombocytopenia, and/or neutropenia)
Fanconi anemia (anemia and/or thrombocytopenia precede neutropenia)
Common variable immunodeficiency
Hyper-IgM syndrome
Hyper-IgE syndrome
Cohen syndrome (with severe mental retardation and dysmorphic features)

9: Immunologic Disorders, Immunodeficiency, and Autoimmunity

Granulocyte Defects>Inherited Neutropenias: Congenital Neutropenia and Cyclic Neutropenia; Chediak-Higashi Syndrome; Shwachman-Diamond Syndrome; Dyskeratosis Congenita; Myelokathexis

- Examination of the bone marrow finds a maturation arrest at the promyelocyte stage. Maturation arrest is intermittent in cyclic neutropenia, but even in intercritical periods, the neutrophil count rarely exceeds 2000/μL.

- Mutations in the *ELA2* (neutrophil elastase) gene, located at 19p13, are responsible for both conditions. Mutations in *GFI1*, a gene whose expression exerts control over that of *ELA2*, can also cause these syndromes.

- There are autosomal recessive and autosomal dominant forms of less severe congenital neutropenia, collectively termed benign familial neutropenias.

Chediak-Higashi Syndrome

- See section on syndromes culminating in fulminant hemophagocytic syndrome.

Shwachman-Diamond Syndrome

- An autosomal recessive disease characterized by neutropenia or pancytopenia, pancreatic dysfunction (see chapter 8), and skeletal anomalies (metaphyseal dysostosis). Note that this syndrome is distinct from Blackfann-Diamond syndrome (pure red cell aplasia, no pancreatic or bone disease).

- The hematologic findings include neutropenia, eventually leading to aplastic anemia, myelodysplasia, and possibly acute leukemia. The bone marrow is hypocellular, usually with paucity of granulocytic precursors, and these may appear dysplastic.

- Neutropenia leads to recurrent infections, particularly skin infections, osteomyelitis, otitis media, and sinusitis.

- Shwachman-Diamond syndrome is caused by mutations in a gene known as *SBDS* (Shwachman-Bodian-Diamond syndrome) on chromosome 7. While the function of the gene is unknown, mutations in it appear to arise as a result of exchange of genetic material with a nearby pseudogene (*SBDSP*) in a manner similar to the mechanism of mutation in congenital adrenal hyperplasia (See Chapter 7).

Dyskeratosis Congenita (Zinsser-Engman-Cole Syndrome)

- Dyskeratosis congenita may initially present with leukopenia, anemia, and/or thrombocytopenia, but invariably these isolated cytopenias progress to pancytopenia. Other findings, many of which may precede cytopenias, include reticulated skin hyperpigmentation, nail dystrophy, oral leukoplakia, lacrimal duct atresia (causing overflow lacrimation), and testicular atrophy.

- Dyskeratosis congenita appears to result from more than 1 genetic basis, because there are X-linked forms (most common) and autosomal forms (recessive and dominant).

- 2 genes associated with dyskeratosis congenita, *DKC1* and *TERC*, encode proteins involved in telomerase. *DKC1*, which encodes the protein dyskerin, is located at Xq28. Telomeres are regions of the chromosome whose function, during mitosis, is to maintain chromosomal stability. Telomerase plays a role in telomere maintenance. The more rapidly a tissue type proliferates, the more sensitive it is to telomerase anomalies; thus, bone marrow is very sensitive.

- The most common causes of death are fatal opportunistic infections (due to leukopenia), fatal hemorrhage (caused by thrombocytopenia), and malignancy.

Myelokathexis (and WHIM Syndrome)

- Myelokathexis is a term that refers to an autosomal dominant disorder, with neutropenia and recurrent bacterial infections, in which circulating neutrophils have characteristic morphologic findings. In peripheral blood smears, neutrophils appear to be degenerating, with pyknotic nuclei, characteristic fine chromatin filaments, and hypersegmentation. Examination of the marrow discloses only hypercellularity with myelocytic hyperplasia.

- WHIM is an acronym that refers to a subset of myelokathexis cases, in which there are warts, hypogammaglobulinemia, infections, and myelokathexis.

- Both syndromes are related to defective release of mature granulocytes from the marrow, reduced expression of bcl-x in granulocytic precursors, and for some reason, enhanced apoptosis in circulating granulocytes.

- Mutations in the *CXCR4* (chemokine receptor) gene have been identified as the cause of WHIM syndrome.

Barth Syndrome

- Barth syndrome is an X-linked recessive syndrome of dilated cardiomyopathy, skeletal myopathy, aminoaciduria of 3-methylglutaconic acid, cardiolipin deficiency, and neutropenia.

- Marrow examination reveals maturation arrest at the myelocytic stage.

- Barth syndrome is caused by mutations in the *TAZ* gene, which encodes taffazin proteins involved in phospholipid biosynthesis.

Autoimmune Neutropenia

- Autoimmune neutropenia rarely occurs in isolation; more often, it occurs as part of a systemic autoimmune condition, particularly rheumatoid arthritis (Felty syndrome).

- Over 90% of those with Felty syndrome are positive for HLA-DR4. Interestingly, this HLA type is shared with large granular lymphocytosis/leukemia, a disorder consistently associated with neutropenia.

Leukocyte Adhesion Deficiency (LAD)

- The first steps in the granulocyte response are margination and migration across an endothelial surface. This is mediated by receptors on the cell surface that interact with ligands on endothelial cells.

- Leukocyte adhesion deficiency type I (LAD I) is caused by deficient cell-surface expression of the β2-integrin subunit (CD18). The number of circulating neutrophils in this disorder is normal or slightly increased. A classic finding is delayed cord separation after birth. LAD I is caused by mutations in the *ITGB2* gene found at 21q22.3.

- LAD type II (LAD II) is caused by defective fucosylation of cell-surface receptors, somewhat analogous to polymorphisms in red cell antigens. In fact, patients also have unmodified H substance on the surface of their red cells and a Bombay phenotype. This very rare disorder is characterized by normal to high numbers of circulating neutrophils and mental retardation.

- LAD type III (LAD III) is caused by defective G-coupled integrin activation.

Lazy Leukocyte Syndrome

- The so-called lazy leukocyte syndrome is associated with chronic neutropenia, an increased risk of infection, and a normal marrow examination. It was described over 30 years ago but has barely been elucidated since.

Chronic Granulomatous Disease (CGD)

- An important component of the immune response is the NADPH oxidase-driven oxidative burst. Superoxide generated in this process is used to generate oxidants, including hydrogen peroxide and hypochlorous acid. These oxidants can directly kill bacteria. There are other mechanisms for producing hydrogen peroxide, but they are weak in comparison and can be overcome by bacterial catalase.

- The CGD phenotype can form on the basis of any 1 of several genetic defects that result in defective intracellular oxidative killing of ingested organisms. This results in a syndrome of chronic recurrent suppurative infections, especially ones caused by organisms that are catalase-producing. At the sites of infection, just as with mycobacterial organisms that cannot be fully killed, there is extensive granuloma formation.

- The clinical manifestations usually begin before the age of 3 years. Affected children are particularly susceptible to *Staphylococcus aureus,* certain gram-negative bacilli (*Serratia, Salmonella, Burkholderia*), *Aspergillus* species, and *Nocardia* species. Such individuals do not suffer from an increased incidence of streptococcal infections. Common sites of infection include skin, lungs, bone, GI tract, liver, and lymph nodes.

- CGD has several genetic causes. About 2 in 3 cases have X-linked inheritance, and 1 in 3 has autosomal recessive inheritance. The enzyme NADPH oxidase is central to these various forms of CGD, each leading in its own way to a deficiency in this enzyme. The active form of NADPH oxidase is composed of 4 polypeptide subunits. In the unstimulated neutrophil, the 4 subunits exist separately; on stimulation, they rapidly assemble and the enzyme becomes active. Mutations in any 1 of the subunit genes can cause NADPH deficiency. X-linked cases result from mutations in the gp91phox subunit of flavocytochrome b, encoded on the X chromosome.

9: Immunologic Disorders, Immunodeficiency, and Autoimmunity

Granulocyte Defects>CGD; Myeloperoxidase Deficiency; May-Hegglin Anomaly; Alder-Reilly Anomaly; Pelger-Huet Anomaly I
Complement Component Deficiencies>Deficiency of Classic Pathway Components; Deficiency of C3

- The screening test is the nitroblue tetrazolium (NBT) test performed on a peripheral blood film, in which phagocytic cells with normal oxidative function can convert the yellow dye to a blue product. Affected leukocytes are also deficient in C3b receptors. Red cells often bear the McLeod phenotype (absence of Kell antigen Kx).

Myeloperoxidase (MPO) Deficiency

- MPO is a component of azurophilic granules and is instrumental in granulocyte-mediated fungal and bacterial killing. MPO deficiency results in a blunted immune response to candidal infections in particular; however, this effect is mitigated by other, still functional, components of the granulocyte, and most cases are clinically mild.

- The incidence of MPO deficiency is about 1 in 4000, making it the most common inherited granulocyte disorder (CGD has an incidence of about 1 in 200,000).

- MPO deficiency is inherited in an autosomal recessive manner. At the genetic level, it is caused by a number of different mutations, all of which have as their end-result a low level of MPO activity. The *MPO* gene itself, located on 17q, is not commonly affected.

May-Hegglin Anomaly

- Autosomal dominant condition manifesting as Döhle-like bodies in granulocytes and monocytes, large platelets, and thrombocytopenia. The Döhle-like bodies can be abolished by addition of ribonuclease.

- About half of patients have an abnormal bleeding history, but bleeding complications have only been documented when the platelet count falls below 80,000/μL. Platelet aggregation studies are usually normal, and there does not appear to be much of an immune defect.

Alder-Reilly Anomaly

- Mainly a morphologic finding, Alder-Reilly anomaly is an autosomal dominant condition manifesting as large azurophilic granules resembling toxic granulation in all white blood cells.

- There is an association with mucopolysaccharidoses.

Pelger-Huet Anomaly

- Autosomal dominant disorder with dysfunctional segmentation of neutrophils. Bilobed neutrophils are seen rather than normally segmented forms.

- In homozygotes, monolobated neutrophils (Stodtmeister cells) are seen. Functionally, the cells are normal.

- Lamin β receptor mutations have been found in some cases.

Complement Component Deficiencies

Deficiency of Classic Pathway Components (C1q, C2, C4)

- Defects in these early classic pathway components are mainly associated with the development of autoimmune conditions such as SLE. The incidence of SLE in C1q deficiency is over 90%.

- Immunodeficiency is mild and a secondary concern in these patients, presumably because the alternate pathway is sufficient for dealing with most infections.

- C1q is composed of 3 separate protein subunits—C1qA, C1qB, and C1qC—encoded separately by highly homologous genes on 1q. Mutations in any subunit can lead to clinically significant C1q deficiency.

- C2 deficiency is the most common inherited complement component deficiency, with an overall incidence of about 1 in 10,000 births. Like most of the complement proteins, the gene for C2 is located within the major histocompatability complex (MHC) on chromosome 6.

- C4 deficiency is very rare, because, like the alpha globin chain gene, each chromosome carries 2 copies of the gene. Unlike the alpha globin chain, all 4 alleles of C4 must be deleted to produce a clinically significant deficiency in C4.

Deficiency of C3

- Because C3 is utilized in both the alternate and classic complement pathways, both are neutralized by an inherited C3 deficiency (or the extremely rare properdin deficiency). Recurrent infections, especially with encapsulated organisms, cause major morbidity in patients with inherited C3 deficiency.

9: Immunologic Disorders, Immunodeficiency, and Autoimmunity

Complement Component Deficiencies>Deficiency of C3; Deficiency of Terminal Complement Components/Membrane Attack Complex Components; C1 Esterase Inhibitor Deficiency | Chromosomal Breakage Syndromes>Ataxia-Telangiectasia

- Autoimmunity is not the major concern, but the incidence of immune complex-mediated glomerulonephritis is high.

- Deficiency of factor I, the physiologic inhibitor of C3 activation, leads to consumption of C3 and, in effect, behaves clinically as a C3 deficiency. Properdin deficiency is associated with an extremely high risk of disseminated meningococcal infection and very high mortality once infected.

Deficiency of Terminal Complement Components/Membrane Attack Complex Components (C5-C9)

- Defects in terminal complement components (C5-C9) are associated with an increased susceptibility to certain gram-negative bacteria, especially *Neisseria meningitidis* and *N gonorrhea*. Autoimmune disease is not a feature.

C1 Esterase Inhibitor (C1 Inh) Deficiency

- A deficiency of C1 esterase inhibitor causes hereditary angioedema (HAE). This autosomal dominant inhibitor deficiency is more common than any of the complement component deficiencies.

- HAE is characterized by episodes of edema affecting skin and the mucosa of the upper respiratory and gastrointestinal tracts. Upper respiratory edema may result in asphyxia, and gastrointestinal edema may lead to vomiting or diarrhea. Classic HAE displays a fairly characteristic temporal and spatial pattern of edema episodes. On average, women have more severe disease than men, and patients with an early onset of symptoms have more severe disease than those with late onset. In most cases, the pattern is as follows: a symptom-free infancy and early childhood is followed by the onset of clinical symptoms, usually in late childhood or adolescence. After onset, the disease persists for the life of the patient, with critical and intercritical periods. With regard to the spatial pattern, swelling is seen most consistently in the skin (upper extremity more than lower) and intestinal tract (abdominal pain episodes). Laryngeal edema, though classic and potentially lethal, is present in only about 1% of episodes but has a lifetime incidence of about 50%. Facial swelling is rare, and while there is swelling of the soft palate and uvula, it spares the tongue. Acute episodes are treated with androgenic agents.

- There are 2 forms: either C1 Inh is absent (type I) or C1 Inh is present but functionally defective (type II). A third type of HAE has been described that is not associated with C1-INH deficiency, and its underlying mechanism is unknown.

Chromosomal Breakage Syndromes

Ataxia-Telangiectasia (Louis-Bar Syndrome)

- Ataxia-telangiectasia (AT) is an autosomal recessive disease that affects approximately 1 in 50,000 births.

- It is characterized by cerebellar ataxia, oculocutaneous telangiectasia, thymic hypoplasia, recurrent sinopulmonary infections, hypogonadism, and a high incidence of malignancy.

- Magnetic resonance imaging shows the cerebellum to be frequently small. Progressive cerebellar ataxia is often the first sign of the disease, manifesting as soon as walking begins. Microscopically, there is a paucity of the 2 main cerebellar neuronal cell types: Purkinje cells and granule cells.

- The immunodeficiency is a combined T-cell and B-cell defect. IgA is usually deficient, and there is impaired antibody response to pneumococcal vaccine.

- Affected individuals have very high serum alpha-fetoprotein and carcinoembryonic antigen levels for unknown reasons.

- The lifetime risk for malignancy is 38%, and hematolymphoid malignancies account for most of these.

- AT is caused by mutations in the *ATM* gene, on 11q22.3, which encodes the ATM protein kinase involved in DNA repair **T9.3**. An immunoblotting assay is available for the ATM protein in nuclear lysate, as well as assays for ATM kinase activity. A radiosensitivity assay determines the survival of lymphoid cells after irradiation, and this is abnormal in more than 95% of affected individuals. Cytogenetic analysis may be performed for chromosome breakage in dividing cells exposed to irradiation. Routine cytogenetics can detect the t(7; 14) in about 10% of cases, but direct sequence analysis of the *ATM* gene is required for a definitive molecular diagnosis in most cases.

T9.3
Chromosomal Breakage Syndromes

Syndrome	Gene (Chromosome)	Chromosome Hypersensitivity Immunodeficiencies	Immunodeficiency	Malignancy
Ataxia-telangiectasia	*ATM* (11q22.3)	Ionizing radiation	IgA deficiency and T-cell dysfunction	Hematolymphoid Breast
Bloom syndrome	*BLM* (15q26.1)	UV irradiation bromodeoxyuridine	IgA	Hematolymphoid Colorectal carcinoma Skin cancer
Fanconi anemia	FANCA (16q24.3) FANCC (9q22.3) FANCG (9p13)	UV irradiation DNA crosslinking agents	Cytopenia	Hematolymphoid Squamous cell carcinoma Medulloblastoma Wilms tumor Breast Hepatocellular
Xeroderma pigmentosum	XPA (9q22.3) XPC (3p25) XPD (19q)	UV irradiation	Immunoglobulin deficiency	Squamous cell carcinoma Basal cell carcinoma Melanoma Sarcoma
Nijmegen breakage syndrome	*NBS1* (8q21)	UV irradiation	Immunoglobulin deficiency	

Bloom Syndrome

- Autosomal recessive disorder characterized by short stature, narrow face with beaked nose, telangiectasia, a photosensitive erythematous skin lesion (usually on the face), chronic infections, and susceptibility to hematolymphoid malignancies, especially acute leukemia.

- Patients with Bloom syndrome have decreased serum IgA. The immunodeficiency leads to repeated episodes of otitis media and bacterial pneumonia. Recurrent respiratory infections lead to bronchiectasis.

- The characteristic skin lesions are absent at birth and develop during the first year of life, following sun exposure, most commonly as a butterfly-pattern facial lesion. Café-au-lait spots and areas of hypopigmentation are common.

- Bloom syndrome is caused by a mutation in the *BLM* gene, on 15q26.1, encoding a DNA helicase.

The classic cytogenetic finding in Bloom syndrome is the quadriradial pattern, a cruciate configuration formed by 2 homologous chromosomes that have broken and rejoined in this way. A large number of sister chromatid exchanges (SCEs) is another characteristic cytogenetic abnormality. The syndrome may be diagnosed by demonstrating a greatly increased frequency of these anomalies in cytogenetic cultures exposed to bromodeoxyuridine (BUDR). Even in cultures not exposed, there may be increased numbers of chromosomal breaks, chromatid gaps, and chromosomal rearrangements. Testing for mutations in the *BLM* gene is clinically available. If the ethnicity of the affected individual is known, targeted mutation analysis can be used; in Ashkenazi Jews, Bloom syndrome is nearly always caused by a particular mutation known as BLMASH whose frequency is about 1% in that population.

147

9: Immunologic Disorders, Immunodeficiency, and Autoimmunity

Chromosomal Breakage Syndromes>Fanconi Anemia; Xeroderma Pigmentosum/DeSanctis-Cacchione Syndrome; Nijmegen Breakage Syndrome I Primary Immunodeficiency: Summary and Approach>Classification

Fanconi Anemia (FA)

- FA is characterized in cell culture by an increased number of chromosomal breaks, gaps, radials, and rearrangements. Instability is enhanced by exposure to mitomycin C (MMC), diepoxybutane (DEB), or cisplatin.

- The overall incidence is about 1 in 100,000. A particularly high incidence is present in descendants of white South Africans.

- The clinical syndrome is characterized by the development of macrocytic anemia, progressing to aplastic anemia (pancytopenia), which may eventually give way to acute leukemia. Growth retardation beginning before or after birth is quite common, and there is a high incidence of physical anomalies, including absent radii, thumb malformations, microcephaly, short stature, and renal malformations. Café-au-lait spots are present in about 1 in 4. About 1 in 3 have no physical findings.

- Molecular testing is complicated by the fact that the underlying genetic defects are numerous. The most commonly affected gene is *FANCA*, implicated in about 2 in 3 cases. In decreasing order, additional gene mutations are found in *FANCC, FANCG, FANCB*, and others. In Ashkenazi Jews, testing is more practical because a single gene, *FANCC*, is usually involved.

Xeroderma Pigmentosum (XP)/ DeSanctis-Cacchione Syndrome

- Patients with XP have extreme photosensitivity and photophobia. Sun exposure is associated with the development of severe sunburn, extensive freckling, poikiloderma, corneal opacification, and telangiectasias. Freckling, which is unusual in children younger than 2 years, may be seen in infants with XP who are exposed to sun. Sun exposure eventually results in an outcropping of numerous epidermal and ocular neoplasms, often before the 10th birthday.

- The underlying defect is dysfunction of an enzyme involved in nucleotide excision repair. Exposure to sunlight (UV irradiation) induces the damage in need of repair. There are presently no laboratory assays available clinically for the diagnosis of XP. In research settings, several assays have been developed which evaluate the ability of cells to repair UV-induced DNA damage. These include post-UV cell survival, post-UV host cell reactivation, and post-UV unscheduled DNA synthesis. Chromosomal breakage in dividing cell cultures exposed to UV light is enhanced in XP.

- While mutations in several genes are known to underlie XP, especially *XPA* (9q22) and *XPC* (3p), both encoding DNA repair proteins, molecular testing is not presently available on a clinical basis.

- XP, severe neurologic impairment, and dwarfism characterize the DeSanctis-Cacchione syndrome. Some individuals manifest an overlapping XP and Cockayne syndrome. These are believed to arise from a different set of genes than those causing pure XP, especially ERCC3 on chromosome 2q.

Nijmegen Breakage Syndrome (Berlin Syndrome, Seemanova Syndrome)

- Autosomal recessive chromosomal breakage syndrome characterized by short stature, microcephaly, mental retardation, premature ovarian failure, immunodeficiency, and an increased risk for malignancy. A characteristic dysmorphic appearance is often present: sloping forehead, prominent nasal root, large ears, and upwardly slanting palpebral fissures. The vast majority of Nimmegen syndrome–associated malignancies are B-cell lymphomas.

- Recurrent sinopulmonary infections are a common problem. Laboratory testing discloses hypo- or agammaglobulinemia, and in some cases, decreased CD3+/CD4+ T cell subsets.

- Chromosomal instability may be noted in cytogenetic cultures.

- Mutations in the *NBS1* gene (8q21–encoding nibrin) underlie all known cases.

Primary Immunodeficiency: Summary and Approach

Classification

- In 2005, a combined National Institutes of Health (NIH)/International Union of Immunological Societies (IUIS) group published a proposed classification of the primary immunodeficiencies. This system is loosely adhered to in the preceding text, and in skeletal summary, the classification is as follows:

- Immunoglobulin defects

  □ Severe reduction in all isotypes (BTK mutations and others)

  □ Severe reduction in at least 2 isotypes (CVI and others)

- □ Severe reduction in IgG and IgA with increased IgM
- □ Isotype or light chain deficiencies with normal numbers of B cells (IgG subclass deficiencies, selective IgA deficiency, and others)
- □ Specific antibody deficiency with normal immunoglobulin concentrations and normal numbers of B cells (inability to make antibodies to specific antigens)
- □ Transient hypogammaglobulinemia of infancy
- Combined T- and B-cell defects
  - □ T⁻B⁺ SCID (CγC deficiency, JAK3 deficiency, and others)
  - □ T⁻B⁻ SCID (RAG1/RAG2 deficiency, ADA deficiency, reticular dysgenesis)
  - □ Omenn syndrome
  - □ DNA ligase IV deficiency
  - □ CD40 ligand (CD40L) deficiency
  - □ CD40 deficiency
  - □ Others: PNP deficiency, MHC class II deficiency, CD3γ deficiency, CD8 deficiency, ZAP-70 deficiency, TAP-1/2 deficiency, winged helix deficiency
- Immune regulation defects
  - □ Immunodeficiency with hypopigmentation (Chediak-Higashi and Griscelli syndromes)
  - □ FHL syndromes (perforin deficiency and others)
  - □ X-linked lymphoproliferative (XLP) syndrome (Duncan disease)
  - □ Syndromes with autoimmunity (autoimmune lymphoproliferative syndrome, APECED, IPEX, and others)
- Phagocyte defects
  - □ Severe congenital neutropenias (ELA2 mutations and others)
  - □ Kostmann syndrome
  - □ Cyclic neutropenia
  - □ X-linked neutropenia (WASP mutations)
  - □ Leukocyte adhesion deficiency types 1-3
  - □ Schwachman-Diamond syndrome
  - □ Chronic granulomatous disease

- □ Others: RAC2 mutation, localized juvenile periodontitis, Papillon-Lefevre syndrome, neutrophil glucose-6-phosphate dehydrogenase deficiency
- Other well-defined syndromes
  - □ Wiskott-Aldrich syndrome
  - □ DNA repair defects (Ataxia-telangiectasia, Nijmegen breakage syndrome, Bloom syndrome)
  - □ Thymic defects (DiGeorge syndrome)
  - □ Immuno-osseous dysplasia (cartilage-hair hypoplasia, Schimke syndrome)
  - □ Hermansky-Pudlak syndrome
  - □ Hyper-IgE syndrome
  - □ Chronic mucocutaneous candidiasis
  - □ WHIM syndrome
- Complement deficiencies

Suspecting a Primary Immunodeficiency

- Primary immunodeficiencies may present insidiously and nonspecifically, for example, as a failure to thrive. Nonetheless, the usual clue is recurrent or recalcitrant infection. However, infections are common in children, and in those with excessive rates of infection, the relatively rare immunodeficiency syndromes are diluted by other causes, such as environment or nonimmune abnormalities like neurologic impairment, cystic fibrosis, congenital anatomic abnormalities, or hematologic diseases.

- Immunodeficiency should be suspected when infections are unusually frequent, unexpectedly severe, or found in unusual sites. It may be suspected on the basis of unusual organisms (P carinii, G lamblia, Cryptosporidium) or ones that are resistant to treatment. For example, it has been recommended that more than 7 episodes of otitis media in 1 year or more than 1 serious infection (pneumonia, deep soft tissue, complicated sinus infection, infection requiring intravenous antibiotics) should raise alarm. Thrush beyond infancy is another clue.

- Most primary immunodeficiencies display X-linked recessive inheritance and therefore affect males, with an overall male to female ratio of 5:1. While the vast majority present at a very young age, it is notable that CVI, which is a relatively common primary immunodeficiency, presents in the second or third decade and affects males and females equally.

9: Immunologic Disorders, Immunodeficiency, and Autoimmunity

Primary Immunodeficiency: Summary and Approach>Suspecting a Primary Immunodeficiency; Suspecting a Particular Group of Primary Immunodeficiencies; Laboratory Screening for Immunologic Defects I Autoimmunity>ADI

- The physical examination may be notable for lymphadenopathy (typical of CVI and others), thrush, or skin lesions (eg, furuncles). Furthermore, specific syndromic features may be noted, such as telangiectasia (AT), albinism (Chediak-Higashi), eczema (WAS), abnormal scalp hair, ataxia, or dysmorphic features. The commonly touted "small lymph glands" are difficult for most examiners to appreciate, but tonsils can be easily viewed (small or absent in Bruton agammaglobulinemia and SCID).

Suspecting a Particular Group of Primary Immunodeficiencies

- Once suspected, physical findings may point to a particular diagnosis or group of disorders. If not, the variety of infectious episodes is important for focusing further inquiry.

- Recurrent infection with *G lamblia, Streptococcus pneumoniae* and/or *Haemophilus influenzae* is indicative of a B-cell (immunoglobulin) defect. *S pneumoniae* and *H influenzae* are also common in complement deficiency.

- A strong personal or family history of autoimmune disorders suggests an early complement component deficiency, CVI, or IgA deficiency.

- Recurrent infection with *P carinii, Cryptosporidium,* opportunistic viruses (or live, attenuated vaccine), fungi, or mycobacteria suggest a T-cell defect.

- Transfusion-associated graft-versus-host disease is a feature of SCID.

- Widespread staphylococcal infections, infections with gram-negative organisms (*Serratia, Burkholderia, Klebsiella*), infections with particular fungal infections (*Aspergillus*), and gingivitis suggest granulocyte defects.

Laboratory Screening for Immunologic Defects

- B-cell defects can be effectively tested by measuring serum immunoglobulins. It is important to measure each immunoglobulin class (isotype), as a global measurement of immunoglobulin (eg, by serum protein electrophoresis) can be misleading. At the very least, IgG, IgM, and IgA should be measured. IgG subclasses should be measured if an immunoglobulin deficiency is suspected but total IgG is normal. Selective deficiencies of IgE and IgD have not been described, but IgE should be measured if the clinical picture fits that of

Job syndrome. More information about B-cell function can be gained by measuring specific antibodies (isohemagglutinin titers), such as antibody against pneumococcal capsular polysaccharide, that are nearly universal in humans. Alternately, one may choose to measure specific antibody raised in response to prior immunization (tetanus, for example). This type of test, like delayed-type hypersensitivity testing (below) is not very useful in neonates or young infants. Additional information may be obtained from reviewing GI or lymph node biopsies.

- Many T-cell defects are associated with a small or aplastic thymus, identified in newborns and young infants as an absent "thymic shadow" on chest X-ray. Because T cells usually represent about 80% of circulating lymphocytes, T-cell defects can produce peripheral blood lymphopenia. Flow cytometry can be used to enumerate T cells and T-cell subsets. T-cell defects may result in an impaired reaction to delayed type hypersensitivity skin tests, and this can be a useful screening assay, so long as inherent limitations are recognized.

- A peripheral blood smear is also a good beginning when neutrophil defects are suspected, because this may display neutropenia, specific morphologic abnormalities, or thrombocytopenia (WAS). More detailed studies of neutrophil function are available, including assays of chemotaxis and bactericidal activity. The nitroblue tetrazolium test is a good way to screen for chronic granulomatous disease.

- The CH50 assay is a screening test for complement component deficiencies.

Autoimmunity

Autoimmune Diseases and Inheritance

- While it is clear that inheritance has a major impact on the development of autoimmune disease, there are only a few monogenetic autoimmune diseases. Most are instead influenced by 1 or several susceptibility loci as well as hormonal milieu (sex), and environmental factors; ie, most are multifactorial.

- The MHC is one such locus, a polymorphism of which is implicated in nearly every major autoimmune condition. For example, there are strong associations with several diseases and particular HLA types:

- □ HLA-DR3 with insulin-dependent diabetes mellitus (IDDM), SLE, Sjögren syndrome, myasthenia gravis, dermatitis herpetiformis, celiac sprue, and Graves disease

- □ HLA-DR4 with IDDM, rheumatoid arthritis (RA), pemphigus vulgaris

- □ HLA-DR2 with multiple sclerosis, narcolepsy; protective for IDDM

- □ HLA-B27 with ankylosing spondylitis and other "reactive" arthritides

- Familial aggregation varies from 1 autoimmune disease to the next, as does concordance among identical twins. Familial aggregation is loose, for example, in rheumatoid arthritis, whereas it is pronounced in SLE and the seronegative spondyloarthropathies (ankylosing spondylitis and Reiter syndrome). In SLE, for example, the recurrence rate (relative risk) is about 50 for blood relatives.

Monogenetic Autoimmune Conditions

- Familial Mediterranean fever (FMF) is an inherited (autosomal recessive) autoimmune disease characterized by episodes of abdominal pain and fever. Abdominal pain is related to an acute neutrophilic serositis and can be the cause of a pseudosurgical abdomen (similar to attacks of porphyria). Atypical presentations can include acute synovitis and something called an "acute scrotum."

- Over time, recurrent inflammation may lead to an AA-type amyloidosis.

- Specific autoantibodies have not been described in this condition.

- FMF is found in greatest prevalence among Sephardic Jews, Armenians, Arabs, and Turks. About 1 in 10 Jews of North African descent are carriers of the disease-associated allele of the *MEFV* gene.

- The product of the *MEFV* gene is called pyrin (or marenostrin). Over 25 different mutations have been described in *MEFV*, which is found on 16p.

- APECED syndrome (autoimmune polyendo-crinopathy with candidiasis and ectodermal dystrophy) is an autoimmune disease affecting the parathyroid glands, adrenal cortex, and thyroid gland associated with chronic mucocutaneous candidiasis. It is caused by mutatins in the AIRE gene (see chapter 7).

- IPEX (immune dysregulation, polyendocrinopathy, enteropathy, X-linked) syndrome is caused by mutations in the *FOXP31*gene. It is characterized by autoimmune enteropathy, type 1 diabetes, autoimmune thyroiditis, and autoimmune hemolytic anemia and thrombocytopenia (see T-cell and combined defects).

Systemic Lupus Erythematosus

- Evidence for a genetic influence on the development of SLE includes:

- □ Family members of patients with SLE are at increased risk for developing SLE.

- □ Even among those unaffected clinically, nearly 20% have antinuclear antibodies.

- □ The concordance rate for identical twins is about 25%. As in nonidentical family members, the concordance is much higher for autoantibodies than for clinical disease.

- HLA haplotypes and extended haplotypes (particular combinations of haplotypes) have been associated with an increased risk of SLE.

- Complement proteins are among several non-HLA genes that influence the risk of SLE. About 5% of patients with SLE have an inherited deficiency of 1 of the early complement components (C2, C4, or C1q); conversely, the likelihood of SLE in these deficiency states is nearly 50%.

Sjögren Syndrome

- Sjögren syndrome is autoimmune destruction of lacrimal and salivary glandular tissue that results in the association of dry eyes (keratoconjunctivitis sicca) and dry mouth (xerostomia). Many cases also have some autoimmunity directed at other organs, such as the lung and pancreas. Sjogren syndrome may be primary or secondary (arising in another autoimmune condition, most commonly rheumatoid arthritis).

- There is a moderate association with HLA-B8, HLA-DR3, HLA-DRW52, HLA-DQA1, and HLA-DQB1 loci.

9: Immunologic Disorders, Immunodeficiency, and Autoimmunity

Autoimmunity>Seronegative Spondyloarthropathies: Ankylosing Spondylitis, Reiter Syndrome, Psoriatic Arthritis, and Enteropathic Arthritis; Rheumatoid Arthritis | References

Seronegative Spondyloarthropathies: Ankylosing Spondylitis, Reiter Syndrome, Psoriatic Arthritis, and Enteropathic Arthritis

- Ankylosing spondylitis (AS) is an inflammatory spondyloarthropathy that, in classic cases, begins in the sacroiliac joint and is generally confined to an axial skeletal distribution. Psoriatic arthritis is an inflammatory spondyloarthropathy that arises in association with psoriasis. Enteropathic arthritis is associated with inflammatory bowel disease, and Reiter syndrome (also called reactive arthritis) arises in association with a localized infection, especially enteric infection by *Shigella, Salmonella, Campylobacter,* or *Yersinia*, or urethral infection with *Chlamydia*.

- Unifying these disorders is an axial-predominant distribution, tenosynovial histology resembling that of rheumatoid arthritis, absence of rheumatoid factor, and a strong association with HLA-B27.

- While only a small proportion (10%-20%) of HLA-B27-positive people develop 1 of these conditions, about 90% of those with a seronegative sponyloarthropathy are HLA-B27-positive. Thus, knowledge of the HLA-B genotype can be helpful when entertaining this diagnosis.

Rheumatoid Arthritis (RA)

- As noted earlier, RA displays a somewhat weaker familial aggregation than some other autoimmune conditions. Environment appears to play a more significant role in RA, with such factors as female sex (8: 1) and smoking influencing disease rates. Nonetheless, there is significantly more-than-chance familial clustering and some well-established genetic associations.

- Interestingly, it has been found that smoking, 1 of the stronger risk factors for RA, is genotype-mitigated. The smoking effect is seen mainly in a subset of patients with particular HLA-DRB1 genotypes.

- The HLA-DRB1 genotypes associated with RA have all been found to share a particular amino acid sequence that has become known as the "shared epitope." Chief among these is the HLA-DRB1*0401 haplotype.

- Several non-HLA loci have been associated with RA as well, including loci on 18q, 1p, and 1q.

References

Aghamohammadi A, Kanegane H, Moein M, et al. Identification of an SH2D1A mutation in a hypogammaglobulinemic male patient with a diagnosis of common variable immunodeficiency. *Int J Hematol* 2003; 78: 45-47.

Alter BP. Bone marrow failure syndromes in children. *Pediatr Clin North Am* 2002; 49: 973-988.

Alter BP. Cancer in Fanconi anemia, 1927-2001. *Cancer* 2003; 97: 425-440.

Ancliff PJ. Congenital neutropenia. *Blood Rev* 2003; 7: 209-216.

Ancliff PJ, Gale RE, Linch DC. Neutrophil elastase mutations in congenital neutropenia. *Hematology* 2003; 8: 165-171.

Ancliff PJ, Gale RE, Liesner R, et al. Mutations in the ELA2 gene encoding neutrophil elastase are present in most patients with sporadic severe congenital neutropenia but only in some patients with the familial form of the disease. *Blood* 2001; 98: 2645-2650.

Ancliff PJ, Gale RE, Watts MJ, et al. Paternal mosaicism proves the pathogenic nature of mutations in neutrophil elastase in severe congenital neutropenia. *Blood* 2002; 100: 707-709.

Arico M, Imashuku S, Clementi R, et al. Hemophagocytic lymphohistiocytosis due to germline mutations in SH2D1A, the X-linked lymphoproliferative disease gene. *Blood* 2001; 97: 1131-1133.

Aprikyan AA, Liles WC, Rodger E, et al. Impaired survival of bone marrow hematopoietic progenitor cells in cyclic neutropenia. *Blood* 2001; 97: 147-153.

Bellanne-Chantelot C, Clauin S, Leblanc T, et al. Mutations in the ELA2 gene correlate with more severe expression of neutropenia: a study of 81 patients from the French Neutropenia Register. *Blood* 2004; 103: 4119-4125.

Berliner N, Horwitz M, Loughran TP Jr. Congenital and acquired neutropenia. *Hematology* 2004: 63-79.

References

Boxer LA, Stein S, Buckley D, et al. Strong evidence for autosomal dominant inheritance of severe congenital neutropenia associated with ELA2 mutations. *J Pediatr* 2006; 148: 633-636.

Breban M, Said-Nahal R, Hugot J, et al. Familial and genetic aspects of spondyloarthropathy. *Rheum Dis Clin North Am* 2003; 29: 575-594.

Burns S, Cory GO, Vainchenker W, et al. Mechanisms of WASP-mediated hematologic and immunologic disease. *Blood* 2004; 104: 3454-3462.

Butch AW, Chun HH, Nahas SA, et al. Immunoassay to measure ataxia-telangiectasia mutated protein in cellular lysates. *Clin Chem* 2004; 50: 2302-2308.

Carlsson G, Aprikyan AA, Tehranchi R, et al. Kostmann syndrome: severe congenital neutropenia associated with defective expression of Bcl-2, constitutive mitochondrial release of cytochrome C, and excessive apoptosis of myeloid progenitor cells. *Blood* 2004; 103: 3355-3361.

Coffey AJ, Brooksbank RA, Brandau O, et al. Host response to EBV infection in X-linked lymphoproliferative disease results from mutations in an SH2-domain encoding gene. *Nat Genet* 1998; 20: 129-135.

Cunningham-Rundles C. Physiology of IgA and IgA deficiency. *J Clin Immunol* 2001; 21: 303-309.

Dadi HK, Simon AJ, Roifman CM. Effect of CD3d deficiency on maturation of α/β and γ/δ T-cell lineages in severe combined immunodeficiency. *N Engl J Med* 2003; 349: 1821-1828.

Dale DC, Person RE, Bolyard AA, et al. Mutations in the gene encoding neutrophil elastase in congenital and cyclic neutropenia. *Blood* 2000; 96: 2317-2322.

D'Andrea AD, Grompe M. The Fanconi anaemia/BRCA pathway. *Nat Rev Cancer* 2003; 3: 23-34.

De Saint Basile G. Chediak-Higashi and Griscelli syndromes. *Immunol Allergy Clin North Am* 2002; 22: 301-317.

Dinauer MC. Chronic granulomatous disease and other disorders of phagocyte function. *Hematology* 2005: 89-95.

Dinauer MC, Coates TD. Disorders of phagocyte function and number. In: Hoffman R, Benz E, Shattil S, et al, eds. *Hematology: Basic Principles and Practice*. 4th ed. Philadelphia, Pa: Churchill Livingstone, 2005.

Dror Y, Sung L. Update on childhood neutropenia: molecular and clinical advances. *Hematol Oncol Clin North Am* 2004; 18: 1439-1458.

Durandy A, Honjo T. Human genetic defects in class-switch recombination (hyper-IgM syndromes). *Curr Opin Immunol* 2001; 13: 543.

Elenitoba-Johnson KS, Jaffe ES. Lymphoproliferative disorders associated with congenital immunodeficiencies. *Semin Diagn Pathol* 1997; 14: 35-47.

Erdos M, Uzvolgyi E, Nemes Z, et al. Characterization of a new disease-causing mutation of SH2D1A in a family with X-linked lymphoproliferative disease. *Hum Mutat* 2005; 25: 506.

Faivre L, Guardiola P, Lewis C, et al. Association of complementation group and mutation type with clinical outcome in fanconi anemia: European Fanconi Anemia Research Group. *Blood* 2000; 96: 4064-4070.

Filipovich AH. Hemophagocytic lymphohistiocytosis. *Immunol Allergy Clin North Am* 2002; 22: 281-300.

Fischer A. Have we seen the last variant of severe combined immunodeficiency? *N Engl J Med* 2003; 349(19): 1789-1792.

Freedman MH, Alter BP. Risk of myelodysplastic syndrome and acute myeloid leukemia in congenital neutropenias. *Semin Hematol* 2002; 39: 128-133.

Gaspar HB, Sharifi R, Gilmour KC, et al. X-linked lymphoproliferative disease: clinical, diagnostic and molecular perspective. *Br J Haematol* 2002; 119: 585-595.

Gatti RA, Petersen K, Novak J, et al. Prenatal genotyping of ataxia-telangiectasia. *Lancet* 1993; 342: 376.

Gazda H, Lipton JM, Willig TN, et al. Evidence for linkage of familial Diamond-Blackfan anemia to chromosome 8p23.3-p22 and for non-19q non-8p disease. *Blood* 2001; 97: 2145-2150.

Germeshausen M, Schulze H, Ballmaier M, et al. Mutations in the gene encoding neutrophil elastase (ELA2) are

References

not sufficient to cause the phenotype of congenital neutropenia. *Br J Haematol* 2001; 115: 222-224.

Gillio AP, Verlander PC, Batish SD, et al. Phenotypic consequences of mutations in the Fanconi anemia FAC gene: an International Fanconi Anemia Registry study. *Blood* 1997; 90: 105-110.

Hirsch B, Shimamura A, Moreau L, et al. Association of biallelic BRCA2/FANCD1 mutations with spontaneous chromosomal instability and solid tumors of childhood. *Blood* 2004; 103: 2554-2559.

Jackson CE, Puck JM. Autoimmune lymphoproliferative syndrome: a disorder of apoptosis. *Curr Opin Pediatr* 1999; 11: 521-527.

Kollner I, Sodeik B, Schreek S, et al. Mutations in neutrophil elastase causing congenital neutropenia lead to cytoplasmic protein accumulation and induction of the unfolded protein response. *Blood* 2006; 108: 493-500.

Kutler DI, Singh B, Satagopan J, et al. A 20-year perspective on the International Fanconi Anemia Registry (IFAR). *Blood* 2003; 101: 1249-1256.

Lamy T, Loughran TP Jr. Clinical features of large granular lymphocyte leukemia. *Semin Hematol* 2003; 40: 185-195.

Landmann E, Bluetters-Sawatzki R, et al. Fanconi anemia in a neonate with pancytopenia. *J Pediatr* 2004; 145: 125-127.

Lewis RF, Lederman HM, Crawford TO. Ocular motor abnormalities in ataxia telangiectasia. *Ann Neurol* 1999; 46: 287-295.

Lopez-Granados E, Perez de Diego R, Ferreira A, et al. A genotype-phenotype correlation study in a group of 54 patients with X-linked agammaglobulinemia. *J Allergy Clin Immunol* 2005; 116: 690-697.

Menasche G, Fischer A, de Saint Basile G. Griscelli syndrome types 1 and 2. *Am J Hum Genet* 2002; 71: 1237-1238.

Mentzer WC. Louis Diamond and his contribution to haematology. *Br J Haemat* 2003; 123: 389-395.

Mueller BU, Pizzo PA. Cancer in children with primary or secondary immunodeficiencies. *J Pediatr* 1995; 126: 1-10.

Notarangelo L, Casanova J, Conley ME, et al. International Union of Immunological Societies Primary Immunodeficiency Diseases Classification Committee. Primary immunodeficiency diseases: an update from the International Union of Immunological Societies Primary Immunodeficiency Diseases Classification Committee Meeting in Budapest. *J Allergy Clin Immunol* 2006; 117: 883-896.

Nowak-Wegrzyn A, Crawford TO, Winkelstein JA, et al. Immunodeficiency and infections in ataxia-telangiectasia. *J Pediatr* 2004; 144: 505-511.

Padeh S. Periodic fever syndromes. *Pediatr Clin North Am* 2005; 52: 577-609.

Padyukov L, Silva C, Stolt P, et al. A gene-environment interaction between smoking and shared epitope genes in HLA-DR provides a high risk of seropositive rheumatoid arthritis. *Arthritis Rheum* 2004; 50: 3085-3092.

Palma-Carlos AG, Palma-Carlos ML. Chronic mucocutaneous candidiasis revisited. *Allerg Immunol* 2001; 33: 229-232.

Rieux-Laucat F, Hivroz C, Lim A, et al. Inherited and somatic CD3ζ mutations in a patient with T-cell deficiency. *N Engl J Med* 2006; 354: 1913-1921.

Riminton DS, Limaye S. Primary immunodeficiency diseases in adulthood. *Intern Med J* 2004; 34: 348-354.

Rosen FS, Cooper MD, Wedgwood RJ. The primary immunodeficiencies. *N Engl J Med* 1995; 333: 431-440.

Rosenberg PS, Greene MH, Alter BP. Cancer incidence in persons with Fanconi anemia. *Blood* 2003; 101: 822-826.

Shimamura A, de Oca RM, Svenson JL, et al. A novel diagnostic screen for defects in the Fanconi anemia pathway. *Blood* 2002; 100: 4649-4654.

Snapper SB, Rosen FS. A family of WASPs. *N Engl J Med* 2003; 348: 350-351.

Starkebaum G. Chronic neutropenia associated with autoimmune disease. *Semin Hematol* 2002; 39: 121-127.

Sumazaki R, Kanegane H, Osaki M, et al. SH2D1A mutations in Japanese males with severe Epstein-Barr virus-associated illnesses. *Blood* 2001; 98: 1268-1270.

References

Sumegi J, Huang D, Lanyi A, et al. Correlation of mutations of the SH2D1A gene and Epstein-Barr virus infection with clinical phenotype and outcome in X-linked lymphoproliferative disease. *Blood* 2000; 96: 3118-3125.

Sun X, Becker-Catania SG, Chun HH, et al. Early diagnosis of ataxia-telangiectasia using radiosensitivity testing. *J Pediatr* 2002; 140: 724-731.

Tabata Y, Villanueva J, Lee SM, et al. Rapid detection of intracellular SH2D1A protein in cytotoxic lymphocytes from patients with X-linked lymphoproliferative disease and their family members. *Blood* 2005; 105: 3066-3071.

Teraoka SN, Malone KE, Doody DR, et al. Increased frequency of ATM mutations in breast carcinoma patients with early onset disease and positive family history. *Cancer* 2001; 92: 479-487.

Turesson C, Matteson EL. Genetics of rheumatoid arthritis. *Mayo Clin Proc* 2006; 81: 94-101.

Van Zelm MC, Reisli I, Van der Burg M, et al. An antibody-deficiency syndrome due to mutations in the CD19 gene. *N Engl J Med* 2006; 354: 1901-1912.

Verbsky JW, Grossman WJ. Cellular and genetic basis of primary immune deficiencies. *Pediatr Clin North Am* 2006; 53: 649-684.

Wagner JE, Tolar J, Levran O, et al. Germline mutations in BRCA2: shared genetic susceptibility to breast cancer, early onset leukemia, and Fanconi anemia. *Blood* 2004; 103: 3226-3229.

Weldon D. Differential diagnosis of angioedema. *Immunol Allergy Clin North Am* 2006; 26: 603-613.

Whitney MA, Saito H, Jakobs PM, et al. A common mutation in the FACC gene causes Fanconi anaemia in Ashkenazi Jews. *Nat Genet* 1993; 4: 202-205.

Winchester R. The genetics of autoimmune-mediated rheumatic diseases: clinical and biologic implications. *Rheum Dis Clin North Am* 2004; 30: 213-227.

Yamashita T, Wu N, Kupfer G, et al. The clinical variability of Fanconi anemia (type C) results from expression of an amino terminal truncated FAC polypeptide with partial activity. *Blood* 1996; 87: 4424.

Zeidler C, Welte K. Kostmann syndrome and severe congenital neutropenia. *Semin Hematol* 2002; 39: 82-88.

Chapter 10

Metabolic, Mitochondrial, and Lipid Disorders

Amino Acid and Organic Acid Disorders

In most systems of classification, amino acids are distinguished from organic acids, the latter referring to non–amino carbon-containing acids. These disorders **T10.1** are generally caused by defects in mitochondrial enzymes that are encoded by genes located in the nucleus. In contrast, mitochondrial enzymes encoded by mitochondrial genes are generally those involved in oxidative metabolism and are thought of as "mitochondrial" diseases (see section on Mitochondrial Diseases).

Phenylketonuria (PKU)

- Phenylalanine is normally ingested in excess of what is required for protein synthesis. The extra phenylalanine is converted to tyrosine by *phenylalanine hydroxylase*, whose cofactors are tetrahydrobiopterin (BH4) and dihydropteridine reductase. Phenylalanine that cannot be converted into tyrosine is shunted into other pathways leading to other products, including phenylacetic acid, which is responsible for the characteristic musty or mousy odor.

- Classic PKU is the most common of several clinical variants, with an incidence in the United States of about 1 in 15,000 births. It is an autosomal recessive disorder that is particularly common in those of Scandinavian descent, in which the deficiency of phenylalanine hydroxylase is severe. Classic PKU presents with marked hyperphenylalaninemia, causing severe mental retardation, seizures, skin hypopigmentation, and eczema. However, neurologic function is normal at birth (because of normal maternal metabolism), and dietary restriction of phenylalanine leads to completely normal brain development. By late in childhood the dietary restriction is often discontinued without major sequelae (however, there appears to be a subtle but definite cognitive impact). Thus, PKU is the prototype for neonatal screening programs.

- Maternal PKU refers to the effects upon a fetus of maternal hyperphenylalaninemia. Because many patients discontinue dietary restrictions by the time they are adults, the developing fetus in such women will be exposed to extremely high phenylalanine levels, leading to mental retardation. About 15% to 20% also have congenital heart defects.

- Benign PKU occurs in those having mutations resulting in mildly decreased phenylalanine hydroxylase activity. Mental retardation does not occur.

Hyperhomocysteinemia

- Homocysteine is an amino acid that is formed in the breakdown of protein. It is normally not an end-product in itself; instead, it is a temporary intermediary in the interconversion of methionine and cysteine, both of which can then go on to be used for other purposes. Whenever the utilization of methionine or cysteine is blocked, excess homocysteine accumulates.

- A point of possible confusion is the relationship between homocystinuria and hyperhomocysteinemia. Homocystinuria is a manifestation of *extreme* hyperhomocysteinemia (>100 μmol/L) that leads to a syndrome characterized by overflow of homocysteine into the urine (homocystinuria), mental retardation, ectopia lentis, premature atherosclerosis, and thrombosis. This syndrome is most commonly caused by *homozygous* cystathionine-β-synthase deficiency and is rare. In contrast, mild to moderate hyperhomocysteinemia (16-100 μmol/L) is *not* associated with homocystinuria, is not found in a dysmorphic clinical syndrome, and is quite common.

- A second point of confusion is the relationship of homocyst*eine* to homocyst*ine*. Homocysteine tends to form disulfide bonds with nearby molecules of homocysteine—2 homocyst*eine*s linked by a disulfide bond are called homocyst*ine*. In addition to free homocysteine and homocystine, homocysteine exists as 2 additional forms in blood: bound to other sulfhydryl groups (mixed disulfides) and bound to albumin (bound homocysteine). Most analytical methods measure all forms of homocysteine: homocysteine, homocystine, mixed disulfides, and bound homocysteine.

- Mild to moderate hyperhomocysteinemia affects 5% to 7% of the population and is an independent risk factor for both atherosclerosis and recurrent arteriovenous thromboembolism. Hyperhomocysteinemia is present in up to 40% of patients with premature atherosclerosis and about 15% to 20% of those with thrombophilia.

Amino Acid and Organic Acid Disorders>Hyperhomocysteinemia

T10.1
Amino Acid Disorders

Syndrome	Defect	Comment
Phenylketonuria	Phenylalanine hydroxylase 12q22-q24.1 (rarely TH$_4$)	Mental retardation and seizures Eczema Mousy odor
Tyrosinemia	Tyrosine aminotransferase, fumaryl acetoacetate hydrolase	Fulminant hepatic failure Cirrhosis, hepatocellular carcinoma Neuropathy with pain crises Renal Fanconi syndrome Boiling cabbage odor High incidence in Quebec
Alkoptonuria	Homogentisic acid oxidase	Ochronosis Black urine
Cystinosis	Cystine transmembrane receptor/transporter *CTNS* gene 17p13	Renal Fanconi syndrome Renal calculi Rickets Corneal opacities Tissue deposition of cystine Urine excretion of cystine
Cystinuria	Branched-chain amino acid receptor/transporter	Renal calculi Urinary excretion of cystine No tissue cystine deposition
Homocystinuria (homocystinemia)	Cystathionie synthase or MTHFR	Marfanoid changes Livedo reticularis Mental retardation Premature atherosclerosis Thrombophilia
Hartnup disease	Neutral amino acid receptor/transporter	Most are asymptomatic Amino aciduria of neutral amino acids (serine, threonine, alanine, valine, leucine, isoleucine, phenylalanine, tyrosine, tryptophan, histidine). Photosensitivity, episodic ataxia.
Maple syrup urine disease	Decarboxylases of branched-chain amino acids (leucine, isoleucine, and valine), eg, α-ketoglutarate dehydrogenase (branched-chain ketoacid dehydrogenase)	Varies in severity Severe form — neonatal hypoglycemia, vomiting, coma, and death. Maple syrup odor Mild forms — neurologic deterioration Thiamin (B6) responsive form
Multiple carboxylase deficiency	Defects in biotin-dependent pathways, eg, holocarboxylase synthetase deficiency, biotinidase deficiency, or biotin deficiency	Vomiting, seizures, failure to thrive Exfoliative erythematous rash Tomcat-like urine odor
Urea cycle disorders	Carbamyl phosphate synthetase Ornithine transcarbamylase (OTC) Argininosuccinate synthetase Argininosuccinate lyase Arginase N-Acetylglutamate synthetase	OTC deficiency is X-linked recessive All present with hyperammonemia and non-anion gap metabolic acidosis
Citrullinemia	Arginosuccinic acid synthase	Hyperammonemia
Canavan disease	Apartoacylase	Accumulation of N-acetylaspartic acid in the brain Spongy degeneration of the white matter (leukodystrophy) Ashkenazi Jews

- The most common cause of mild to moderate hyperhomocysteinemia is the common *MTHFR* (methylene tetrahydrofolate reductase) gene mutation. The Cys677Thr substitution, resulting in a valine for alanine substitution, is present in 10% to 50% of various populations (highest in Europe, lowest in Africa). Homozygosity (the so-called TT genotype) results in mildly reduced enzyme activity and mild hyperhomocysteinemia; heterozygosity has no known consequences (thus the trait is autosomal recessive). The effect of homozygosity is worsened by folate deficiency and ameliorated by folate supplementation. A second *MTHFR* alteration, Ala298Cys, acts as a true polymorphism, causing no clinical consequences even in the homozygous state. The *MTHFR* gene is found at 1p36.3. Genetic testing for the Ala677Val (C677T) mutation in *MTHFR* is clinically available.

- The second most common cause of mild to moderate hyperhomocysteinemia is heterozygosity for the *CBS* (cystathionine-β-synthase) mutation. Homozygosity for this mutation causes homocystinuria and severe hyperhomocysteinemia. Cystathionine β-synthase deficiency occurs in 2 forms: one that is vitamin B6-responsive, and one that is B6-unresponsive. Affected individuals are often tall and slender with an asthenic (marfanoid) habitus. In addition to biochemical assays for determining the activity of cystathionine β-synthase, molecular genetic testing is clinically available (direct sequence analysis of the *CBS* gene on 21q).

- Hyperhomocysteinemia is usually diagnosed by measuring plasma levels of homocysteine using high-pressure liquid chromatography. Hyperhomo-cysteinemia is classified as mild (16-24 μmol/L), moderate (25-100 μmol/L), or severe (>100). Plasma measurements are insensitive to very mild defects, but these can be amplified by demonstrating an abnormal increase in plasma homocysteine after an oral methionine load.

Alkaptonuria (Ochronosis)

- It was in describing alkoptonuria that, in 1908, Archibald Garrod coined the term *inborn error of metabolism*. Lack of homogentisic oxidase leads to accumulation of homogentisic acid, an endogenous pigment formed, usually temporarily, in the breakdown of tyrosine.

- Some of it makes its way into urine, imparting a black color to the urine on standing, and into soft tissue, including articular cartilage. Deposition of homogentisic acid in joints causes discoloration (ochronosis) and accelerated degenerative joint disease (often presenting in the fourth decade), most profoundly affecting the intervertebral discs and knees. Deposition in heart valves leads to valve dysfunction.

- Alkaptonuria is most common in persons of Slovak descent and those from the Dominican Republic.

- The *HGO* gene for homogentisic oxidase is found on 3q21. *HGO* mutations are heterogeneous, the most common among them being the M368V mutation, followed by H80Q. A biochemical assay is available for the detection of homogentisic acid in the urine. Targeted mutation analysis is available for the most common mutations.

Urea Cycle Disorders

- The end-product of amino acid metabolism is urea. Ammonia is an intermediate by-product of amino acid metabolism that normally is metabolized to urea through the urea cycle. Several enzymes are involved in this pathway, each of which may be congenitally deficient, resulting in hyperammonemia. The urea cycle disorders include enzyme defects, eg, carbamyl phosphate synthetase (CPS) deficiency, ornithine transcarbamylase (OTC) deficiency, argininosuccinate synthetase (AS) deficiency, that result in failure to adequately metabolize ammonia.

- The clinical presentation is primarily related to the effects of hyperammonemia. Most profoundly affected are the brain and liver. Severe enzyme deficiencies present soon after birth with lethargy, vomiting, seizures, and coma. Milder deficiency may present later, especially during stress such as infection. The common metabolic finding is metabolic acidosis with a normal anion gap.

- OTC deficiency is the most common urea cycle disorder, with an incidence of about 1 in 10,000 births. OTC deficiency displays X-linked inheritance, with severely affected males presenting as neonates with a fulminant syndrome of hepatic failure, coma, and death. Males with a mild enzyme defect may only come to clinical attention when increased metabolic demands (infection or other stress) expose the enzyme defect. For example, OTC deficiency may present as cyclic vomiting, recurrent gastroenteritis, Reye-like syndrome, or apparently cryptogenic hepatitis.

10: Metabolic, Mitochondrial, and Lipid Disorders

Amino Acid and Organic Acid Disorders>Organic Acid Disorders | Nucleic Acid (Purine and Pyrimidine) Metabolism Disorders>Nucleic Acid Metabolism; Lesch-Nyhan Syndrome | Carbohydrate Disorders>Galactosemia

Organic Acid Disorders (Organic Acidemias)

- This group of disorders is closely related to the amino acid disorders, because they too are defects in amino acid metabolism. They are characterized by accumulation of (and increased urinary secretion of) organic acid intermediates that are formed in the metabolism of amino acids, without an accumulation of (or increased urinary excretion of) amino acids.

- Classic cases of organic acidemias present soon after birth, in a previously well infant who develops lethargy, vomiting, metabolic acidosis, ketosis, and coma. If recognized, these disorders can be treated with protein restriction.

- In other cases, the disease may present later, still usually in childhood, with neurologic dysfunction, Reye-like syndrome, or recurrent ketoacidosis.

- Laboratory findings usually include metabolic acidosis with increased anion gap (because of unmeasured organic acid), ketosis (because of β-hydroxybutyrate and acetoacetate), hyperammonemia, hypoglycemia, neutropenia, and abnormal liver function tests. A urine organic acid analysis (gas chromatography–mass spectrometry) will disclose the abnormal presence of specific organic acids, as will plasma amino acid analysis.

- Biochemical assays are available for the activity of specific enzymes.

Nucleic Acid (Purine and Pyrimidine) Metabolism Disorders

Nucleic Acid Metabolism

- The end-product of *purine* metabolism is uric acid (urate). Urate is poorly soluble and even a small increase in serum urate can lead to soft tissue deposition. These increases may result from either increased production (increased degradation of purines) or decreased excretion (renal insufficiency).

- The end-product of *pyrimidine* metabolism is citric acid (citrate), which is far less problematic.

- 2 pathways are available for the synthesis of nucleic acids—1 capable of *de novo* synthesis and the other a salvage (recycling) pathway. Under normal circumstances, the salvage pathway is the source of most nucleotide synthesis. 2 pathways exist for the catabolism of nucleotides—1 for pyrimidines (citric acid pathway) and 1 for purines (uric acid).

- Metabolic disorders of nucleic acid metabolism include defects in the biosynthetic pathways (eg, adenylosuccinase deficiency, pyrimidine 5′-nucleotidase deficiency), defects in the salvage pathway (eg, hypoxanthine-guanine phosphoribosyl transferase [HGPRT] deficiency), and defects in the catabolic pathways (eg, adenosine deaminase [ADA] deficiency, purine nucleoside phosphorylase [PNP] deficiency, hereditary orotic aciduria).

Lesch-Nyhan Syndrome (HGPRT Deficiency)

- Lesch-Nyhan is an X-linked recessive disorder in which a defect in the salvage pathway leads to increased catabolic pathway activity and persistent hyperuricemia, resulting in neurologic dysfunction. A developmental delay becomes evident by 1 year of age, and walking is rarely achieved. By 2 to 3 years of age, extrapyramidal symptoms (such as choreoathetosis) and self-mutilating behavior (biting, head-banging) arise. Deposition of urate leads to renal stones and sometimes gout. The overproduction of urate can be controlled with allopurinol; however, urate control appears to have no effect on neurologic symptoms.

- Megaloblastic anemia (with normal levels of folate and B_{12}) is common.

- Because Lesch-Nyhan is a disease of urate overproduction, affected individuals are found to have an increased urinary urate:creatinine ratio. The serum urate itself is not always elevated, because of adequate urinary excretion.

- An assay for the deficient enzyme—HGPRT—is clinically available. Molecular testing of the *HPRT1* gene, found at Xq26-27.2 and encoding HGPRT, is also available.

Carbohydrate Disorders T10.2

Galactosemia

- Lactose, the major sugar in milk, is normally converted into glucose and galactose by the enzyme lactase (present along the intestinal brush border). Galactose is converted into glucose by the action of several enzymes, including galactose-1-phosphate uridyl transferase (GALT) and galactokinase. Galactosemia is an autosomal recessive disorder caused almost always by deficiency of GALT and rarely by deficiency of galactokinase. Clinical sequelae result from the

Carbohydrate Disorders>Galactosemia

T10.2
Carbohydrate Disorders

Syndrome	Defect	Comment
Glycogen storage disease type Ia (von Gierke disease)	Glucose-6-phosphatase deficiency	Hypoglycemia Hyperlipidemia Hyperuricosemia Hepatomegaly Renomegaly
Glycogen storage disease type Ib	Glucose-6-phosphate translocase	Finding similar to Ia, plus neutropenia
Glycogen storage disease type II (Pompe disease)	α-1,4-Glucosidase (lysosomal glucosidase, acid maltase) deficiency	Lysosomal storage disease with cardiomegaly and heart failure
Glycogen storage disease type III (Cori disease)	Debrancher (-1,6-glucosidase)	Hepatomegaly Hypoglycemia Hyperlipidemia
Glycogen storage disease type IV (Anderson disease)	Branching enzyme	Hepatomegaly Cirrhosis
Glycogen storage disease type V (McArdle's syndrome)	Muscle phosphorylase deficiency	Skeletal muscle cramps Elevated CK Myoglobinuria Failure to make lactate with exercise
Galactosemia	GALT deficiency	Vomiting, jaundice (on exposure to lactose) Hepatomegaly, steatosis, steatohepatitis Cirrhosis Neurologic deterioration *Escherichia coli* septicemia
Essential fructosuria	Fructokinase	Increased urine reducing substances Clinically benign
Hereditary fructose intolerance	Fructose-1-phosphate aldolase	Vomiting, lethargy, hepatic failure

accumulation of galactose-1-phosphate in tissue, especially the liver, myocardium, brain, lens, and spleen.

- Various mutations in the GALT gene result in a range of enzyme activity and of disease severity. Normal persons have a homozygous NN genotype, heterozygous NG genotype, or heterozygous ND. Classic (severe) galactosemia is associated with the homozygous GG genotype, and less severe (Duarte) galactosemia has the DD phenotype.

- The classic presentation is as follows: on the instigation of milk feedings, vomiting develops, followed by jaundice and hepatomegaly. In the liver, steatosis and steatohepatitis leads eventually to cirrhosis. Cataracts form in infancy or early childhood.

In the brain, there is neuronal loss and gliosis. For unclear reasons, there is an increased susceptibility to severe *Escherichia coli* septicemia.

- The diagnosis can be made with an assay of enzyme activity. In fact, prenatal diagnosis can be made by this assay. Newborn screening is based on a GALT enzyme activity assay performed on a blood spot. Galactosemia also produces a positive "reducing substance" test in urine, with a negative urine glucose. 2 mutations in the GALT gene, Gln188Arg (more Americans of European descent) and Ser135Leu (more common in African Americans) account for most cases of galactosemia, permitting targeted mutation analysis.

10: Metabolic, Mitochondrial, and Lipid Disorders

Carbohydrate Disorders>Glycogen Storage Diseases | Lysosomal Disorders>Lysosomes; I-Cell Disease | Peroxisomal Disorders and Disorders of Fatty Acid Oxidation>Peroxisomal Disorders

Glycogen Storage Diseases (Glycogenoses)

- In normal physiology, extracellular glucose is in flux with intracellular glucose, which is in flux with glycogen (the main storage form of glucose, found predominantly in hepatocytes and muscle). In the proper metabolic milieu, the hepatocyte seeks to make glycogen; glucose is first converted into glucose-6-phosphate (by glucokinase also known as *hexokinase*), then into glucose-1-phosphate (by phosphoglucomutase). Glucose-1-phosphate moieties can be sequentially added to one another linearly (by glycogen synthase) or with branches (by branching enzyme) to form the branched chain molecule glycogen. When more glucose is needed, glycogen can be broken down to glucose by a series of phosphorylases and a debranching enzyme.

- Some glycogen is metabolized in lysosomes by the enzyme acid maltase (when acid maltase is deficient, this leads to a lysosomal storage disease instead of a glycogen storage disease).

- Just as there are multiple steps in the interconversion of glucose and glycogen, there are multiple inherited enzyme deficiencies. The manifestations are either largely hepatic (hypoglycemia, hepatomegaly), largely muscular (cramping), or a combination of the 2.

Lysosomal Disorders

Lysosomes

- These are organelles composed of a lipid bilayer membrane enclosing a low pH environment rich in enzymes. Lysosomes contain a variety of enzymes responsible for the degradation of material from either within the cell or without; usually this is complex cell membrane material. When a deficiency is inherited in 1 of the lysosomal enzymes T10.3, its substrate accumulates in the lysosome, ultimately leading to the death of the cell.

- The particular manifestations of a lysosome storage disease depend on what cells are affected, and this depends on where the material is primarily formed or where it is primarily degraded.

- The examination of blood films may provide clues to lysosomal and other metabolic diseases. In some of these disorders, one may find lymphocyte vacuoles and/or Alder-Reilly anomaly.

I-Cell Disease

- Enzymes destined to be for the lysosome are post-translationally modified in the Golgi apparatus, with the addition of a mannose-6-phosphate tag. This tag guides their inclusion in lysosomes when they bud from the far end of the Golgi complex.

- I-cell disease results from an inborn error in the attachment of the mannose-6-phosphate tag, resulting in lysosomes devoid of enzymes. Instead, what results are cells that appear to contain inclusions (I), which are big, empty, lysosomes, and lysosomal enzymes that are misdirected into the extracellular space.

Peroxisomal Disorders and Disorders of Fatty Acid Oxidation

Peroxisomal Disorders (Zellweger Syndrome and X-Linked Adrenoleukodystrophy)

- Peroxisomes are relatively small, dense organelles that are enclosed by a trilaminar membrane. They are the site of a wide variety of metabolic activities, both anabolic and catabolic. Peroxisomes neutralize hydrogen peroxide with peroxisomal catalase. Other peroxisomal activities include the biosynthesis of lipid and the catabolism of purines, ethanol, and very-long-chain fatty acids (VLCFA)—fatty acids with more than 24 carbons.

- Defects of VLCFA metabolism are present in several peroxisomal disorders; thus, there is this point of overlap with the fatty acid oxidation disorders. In fact, measurement of plasma VLCFA is a commonly used assay to screen for peroxisomal disorders.

- Zellweger syndrome
  - Traditionally, 4 phenotypes have been distinguished: classic Zellweger syndrome, neonatal adrenoleukodystrophy (distinct from X-linked adrenoleukodystrophy), infantile Refsum disease, and rhizomelic chondrodysplasia punctata (Conradi syndrome).
  - Classic Zellweger syndrome describes the most severe phenotype and is characterized by neonatal hypotonia, poor feeding, seizures, hepatic dysfunction, liver cysts, characteristic facial dysmorphism (flattened facies, abnormally large anterior fontanelle, broad nasal bridge), and chondrodysplasia punctata.

T10.3
Lysosomal Storage Disease

	Syndrome	Defect	Comment
Sphingolipidoses	GM1 gangliosidosis	GM1 ganglioside β-galactosidase	Type 1—infantile, generalized Type 2—juvenile
	GM2 gangliosidosis: Tay-Sachs disease	Hexosaminidase-α *HEXA* gene 15q	Ashkenazi Jews
	GM2 gangliosidosis: Sandhoff disease	Hexosaminidase-β	
Glycogenoses	Glycogen storage disease type II (Pompe disease)	α-1,4-Glucosidase (lysosomal glucosidase, acid maltase)	Cardiomegaly and heart failure
Sulfatidoses	Metachromatic leukodystrophy	Arylsulfatase A	
	Multiple sulfatase deficiency	Arylsulfatases A, B, C; steroid sulfatase; iduronate sulfatase; heparan N-sulfatase	
	Krabbe disease (globoid cell leukodystrophy)	Galactosylceramidase / galactocererbrosidaseGALC gene 14q31	Neurologic deterioration
	Fabry disease	α-Galactosidase A *GLA* gene Xq22	Pain in distal extremities, Angiokeratomas, Hypohidrosis, Corneal and lenticular opacities, Death from renal failure, cardiovascular disease, or cerebrovascular disease XLR
	Gaucher disease	Glucocerebrosidase / glucosylceramidase *GBA* gene 1q21	Type 1—non-neuronopathic—most common Ashkenazi Jews Bone deformity Hepatosplenomegaly Cytopenias
	Niemann-Pick disease: types A and B	Sphingomyelinase	Neurologic deterioration
Mucopolysaccharidoses (MPS)	MPS I (Hurler)	α-l-Iduronidase	
	MPS II (Hunter)	l-Iduronosulfate sulfatase	
Mucolipidoses	I-cell disease (ML II) and pseudo-Hurler polydystrophy	Deficiency of phosphorylating enzymes essential for the formation of mannose-6-phosphate recognition marker; acid hydrolases lacking the recognition marker cannot be targeted to the lysosomes but are secreted extracellularly	
Miscellaneous	Fucosidosis	α-Fucosidase	
	Mannosidosis	α-Mannosidase	
	Wolman disease	Acid lipase	
	Acid phosphate deficiency	Lysosomal acid phosphatase	

□ When the presentation is that of neonatal adrenoleukodystrophy or Refsum disease, manifestations may develop later in such ways as developmental delays or hearing loss.

□ Biochemical assays of VLCFA in plasma are elevated. A diagnosis of Zellweger syndrome is suggested by any of the following: increased C26:0 VLCFAs, increased C26:1 VLCFAs, an increased ratio of C24:C22, or an increased ratio of C26:C22.

□ This group of disorders arises because of defects of peroxisome import. While numerous genes have been implicated, *PEX1* mutations are responsible for about 70% of cases. *PEX1* is located at 7q21 and encodes peroxisome biogenesis factor.

■ X-linked adrenoleukodystrophy (XLA)

□ XLA is believed to be the most common of the peroxisomal disorders, with an overall incidence of about 1 in 20,000. As implied in the name, this is an X-linked recessive disorder, affecting only boys, that causes deterioration in the adrenal gland and white matter of the brain. Patients present, usually in childhood, with neurologic findings, seizures, or adrenal cortical insufficiency (Addison disease). These effects are caused by accumulation of VLCFA in blood and tissue.

□ The underlying defect is the impaired function of peroxisomal lignoceroyl-CoA ligase, encoded by the *ABCD1* gene on Xq28.

□ Histologically, the brain shows demyelinative lesions, replete with inflammatory cells and histiocytes. Characteristic lamellar cytoplasmic inclusions are present ultrastructurally within adrenal cortex and brain.

□ As in Zellweger syndrome, the key laboratory finding is a high level of VLCFA; most peculiar to this condition is hexacosanoic acid (C26:0).

Fatty Acid Oxidation Disorders

■ Mitochondrial oxidation of fatty acids is essential for production of cellular energy. In the carnitine cycle, fatty acids are carried across the inner mitochondrial membrane and into the mitochondrial matrix linked to carnitine. There they are converted by β-oxidation to acetyl-coenzyme A (acetyl CoA). Because the fatty acids that enter this pathway are of several different

lengths, the mitochondrion is equipped with chain length–specific enzymes; eg, medium chain acyl-CoA dehydrogenase, long chain acyl-CoA dehydrogenase, and very long chain acyl-CoA dehydrogenase. The electron transfer chain carries some of the electrons generated in this process into adenosine triphosphate (ATP). The acetyl-CoA is used to make ketones (β-hydroxybutyrate and acetoacetate). This is a multi-step process, and autosomal recessive defects have been documented for nearly every enzymatic step **T10.4**.

■ The clinical manifestations are largely similar for all of these defects: skeletal and cardiac myopathy (which prefer fatty acids as an energy source) and difficulty dealing with prolonged fasts (in which the rest of the body switches from utilization of glycogen and glucose to utilization of fatty acids).

■ 1 clue to the diagnosis of a defect in mitochondrial β-oxidation is the absence of urinary ketones in an infant who has hypoglycemia. Furthermore, newborn screening programs that use tandem mass spectrometry can readily detect the abnormal acylcarnitines thay typify these disorders.

■ Medium-chain acyl-CoA dehydrogenase (MCAD) deficiency

□ MCAD deficiency is the most common of these disorders. Most affected persons are of northern European ancestry. The estimated incidence is 1 in 5000. The disease presents most commonly in infants with episodes, brought on by prolonged fasting, of hypoglycemia, vomiting, and lethargy. These may progress to coma and death. At autopsy, the liver shows microvesicular steatosis. The overall picture resembles Reye syndrome. During these episodes, hypoglycemia is not accompanied by passage of urinary ketones. Mass spectrometry, performed as part of newborn screening, can detect this condition by finding octanoylcarnitine.

□ Most cases are the result of a single point mutation in the MCAD gene: an A to G substitution at nucleotide 985. Targeted mutation analysis is clinically available to detect the A985G mutation. Rare cases are caused by a G583A mutation. A very common polymorphism is T199C. This mutation, while picked up on neonatal screening (because it produces an increase in octanoylcarnitine) does not appear to cause clinical disease.

10: Metabolic, Mitochondrial, and Lipid Disorders

Peroxisomal Disorders and Disorders of Fatty Acid Oxidation>Fatty Acid Oxidation Disorders |
Mitochondrial Disorders>Mitochondria

T10.4
Defects in Mitochondrial Fatty Acid Oxidation

Syndrome	Enzyme	Comment
Medium-chain acyl-CoA dehydrogenase (MCAD) deficiency	MCAD	See text
Long-chain/very long chain acyl-CoA dehydrogenase (LCAD/VLCAD) deficiency	LCAD/VLCAD	More severe than MCAD Skeletal and cardiac myopathy
Long-chain 3-hydroxyacyl-CoA dehydrogenase (LCHAD) deficiency	LCHAD	Mutation in the fetus associated with acute fatty liver of pregnancy in the mother
Carnitine Deficiency	Carnitine	Cardiomyopathy

MCAD = medium-chain acyl-CoA dehydrogenase; LCAD = long-chain acyl-CoA dehydrogenase; LCHAD = long-chain 3 hydroxyacyl-CoA dehydrogenase; VLCAD = very-long-chain acyl-CoA dehydrogenase.

☐ The treatment is avoidance of prolonged (>12-hour) fasting. Patients so treated can live a normal lifespan, because unlike other fatty acid oxidation disorders there is no associated myopathy, and tolerance for fasting appears to improve with age.

Mitochondrial Disorders

Mitochondria

■ Mitochondria are derived from symbiotic intracellular bacteria that came complete with their own genome and capacity to divide. The genome and faculty to reproduce persist, but many mitochondrial constituents are now encoded in the nucleus. Thus, inherited mitochondrial diseases may follow mendelian or mitochondrial inheritance.

■ Mitochondrial inheritance, also called maternal inheritance, is simple in some respects but complicated in others.

☐ The sperm provides the fertilized ovum with no mitochondria. All mitochondria, and therefore all mitochondrial DNA (mtDNA), are passed on to the offspring from the mother. Furthermore, only affected daughters can pass an mtDNA trait on to the next generation.

☐ What complicates this simple scheme is that, unlike the nucleus which contains 2 copies of each chromosome for a total of 46 discrete DNA molecules, each mitochondrion contains thousands of DNA molecules. Thus, whereas

a mutation in nuclear DNA can be present in 1 or 2 of 2 gene copies, a mutation may be present in the mitochondrial genome in a very wide range of dilutions. These mutations become clinically significant when they reach a certain concentration (the threshold effect).

☐ Also, when mitochondria divide (in order to provide sufficient mitochondria for both products of a cell division) these mtDNA molecules are randomly divided among the newly formed mitochondria. So different cells in the body (and different organs in the body) can end up with genetically very different mitochondria, a situation called *heteroplasmy*. The cells of normal individuals usually contain a single clone of mitochondria (with identical genomes, inherited from the mother, also known as *homoplasmy*). Heteroplasmy is the basis for the broad phenotypic variability observed in mitochondrial disease.

☐ The effect of mutations in mitochondrial genes, whether affecting a gene located in the nucleus or in the mitochondrion, is manifested most profoundly in those tissues that participate in a lot of oxidative metabolism; in decreasing order, these are the brain, myocardium, skeletal muscle, liver, kidneys, and other organs.

■ Mitochondria carry out a restricted set of essential cellular functions: the aerobic (oxidative) generation of energy (ATP), the removal of reactive oxygen species, portions of the urea cycle, Krebs cycle, and the oxidation of fatty acids and pyruvate. Tissues

10: Metabolic, Mitochondrial, and Lipid Disorders

Mitochondrial Disorders>Mitochondria; Disorders Caused by Structural Mitochondrial DNA Defects: Kearns-Sayre Syndrome, Pearson Syndrome, and Progressive External Ophthalmoplegia; MELAS

that depend greatly on the aerobic generation of energy (brain, skeletal muscle, cardiac muscle) are particularly sensitive to mitochondrial dysfunction. Aerobic oxidation is the process by which electrons obtained from organic metabolites are passed down the electron-transfer chain to oxygen. The energy from this gradient is used to generate an electrical gradient which, in turn, is used to phosphorylate adenosine diphosphate to produce ATP (oxidative phosphorylation). During this process, reactive oxygen species are created which must be detoxified, the function of superoxide dismutase. Pyruvate oxidation provides acetyl-CoA for entry into Krebs cycle, the enzymes for which are contained in mitochondria. Portions of the urea cycle take place in mitochondria.

- Mitochondrial dysfunction results in a heterogeneous group of disorders that usually affect the neuromuscular system at some level, tending to produce such manifestations as ophthalmoplegia, ptosis, retinopathy, optic atrophy, skeletal myopathy, cardiomyopathy, sensorineural deafness, and encephalopathy.

- Mitochondrial diseases caused by mutations in nuclear DNA tend to present in childhood, while those caused by mutations in mitochondrial DNA often present later.

- Also, point mutations in mitochondrial DNA are usually inherited (maternally), while gross deletions in mitochondrial DNA usually arise sporadically (de novo).

- Mitochondrial diseases should be considered in the differential whenever there is an unexplained multilevel neuromuscular disorder. Screening tests that should be abnormal in mitochondrial diseases include plasma or cerebrospinal fluid (CSF) lactic acid, ketones, acylcarnitines, and urinary organic acids. If these are abnormal, one should next consider muscle biopsy.

- In classic cases, the muscle biopsy displays ragged red fibers (trichrome stain). The succinate dehydrogenase stain, in addition to highlighting the muscle fibers, shows stronger than usual staining in blood vessels, because of an abundance of mitochondria. Ultrastructural examination shows characteristic ("parking lot") inclusions.

Disorders Caused by Structural Mitochondrial DNA Defects: Kearns-Sayre Syndrome, Pearson Syndrome, and Progressive External Ophthalmoplegia

- Kearns-Sayre has the following features: presentation before the age of 20 years, pigmentary (salt and pepper) retinopathy, external ophthalmoplegia, elevated CSF protein, cerebellar ataxia, cardiac conduction block, sensorineural hearing loss, skeletal myopathy, diabetes mellitus, and hypoparathyroidism. Progressive external ophthalmoplegia (PEA) and maternally inherited diabetes mellitus (MIDM) are syndromes that present after age 20 years with the limited manifestations that their names describe.

- Pearson syndrome presents in childhood and is uniformly fatal. Its manifestations include sideroblastic anemia, progressing to pancytopenia, and pancreatic exocrine insufficiency.

- These syndromes are caused by major defects—gross deletions or large rearrangements—in mtDNA. Such defects are usually sporadic (de novo), but they are sometimes maternally derived. Heteroplasmy leads to the variety of clinical presentations.

Mitochondrial Encephalopathy with Lactic Acidosis and Strokelike Episodes (MELAS)

- MELAS presents in childhood, between 2 and 10 years of age. Initial development is normal, but this is followed by progressive neurologic deterioration.

- It presents with strokelike neurologic deficits (transient hemiparesis or cortical blindness), often accompanied by seizures. Additional features are diabetes mellitus, cardiomyopathy, sensorineural hearing loss, pigmentary retinopathy, cerebellar ataxia, and lactic acidosis (causing easy fatigueability). Interestingly, during strokelike episodes, magnetic resonance imaging of the brain shows lesions inconsistent with a vascular distribution. The basal ganglia often show calcifications.

- MELAS is caused by mutations in the *MT-TL1* gene, which is located within the mitochondrial DNA and encodes tRNA^{Leu}. Because a single mutation—an A to G substitution at nucleotide 3243 (A3243G)—is responsible for more than 80% of cases, this disease lends itself to targeted mutation analysis.

10: Metabolic, Mitochondrial, and Lipid Disorders

Mitochondrial Disorders>Myoclonic Epilepsy with Ragged Red Fibers; MNGIE; Leigh Syndrome I
Classification and Approach to Metabolic Disorders>Classification; Suspecting a Metabolic Disorder

Myoclonic Epilepsy with Ragged Red Fibers (MERRF)

- MERRF manifests as myoclonic seizures, cerebellar ataxia, dementia, optic atrophy, sensorineural hearing loss, skeletal myopathy, and cardiomyopathy. Symmetrical lipomas affect the neck and shoulders in some cases.

- Like MELAS, a single mutation is responsible for more than 80% of cases—an A to G substitution at nucleotide 8344 (A8344G)—in the mitochondrial *MT-TK* gene which encodes tRNA^{Lys}. Targeted mutation analysis for this and 2 to 3 other mutations can detect more than 90% of cases.

Mitochondrial Neurogastrointestinal Encephalomyopathy (MNGIE)

- MNGIE is inherited as an autosomal recessive trait, as it results from nuclear DNA mutations. It presents in late childhood, adolescence, or early adulthood (average age, 19 years).

- It is characterized by episodes of abdominal pain accompanied by nausea, vomiting, and/or diarrhea. These symptoms are the result of a function bowel obstruction (pseudo-obstruction). In addition, there are neurologic manifestations that include progressive external ophthalmoplegia, leukodystrophy, skeletal myopathy, and peripheral neuropathy.

Leigh Syndrome

- Leigh syndrome presents in childhood, usually before the second birthday, initially with failure to thrive, developmental delay, hypotonia, and eventual developmental regression, external ophthalmoplegia, optic atrophy, and seizures. Death results from pneumonia or apnea.

- Also called subacute necrotizing encephalomyelitis, Leigh syndrome is characterized by scattered but symmetric foci of spongy degeneration and vascular proliferation, located predominantly in the cerebellum, basal ganglia, and thalamus.

- Leigh syndrome is genetically heterogeneous, being caused by mutations in several mitochondrial and nuclear genes.

Classification and Approach to Metabolic Disorders

Classification

- Deciding what is and is not a metabolic disorder is somewhat arbitrary. The inability to synthesize cortisol (in congenital adrenal hyperplasia) and the defects that underlie a wide range of other disorders are clearly metabolic defects; however, these are not listed as traditional metabolic disorders.

- The characteristics shared by *most* diseases in this category are (1) Mendelian inheritance with a recessive pattern (autosomal or X-linked), (2) systemic effects (more or less), and (3) presentation at a very young age. In the foregoing discussion, all X-linked recessive disorders are indicated; the remainder should be assumed to be autosomal recessive.

- A source of much confusion are the several somewhat overlapping bases applied to classification of metabolic disorders. The first is the nature of the substrate affected (such as carbohydrate, amino acid, or lipid). The second is the location of the defect in the cell (cell membrane, lysosome, peroxisome, mitochondrion, cytosol). Cell membrane receptor/transporter diseases are scattered throughout this chapter and the remainder of the book T10.5. The third is the nature of the offending by-product (hyperammonemia, hyperuricosuria, or amino aciduria) or deficient product (glucose or melanin). The fourth is the predominantly offended organ (neuropathic or hepatopathic). Accepting that these classifications are somewhat arbitrarily and inconsistently applied may make their study less frustrating.

Suspecting a Metabolic Disorder

- Metabolic disorders usually present in neonates or infants, but occasionally present later in life. Common clinical findings in neonatal/infantile presentations include lethargy, dehydration, metabolic acidosis, vomiting, hyperammonemia, hypoglycemia, or seizures (sepsis must be excluded). Many appear normal at birth and progressively deteriorate.

- Some metabolic disorders present instead with dysmorphic features and hepatosplenomegaly, especially the lysosomal defects (mucopolysaccharidoses, sphinogolipidoses, and other lysosomal storage diseases).

T10.5
Selected Diseases Caused by Mutations in Membrane Receptors or Transporters

Syndrome	Receptor/Transporter	Comment
Long QT syndrome	Chloride channel	See Chapter 6
Cystic fibrosis	Chloride (CFTR) channel	Pulmonary disease, pancreatic insufficiency
Cystinuria	Cystine, ornithine, lysine, arginine (COLA) receptor/transporters in renal tubular epithelium and intestinal epithelium	Cystine stones
Hartnup	Neutral amino acid receptor/transporter, renal tubular epithelium and intestinal epithelium	
Renal tubular acidosis, type 1	Cation (H+) channel, distal renal tubular epithelium	Metabolic acidosis, Hypokalemia, nephrocalcinosis
Renal tubular acidosis, type 2	Bicarbonate channel, proximal renal tubular epithelium	Metabolic acidosis Hypokalemia
Blue diaper syndrome	Intestinal tryptophan receptor/transporter	Hypercalcemia
Familial hypophosphatemic rickets	Phosphate receptor transporter, renal tubular epithelium and intestinal epithelium	Rickets X-linked dominant
Iminoglycinuria	Glycine, proline, hydroxyproline receptor/transporter, renal tubular epithelium and intestinal epithelium	

- Beyond the neonatal/infantile period, an inborn error of metabolism may present with mental retardation, developmental delay, seizures, nephrolithiasis, cardiomyopathy, skeletal myopathy, or episodes in association with acute stress (eg, infection) that include vomiting, acidosis, or altered mental status.

- Hyperammonemia is a manifestation of several metabolic disorders, including urea cycle disorders, organic acidemias, fatty acid oxidation disorders (MCAD), and hepatic dysfunction (which may itself be caused by other metabolic diseases). At high concentrations, ammonia is a neurotoxin, capable of producing clinical manifestations including lethargy, vomiting, asterixis, coma, and death.

- The infant in whom a metabolic disease is suspected should be given nothing by mouth. Serum and urine samples should be obtained. In suspected mitochondrial disorders, muscle biopsy or fibroblast cultures may be needed.

- State-mandated neonatal screening tests help eliminate consideration of some metabolic disorders. Screening tests are available for phenylketonuria, hypothyroidism, galactosemia, biotinidase deficiency, cystic fibrosis, maple syrup urine disease, congenital adrenal hyperplasia, hemoglobinopathies, and others, but the extent of newborn screening programs differ from state-to-state.

Lipid Disorders

Lipids and Classification of Lipid Disorders T10.6

- The major lipids found in plasma are cholesterol, triglyceride (TG), and phospholipid.

- Lipids are insoluble in aqueous media such as plasma and therefore must be packaged into *lipoprotein* particles. In the external phospholipid layer are the various *apolipoproteins*. In the center of the lipoprotein particle are cholesterol and TG. Every lipoprotein contains cholesterol, TG, phospholipids, and apolipoproteins. However, 5 different lipoprotein classes are identified based on the various proportions of these 4 constituents and the particular apolipoproteins they possess.

   □ Chylomicrons contain mainly TG, being carried from the gut to the liver, and the apolipoproteins Apo B-48, Apo A-1, Apo C, and Apo E

169

T10.6

Classification of Lipid Disorders by Predominant Lipids

Disorder	Phenotype	Cholesterol	Triglyceride	Clinical Features
Familial lipoprotein lipase deficiency	I	↑	↑↑↑	Eruptive xanthomas, pancreatitis
Familial apo C-II deficiency	I or V	↑	↑↑↑	Pancreatitis
Familial hypercholesterolemia	IIa	↑↑↑	→↑	Tendinous xanthomas, premature atherosclerosis
Apolipoprotein E deficiency	IIb or III	↑↑↑	↑	
Familial dysbetalipoproteinemia	III	↑↑↑	↑↑↑	Eruptive xanthomas, premature atherosclerosis
Familial combined hyperlipidemia	II or IV	↑	↑	Premature atherosclerosis
Familial hypertriglyceridemia	IV	↑	↑↑↑	Eruptive xanthomas, pancreatitis

- ☐ Very-low-density lipoprotein (VLDL) contains mainly TG, being carried from the liver to the peripheral tissues, and the apolipoproteins Apo-B100, Apo C, and Apo E

- ☐ Intermediate density lipoprotein (IDL) contains mainly cholesterol and the apolipoproteins Apo-B100 and Apo E

- ☐ Low-density lipoprotein (LDL) contains mainly cholesterol and the apolipoprotein Apo-B100

- ☐ High-density lipoprotein (HDL) contains mainly cholesterol and the apolipoproteins Apo A-1, Apo C, and Apo E

- Ingested lipids are internalized by small bowel enterocytes and packaged into chylomicrons, in which they are transported to the liver. These have very low density because of a large TG component. In the liver, cholesterol and TG are packaged as VLDL and secreted into blood. In the blood, the TG undergoes progressive hydrolysis by the endothelium-based enzyme, lipoprotein lipase (LPL). Over time, enough TG is removed from VLDL to increase its density to that of IDL and, eventually, LDL. The typical LDL particle has lost most of its TG and a good bit of its apolipoproteins C and E, leaving predominantly phospholipid, cholesterol, and Apo-B100. LDL is the main vehicle for transporting cholesterol to somatic cells where LDL particles undergo endocytosis mediated by the LDL receptor and Apo-B100. The function of HDL appears to be the scavenging of cholesterol from the periphery and returning it to the liver.

- There are 2 main sources of human cholesterol: diet and endogenous production in hepatocytes. Of the lipoproteins, LDL is the richest in cholesterol.

- There are several ways of classifying lipid disorders: by the patient's lipoprotein profile (the relative proportions of VLDL, LDL, HDL, etc), by the lipid profile (relative concentration of cholesterol and TG), or by the genetic defect.

Familial Hypercholesterolemia (FH)

- The LDL receptor is capable of binding either to apoprotein B100 or apoprotein E, both of which are on the surface of lipoproteins such as LDL. When LDL is bound to the cell, a process of receptor-mediated endocytosis internalizes the contents of the LDL particle into it. The presence of cholesterol in the hepatocyte then exerts negative feedback on hepatocytic (endogenous) cholesterol production in 2 ways: it inhibits the enzyme HMG CoA reductase (3-hydroxy-3-methylglutaryl coenzyme A reductase), which catalyzes the rate-limiting step in cholesterol biosynthesis; and it enhances the activity of the enzyme ACAT (acyl-coenzyme A:cholesterol acyltransferase), which catalyzes the incorporation of cholesterol into cholesterol esters for storage. Furthermore, cholesterol suppresses the production of LDL receptors.

- FH results from a mutation in the gene encoding the LDL receptor gene (*LDLR*) found on chromosome 19. This causes (1) loss of the main mechanism by which cholesterol is removed from serum, and (2) loss of the negative feedback normally exerted through LDL on the endogenous production of cholesterol. The net effect is hypercholesterolemia (type II hyperlipidemia). Heterozygosity for the mutant allele, with an incidence of 1 in 500, results in an increase of 2 to 3 times in serum cholesterol. Homozygosity is much more severe. *LDLR* is an extremely large gene, composed of 18 exons (45 kilobases) that encode 5 domains. Many different disease-causing mutations have been described.

- A similar phenotype results from mutations in the *APO-B100* gene (familial defective Apo-B100). The incidence of familial defective Apo-B100 is roughly that of heterozygous LDL receptor defects, occurring in about 1 in 500 Caucasian Americans. The 2 defects are clinically indistinguishable, with the exception that the coronary artery disease (CAD) risk is significantly higher in LDL receptor defects.

- The diagnosis of LDL receptor defects and Apo-B100 defects is suspected in patients with tendonous xanthomas and a family history of premature CAD. The diagnosis is supported by the finding of increased plasma LDL-C with normal TG levels. Cases of familial defective apo-B100 are usually caused by a single mutation (in contrast to the multitude of mutations in LDLR causing FH), so the 2 are most easily distinguished by screening for the APO-B100 mutation.

- More rarely, familial hypercholesterolemialike phenotypes may also be produced by mutations in the *ABC* (ATP-binding cassette) genes, causing sitosterolemia, and the *ARH* gene.

- 1 of the ways the body has to compensate for this is the so-called scavenger receptor on the surface of histiocytes and monocytes. This leads to the formation of xanthomas, which are essentially nodules of lipid-laden histiocytes.

- Elevated levels of LDL cholesterol have a direct impact on the risk of CAD.

Familial Hyperchylomicronemia

- Apo-CII is a cofactor for LPL. Familial hyperchylomicronemia results from reduced or absent LPL activity or less commonly from the absence Apo CII. Apo-CII deficiency is a rare autosomal recessive disorder, with an incidence of about 1 in 1 million.

- Phenotypically, it is associated with hyperchyoironemia, and therefore increased TG (type I hyperlipidemia) syndrome similar to what is seen in LPL deficiency.

- As in other causes of hypertriglyceridemia, the features include recurrent pancreatitis. Hypertriglyceridemia alone does not appear to cause a significant increase in the risk of CAD.

Familial Hypertriglyceridemia

- Familial hypertriglyceridemia is characterized by increased plasma concentrations of VLDL (type IV hypertriglyceridemia) and therefore increased TG. The LDL cholesterol is normal, but HDL is reduced.

- Recurrent pancreatitis, obesity, and insulin resistance are common manifestations. Hypertriglyceridemia alone does not appear to cause a significant increase in CAD risk, but the low HDL may.

- The genetic defect in familial hypertriglyceridemia is unknown. Until it is, familial hypertriglyceridemia is diagnosed in persons with high triglyceride levels, normal plasma cholesterol, and hypertriglyceridemia in over half of first-degree relatives. The triglyceride abnormality does not arise until adulthood.

Elevated Plasma Lp(a)

- An elevated level of Lp(a) is a relatively common disorder that appears to be associated with an increased CAD and peripheral vascular disease risk. Lp(a) is a modified LDL particle in which Apo-B has been attached, via disulfide bonds, to Apo(a). Apo(a) is a protein that shares significant sequence homology with plasminogen. Unlike plasminogen, however, the serine proteaselike domain of apo(a) is nonfunctional; thus, it is thought that it may competitively inhibit plasminogen, thereby interfering with fibrinolysis.

- Lp(aw) levels are heavily influenced by heredity. The Apo (a) gene has multiple repeats of 1 of the plasminogenlike kringle motifs (kringle IV). The number of repeats varies from 12 to 40 in different polymorphisms of the Lp (a) gene, and the Lp (a) level correlates inversely with the number of kringle repeats. However, the Lp (a) level appears to be largely but not entirely dependent on the Lp (a) genotype, and the impact of Lp (a) genotype on Lp (a) levels seems to be affected by race. At this time, genotype-phenotype correlations are still being elucidated.

Familial Dysbetalipoproteinemia

- Dysbetalipoproteinemia (type III hyperlipidemia) is associated with accumulation in plasma of remnant lipoprotein particles (partially hydrolyzed chylomicrons and VLDL). The patients have increased cholesterol and TG levels. On lipoprotein electrophoresis, this produces a typical pattern of a broad band extending from pre-β to β; so the disease is sometimes called "broad beta disease."

- In addition to an increased CAD risk, these patients manifest tuberous xanthomas and palmar striated xanthomas.

- This disorder is the result of apolipoprotein E deficiency, caused by mutations in the *APOE* gene on 19q13.2. ApoE is the major apolipoprotein of the chylomicron, and its function is to bind to a specific receptor on the surface of hepatocytes, initiating reuptake.

- There are 3 major isoforms of human apolipoprotein E (apoE2, apoE3, apoE4), with E3 being the normal (wild) type. The E2 allele encodes an apolipoprotein that binds poorly to its receptor, leading to dysbetalipoproteinemia. However, not every person homozygous for E2/E2 manifests this or any lipid abnormality; thus, other factors are thought to be involved in developing overt disease.

Familial Combined Hyperlipidemia

- This is one of the most common inherited disorders of lipid metabolism, with an incidence of over 1 in 100. Both cholesterol and triglyceride are increased, in a pattern similar to dysbetalipoproteinemia. This is commonly accompanied by obesity, glucose intolerance, premature CAD, and hyperuricemia.

- The precise genetic basis is unknown, but it appears to be inherited as an autosomal dominant trait. The diagnosis depends on finding the abnormal lipid profile in at least 1 first-degree relative.

Lecithin Cholesterol Acyl Transferase (LCAT) Deficiency

- LCAT is the enzyme that catalyzes the conversion of cholesterol (acquired by HDL) to cholesteryl esters. LCAT deficiency is an autosomal recessive disorder characterized by extremely low levels of HDL cholesterol and severe corneal opacities producing a so-called "fish eye" appearance.

Tangier Disease

- Tangier disease is a rare autosomal dominant disorder associated with very low HDL levels and an elevated CAD risk. Foam cells accumulate in the body, leading to large orange tonsils, hepatosplenomegaly, and peripheral neuropathy.

- Tangier disease is caused by mutations of an ATP-binding cassette recorder gene (ABC1).

References

References

Amir G, Ron N. Pulmonary pathology in Gaucher's disease. *Hum Pathol* 1999; 30: 666-670.

Anderson G, Smith VV, Malone M, et al. Blood film examination for vacuolated lymphocytes in the diagnosis of metabolic disorders: retrospective experience of more than 2500 cases from a single centre. *J Clin Pathol* 2005; 58: 1305-1310.

Anikster Y, Lacbawan F, Brantly M, et al. Pulmonary dysfunction in adults with nephropathic cystinosis. *Chest* 2001; 119: 394-401.

Arad M, Maron BJ, Gorham JM, et al. Glycogen storage diseases presenting as hypertrophic cardiomyopathy. *N Engl J Med* 2005; 352: 362-372.

Barness LA. An approach to the diagnosis of metabolic diseases. *Fetal Pediatr Pathol* 2004; 23: 3-10.

Bendavid C, Kleta R, Long R, et al. FISH diagnosis of the common 57-kb deletion in CTNS causing cystinosis. *Hum Genet* 2004; 115: 510-514.

Beutler E, Beutler L, West C. Mutations in the gene encoding cytosolic beta-glucosidase in Gaucher disease. *J Lab Clin Med* 2004; 144: 65-68.

Borm B, Moller LB, Hausser I, et al. Variable clinical expression of an identical mutation in the ATP7A gene for Menkes disease/occipital horn syndrome in three affected males in a single family. *J Pediatr* 2004; 145: 119-121.

Boushey CJ, Beresford SA, Omenn GS, et al. A quantitative assessment of plasma homocysteine as a risk factor for vascular disease. *JAMA* 1995; 274: 1049-1057.

Brusilow SW. Hyperammonemic encephalopathy. *Medicine* 2002; 81: 240.

Chace DH, Kalas TA, Naylor EW. Use of tandem mass spectrometry for multianalyte screening of dried blood specimens from newborns. *Clin Chem* 2003; 49: 1797-1817.

Chinnery PF, Andrews RM, Turnbull DM, et al. Leber hereditary optic neuropathy: does heteroplasmy influence the inheritance and expression of the G11778A mitochondrial DNA mutation? *Am J Med Genet* 2001; 98: 235-243.

Chinnery PF, DiMauro S, Shanske S, et al. Risk of developing a mitochondrial DNA deletion disorder. *Lancet* 2004; 364: 592-596.

Chinnery PF, Howell N, Lightowlers RN, et al. Molecular pathology of MELAS and MERRF: the relationship between mutation load and clinical phenotypes. *Brain* 1997; 120: 1713-1721.

Chinnery PF, Johnson MA, Wardell TM, et al. The epidemiology of pathogenic mitochondrial DNA mutations. *Ann Neurol* 2000; 48: 188-193

Chinnery PF, Turnbull DM. Epidemiology and treatment of mitochondrial disorders. *Am J Med Genet* 2001; 106: 94-101.

References

Clarke R, Daly L, Robinson K. Hyperhomocysteinemia: an independent risk factor for vascular disease. *N Engl J Med* 1991; 324: 1149-1155.

Collins CS, Gould SJ. Identification of a common PEX1 mutation in Zellweger syndrome. *Hum Mutat* 1999; 14: 45-53.

Corzo D, Gibson W, Johnson K, et al. Contiguous deletion of the X-linked adrenoleukodystrophy gene (ABCD1) and DXS1357E: a novel neonatal phenotype similar to peroxisomal biogenesis disorders. *Am J Hum Genet* 2002; 70: 1520–1531.

Darin N, Oldfors A, Moslemi AR, et al. The incidence of mitochondrial encephalomyopathies in childhood: clinical features and morphological, biochemical, and DNA abnormalities. *Ann Neurol* 2001; 49: 377-383.

De Baulny HO, Benoist JF, Rigal O, et al. Methylmalonic and propionic acidaemias: management and outcome. *J Inherit Metab Dis* 2005; 28: 415-423.

Desnick RJ, Brady R, Barranger J, et al. Fabry disease, an under-recognized multisystemic disorder: expert recommendations for diagnosis, management, and enzyme replacement therapy. *Ann Intern Med* 2003; 138: 338-346.

DiDomenico P, Berry G, Bass D, et al. Noncirrhotic portal hypertension in association with juvenile nephropathic cystinosis: case presentation and review of the literature. *J Inherit Metab Dis* 2004; 27: 693-699.

Dimauro S, Davidzon G. Mitochondrial DNA and disease. *Ann Med* 2005; 37: 222-232.

DiMauro S, Schon EA. Mitochondrial DNA mutations in human disease. *Am J Med Genet* 2001; 106: 18-26.

Frosst P, Blom HJ, Milos R, et al. A candidate genetic risk factor for vascular disease: a common mutation in methylenetetrahydrofolate reductase. *Nature Genet* 1995; 10: 111-113.

Fu L, Inui K, Nishigaki T, et al. Molecular heterogeneity of Krabbe disease. *J Inherit Metab Dis* 1999; 22: 155-162.

Gahl WA, Thoene JG, Schneider JA. Cystinosis. *N Engl J Med* 2002; 347: 111-121.

Harris JC. Disorders of purine and pyrimidine metabolism. In: *Nelson Textbook of Pediatrics.* Philadelpha, Pa: WB Saunders, 2007; chap 78.

Hoffmann GF, Zschocke J. Glutaric aciduria type I: from clinical, biochemical and molecular diversity to successful therapy. *J Inherit Metab Dis* 1999; 22: 381-391.

Iizuka T, Sakai F, Kan S, et al. Slowly progressive spread of the stroke-like lesions in MELAS. *Neurology* 2003; 61: 1238-1244.

References

Kumps A, Duez P, Mardens Y. Metabolic, nutritional, iatrogenic, and artifactual sources of urinary organic acids: a comprehensive table. *Clin Chem* 2020; 48: 708-717.

Lee R, Frenkel EP. Hyperhomocysteinemia and thrombosis. *Hematol Oncol Clin North Am* 2003; 17: 85-102.

Leonard JV, Dezateux C. Screening for inherited metabolic disease in newborn infants using tandem mass spectrometry. *BMJ* 2002; 324: 4.

Leonard JV, Schapira AV. Mitochondrial respiratory chain disorders: I, mitochondrial DNA defects. *Lancet* 2000; 355: 299-304.

Leonard JV, Schapira AV. Mitochondrial respiratory chain disorders: II, neurodegenerative disorders and nuclear gene defects. *Lancet* 2000; 355: 389-394.

Li Y, Brockmann K, Turecek F, et al. Tandem mass spectrometry for the direct assay of enzymes in dried blood spots: application to newborn screening for Krabbe disease. *Clin Chem* 2004; 50: 638-640.

Longo N. Mitochondrial encephalopathy. *Neurol Clin North Am* 2003; 21: 817-831.

Marcovina SM, Koschinsky ML, Albers JJ, et al. Report of the National Heart, Lung, and Blood Institute Workshop on Lipoprotein(a) and Cardiovascular Disease: recent advances and future directions. *Clin Chem* 2003; 49: 1785-1796.

Marti R, Spinazzola A, Tadesse S, et al. Definitive diagnosis of mitochondrial neurogastrointestinal encephalomyopathy by biochemical assays. *Clin Chem* 2004; 50: 120-124.

Meikle PJ, Hopwood JJ, Clague AE, et al. Prevalence of lysosomal storage disorders. *JAMA* 1999; 281: 249-254.

Meschia JF, Brott TG, Brown RD Jr. Genetics of cerebrovascular disorders. *Mayo Clin Proc* 2005; 80: 122-132.

Mignot C, Gelot A, Bessieres B, et al. Perinatal-lethal Gaucher disease. *Am J Med Genet* 2003; 120: 338-344.

Moat SJ, Ashfield-Watt PAL, Powers HJ, et al. Effect of riboflavin status on the homocysteine-lowering effect of folate in relation to the MTHFR (C677T) genotype. *Clin Chem* 2003; 49: 295-302.

Moser HW. Genotype-phenotype correlations in disorders of peroxisome biogenesis. *Mol Genet Metab* 1999; 68: 316-327.

Munnich A, Rustin P. Clinical spectrum and diagnosis of mitochondrial disorders. *Am J Med Genet* 2001; 106: 4-17.

Neudorfer O, Pastores GM, Zeng BJ, et al. Late-onset Tay-Sachs disease: phenotypic characterization and genotypic correlations in 21 affected patients. *Genet Med* 2005; 7: 119-123.

Phornphutkul C, Introne WJ, Perry MB, et al. Natural history of alkaptonuria. *N Engl J Med* 2002; 347: 2111-2121.

References

Pitkanen ST, Salo MK, Heikinheimo M. Hereditary tyrosinemia type I: from basic to progress in treatment. *Ann Med* 2000; 32: 530.

Refsum H, Smith AD, Ueland PM, et al. Facts and recommendations about total homocysteine determinations: an expert opinion. *Clin Chem* 2004; 50: 3-32.

Rezvani I. An approach to inborn errors of metabolism. In: *Nelson Textbook of Pediatrics*. Philadelphia, Pa: WB Saunders, 2007; chap 73.

Rowe PC, Newman SL, Brusilow SW. Natural history of symptomatic partial ornithine transcarbamylase deficiency. *N Engl J Med* 1986; 314: 541-547.

Sachdev B, Takenaka T, Teraguchi H, et al. Prevalence of Anderson-Fabry disease in male patients with late onset hypertrophic cardiomyopathy. *Circulation* 2002; 105: 1407-1411.

Schultz RE, Salo MK. Under recognition of late onset ornithine transcarbamylase deficiency. *Arch Dis Child* 2000; 82: 390-391.

Steinberg S, Chen L, Wei L, et al. The PEX gene screen: molecular diagnosis of peroxisome biogenesis disorders in the Zellweger syndrome spectrum. *Mol Genet Metab* 2004;83: 252-263.

Steiner RD, Cederbaum SD. Laboratory elevation of urea cycle disorders. *J Pediatr* 2001; 138: S21.

Summar M. Current strategies for the management of neonatal urea disorders. *J Pediatr* 2001; 138: S30.

Tatsumi N, Inui K, Sakai N, et al. Molecular defects in Krabbe disease. *Hum Mol Genet* 1995; 4: 1865-1868.

Thorburn DR, Dahl HH. Mitochondrial disorders: genetics, counseling, prenatal diagnosis and reproductive options. *Am J Med Genet* 2001; 106: 102-114.

Vlay SC, Hartman AR, Culliford AT. Alkaptonuria and aortic stenosis. *Ann Intern Med* 1986; 104: 446.

Walter C, Gootjes J, Mooijer PA, et al. Disorders of peroxisome biogenesis due to mutations in PEX1: phenotypes and PEX1 protein levels. *Am J Hum Genet* 2001; 69: 35-48.

Walter JH. Inborn errors of metabolism and pregnancy. *J Inherit Metab Dis* 2000; 23: 229-236.

Wilcken B, Bamforth F, Li Z, Zhu H, et al. Geographical and ethnic variation of the 677C-T allele of 5,10 methylenetetrahydrofolate reductase (MTHFR): findings from over 7000 newborns from 16 areas world wide. *J Med Genet* 2003; 40: 619-625.

Wilcken B, Wiley V, Hammond J, Carpenter K. Screening newborns for inborn errors of metabolism by tandem mass spectrometry. *N Engl J Med* 2003; 348: 2304-2312.

Willinger M, James LS, Catz C. Defining the sudden infant death syndrome (SIDS): deliberations of an expert panel convened by the National Institute of Child Health and Human Development. *Pediatr Pathol* 1991; 11: 677.

Chapter 11

Neurolomuscular Diseases

Central Neurodegenerative Diseases

Alzheimer Disease

- Alzheimer disease **T11.1** is by far the most common cause of dementia in the United States, with an incidence of 5% to 10% in persons older than 70 years and 15% to 20% in persons older than 85 years. About 25% of cases are familial, some with early-onset and others with usual (late) onset.

- About 5% of all cases of Alzheimer disease have an early onset (<60 years), and about half of these are familial or so-called *early-onset familial Alzheimer disease* (EOFAD). 1 of the consistent findings in Alzheimer disease is accumulation of a type of amyloid (Aβ amyloid), which is derived from amyloid precursor protein (APP), the gene for which (*APP*) is found on chromosome 21. Interestingly, histopathologic features of Alzheimer disease are universal in those with trisomy 21 by the age of 40 years, and the first mutation to be identified in familial Alzheimer disease was in the *APP* gene. Subsequently, EOFAD was found in association with mutations in 2 additional genes—*PSEN1* and *PSEN2*. *PSEN1* is found at 14q24 and encodes presenilin 1. *PSEN2* is on 1q and encodes presenilin 2. The *APP* gene is located on 21q21.

- There is an association of usual (late) onset Alzheimer disease with the E4 allele at the *APOE* gene locus at 19q13.2; however, the correlation is not 100%.

T11.1
Central Neurodegenerative Diseases

Condition	Clinical Features	Morphologic Features	Genetic Basis
Alzheimer disease	Memory loss Slowly progressive	Global atrophy, Neurofibrillary tangles (tau protein) in neurons Amyloid plaques in white matter Granulovacuolar degeneration in hippocampus Hirano bodies Often cerebral amyloid angiopathy	Yes (familial Alzheimer disease) *APP* on 21 *Apo E* on 19 *Presenilin-1* on 14 *Presenilin-2* on 1
Frontotemporal dementia (Pick disease)	Personality change, disinhibition Slowly progressive	Frontal lobe atrophy	Yes, rare, see text
Lewy body disease/Parkinson disease	Motor instability Slowly progressive, fluctuating course	Loss of pigmentation in substantia nigra and locus ceruleus. Lewy bodies in substantia nigra and/or cerebral cortex	Yes, rare, see text
Huntington disease	Memory loss, psychotic symptoms	Atrophy of caudate nucleus. Neuronal loss and astrogliosis in basal ganglia	Yes, expanded trinucleotide repeat on 4p
Progressive supranuclear palsy	Akinesia and rigidity Paralysis of upward gaze Slowly progressive	Neurofibrillary tangles (tau protein), tufted astrocytes	Unknown (?H1 haplotype of *tau* gene)
Vascular dementia: Multi-infarct dementia (MID), CADASIL, and Binswanger disease	Stepwise progression	Multiple lacunes (MID) Eosinophilic vascular depositis (CADASIL) Vascular mineralization (Binswanger disease)	*NOTCH3* gene on 19p (CADASIL)
Normal-pressure hydrocephalus (NPH)	Memory loss, urinary incontinence, gait instability Slowly progressive	Massive ventricular enlargement	Unknown
Prion disease (Creutzfeldt-Jakob disease and variants)	Cerebellar ataxia	Spongiform change, neuronal loss	Yes, rare, *PRNP* (PrP) gene mutation

- About 1% of all cases of Alzheimer disease are associated with Down syndrome. Essentially everybody with trisomy 21 (Down syndrome) develops Alzheimer disease if they live beyond the age of 40 years. This is believed to be because of overexpression of the APP gene on chromosome 21.

Familial Pick Disease (Frontotemporal Dementia with Parkinsonism, Disinhibition-Dementia-Parkinsonism-Amyotrophy Complex (DDPAC), Wilhelmsen-Lynch Disease)

- Pick disease disproportionately involves the frontal cortex; thus disinhibition and loss of initiative are prominent features. Subcortical involvement is also present, leading to Parkinson-like rigidity and bradykinesia. The onset of symptoms is often in the mid 40s, and the disease progresses to dementia and death, frequently within 10 years.

- Computed tomography (CT) and magnetic resonance imaging (MRI) reveal cortical atrophy, most pronounced in the anterior frontal and temporal lobes.

- The characteristic anatomic finding is atrophy that is quite noticeably limited to the frontotemporal region. Histologically, argyrophilic intraneuronal inclusions (Pick bodies) and achromatic neurons (Pick cells) are classically found in these regions. Cases having similar clinical findings and macroscopic anatomy, some with and some without these histologic findings, have been classified as frontotemporal dementia (FTD).

- The gene implicated is *MAPT*, on 17q, which encodes the microtubule-associated protein tau. The tau protein is a member of the microtubule-associated protein (MAP) family that is found mainly in neurons. Disease-associated mutations appear to exert their effects by causing altered binding of the tau protein to the microtubule. Pick disease (or FTD) is not the only so-called tauopathy; other conditions associated with tau abnormalities include Alzheimer disease, progressive supranuclear palsy, amyotrophic lateral sclerosis-Parkinsonism-dementia complex of Guam, and dementia pugilistica. Both targeted mutation analysis and direct sequence analysis are clinically available for the detection of mutations.

Parkinson Disease and Lewy Body Disease

- Parkinson disease is the most common cause of Parkinsonism, a movement disorder characterized by bradykinesia, rigidity, and resting tremor. Dementia develops in a significant proportion of cases. Lewy body disease (or dementia with Lewy bodies), is a term that denotes clinical dementia in conjunction with the histopathologic finding of Lewy bodies; thus Lewy body disease encompasses Lewy body variant of Alzheimer disease, dementia associated with Parkinson disease, and isolated dementia with Lewy bodies. There is a clinical continuum between these entities, with most cases exhibiting variable degrees of characteristic clinical features: progressive and fluctuating cognitive impairment, Parkinsonism, delusions, and visual hallucinations.

- The Lewy body is the unifying histopathologic feature of this group of diseases. The distribution of Lewy bodies correlates reasonably well with the clinical manifestations; thus Lewy bodies in the neocortex correlate with dementia and neuropsychiatric manifestations, and Lewy bodies in the subcortical white matter correlate with the movement disorder.

- Rare cases of Lewy body disease are familial, but no responsible gene has yet been identified. Some cases of Parkinson disease are also familial, and several genetic anomalies have been identified in these families, including mutations in the *SCNA* (PARK1), *PARK2*, *PARK3*, *UCHL1* (PARK5), *PINK1* (PARK6), *DJ-1* (PARK7), and *LRRK2* (PARK8) genes. Currently, molecular testing is available for only some of these.

Huntington Disease (Huntington Chorea)

- Huntington disease is an autosomal dominant trinucleotide repeat disorder that causes neurologic impairment in the form of a choreiform movement disorder with eventual dementia and/or psychosis. As is usual for trinucleotide repeat disorders, anticipation is a feature (earlier presentation and/or more severe disease in successive generations). Most patients present with a movement disorder; however about one fourth present with psychiatric disturbances. Over time, a debilitating chorea develops, along with dysarthria and dysphagia.

- Imaging (CT and MRI) shows a highly characteristic atrophy of the caudate and putamen. Median survival is about 15 years after onset.

- The *HD* (*IT15*) gene, found at 4p16, is the site of the disease-causing CAG trinucleotide repeat. In normal persons, there are less than 26 GAG repeats **T11.2**, whereas in affected individuals there are more than 36. Between 26 and 36 is considered a premutation, capable of having an affected offspring. Targeted mutation analysis is available for detecting these expansions. In general, the greater the number of CAG repeats, the earlier the onset. More than 60 repeats usually results in juvenile-onset disease.

- There appears to be a strong correlation between paternal inheritance and early disease onset. Nearly 90% of cases with juvenile onset have both numerous CAG repeats and paternal inheritance.

Cerebral Autosomal Dominant Arteriopathy with Subcortical Infarcts and Leukoencephalopathy (CADASIL)

- CADASIL is an autosomal dominant condition of the cortical and subcortical white matter that presents with migraines, usually with aura, in almost half of cases. Transient ischemic attacks and strokelike events occur in nearly all cases, with a mean age at onset of 45 years. Progressive deterioration of cognitive function follows, with dementia by age 60 years. The dementia is subcortical in nature, characterized by disturbances of memory, motivation, and mentation. MRI reveals multiple hyperintense lesions in the periventricular white matter (particularly in the frontal lobes), basal ganglia, and brain stem. Highly characteristic are subcortical lacunar lesions, appearing as grouped lacunar lesions arranged linearly at the gray-white interface.

T11.2
Effect of Repeat Expansion Size on Clinical Expression of Huntington Disease

Size (Number of Repeats)	Clinical
<26	Normal
26-36	Premutation
37-55	Adult-onset disease
>60	Juvenile-onset disease

- Within the white matter and basal ganglia are found abnormal blood vessels having eosinophilic granular deposits in the media. Multiple lacunar infarcts, mainly in the white matter, are found in association. In addition, skin biopsy can prove diagnostic, showing similar deposits in vascular media.

- More than 90% of individuals with CADASIL have mutations in the *NOTCH3* gene, found at 19p13.2-p13.1. Direct sequence analysis of the NOTCH3 gene is clinically available.

Pantothenate Kinase-Associated Neurodegeneration (formerly known as Hallervorden-Spatz Syndrome)

- A neurodegenerative disease in which there is iron accumulation in the basal ganglia, leading to choreoathetosis, dystonia, rigidity, and pigmentary retinopathy. Systemic iron metabolism is normal.

- Onset is usually in childhood, and MRI shows a classic "eye of the tiger" sign, in which the globus pallidus has a central region of hyperintensity and a rim of hypointensity. The sign is apparently quite sensitive and specific.

- Histopathologically, there is a rust-brown discoloration in the globus pallidus and substantia nigra, because of accumulated iron. Microscopically, areas of iron accumulation display axonal spheroid bodies.

- The responsible gene is *PANK2*, found at 20p13, which encodes pantothenate kinase 2. Direct sequence analysis is capable of detecting more than 98% of disease-causing mutations.

- Drs Hallervorden and Spatz, in honor of whom this condition was eponymously named, based the seminal description of this and other neuropathologic conditions on autopsies performed on murdered mentally ill patients in Germany during world war II. The policy of extermination was one in which these physicians were later deemed at least complicit. The descriptive term of *pantothenate kinase-associated neurodegeneration* has been widely adopted in rebuke of this policy.

McLeod Syndrome (Neuroacanthocytosis)

- McLeod syndrome is an X-linked recessive syndrome in which there is peripheral blood acanthocytosis, reduced expression of Kell antigens (McLeod phenotype), and neurologic dysfunction particularly of the basal ganglia.

- The McLeod blood group phenotype is caused by absence of erythrocyte expression of the Kx antigen and reduced expression of Kell antigens.

- Red blood cell acanthocytosis and a mild hemolysis are found in virtually all affected males.

- There is sometimes a peripheral or cardiac myopathy, but nearly all affected males have an elevated serum creatine phosphokinase (CPK).

- The disease is caused by mutations in the *XK* gene, found at Xp21.

- Other disorders with combined neurologic disease and acanthocytosis exist, including abetalipoproteinemia, some examples of Huntington disease, choreoacanthocytosis, some cases of pantothenate kinase-associated neurodegeneration, and some cases of Wilson disease.

Copper Disorders (Menkes Disease, Occipital Horn Syndrome)

- These diseases are caused by a defect in the copper-transporting ATPase gene, *ATP7A*, on Xq12-q13, resulting in imbalances in copper metabolism, both accumulation of copper in tissues and under-availability of copper for copper-dependent enzymes such as dopamine beta hydroxylase (DBH) and lysyl oxidase.

- Menkes disease presents as cognitive neurologic impairment and characteristic hair changes (lightly colored, short, coarse, twisted, and sparse) in an infant. When examined microscopically, the hair shaft displays pili torti (180° twists), trichoclasis (transverse breaks), and trichoptilosis (longitudinal splits). Seizures ensue, and death usually occurs by 3 years of age.

- Occipital horn syndrome presents with calcifications at the sites of attachment of the trapezius and sternocleidomastoid muscles to the occipital bone (occipital horns), along with laxity of skin and joints, bladder diverticula, inguinal hernias, vascular tortuosity, and dysautonomia.

- A multiplex polymerase chain reaction (PCR) assay is available to detect deletions in *ATP7A*. Direct sequence analysis is also available for detecting point mutations.

Familial Prion Disease (Familial Spongiform Encephalitis, Familial Creutzfeldt-Jakob Disease [CJD], Gerstmann-Sträussler-Scheinker Disease, Fatal Familial Insomnia)

- Familial prion disease is connected with a spectrum of disease phenotypes (Creutzfeldt-Jakob type, Gerstmann-Sträussler-Scheinker type, fatal familial insomnia), all attributed to defects in a single gene, *PRNP*. Common features include dementia, myoclonus, ataxia, dysarthria, autosomal dominant inheritance, and onset adulthood.

- The familial CJD phenotype usually manifests between the age of 30 and 50 years, with dementia, ataxia, and myoclonus. Death occurs within a few months to a few years. The brain biopsy shows typical spongiform change.

- The familial Gerstmann-Sträussler-Scheinker syndrome phenotype also presents between 30 and 50 years, initially with cerebellar dysfunction. Dementia occurs at a later stage, and the course is slower, with death in 7 to 10 years. Amyloid plaques are more common than spongiform change.

- Fatal familial insomnia presents in adulthood with the insidious onset of insomnia. Over time, autonomic disturbances and ataxia develop, and dementia arises late in the course of disease. Histopathologically, one finds thalamic neuronal loss and gliosis.

- Kuru, the original prion disease, was found in those who acquired prions through the practice of cannibalism in New Guinea. Sporadic (acquired) prion diseases are far more common than the familial types, with features that are fairly similar. The prion protein closely recapitulates the sequence of the *PRNP* gene product. Usually, however, the course of acquired CJD is much faster than that of familial CJD.

- Direct sequence analysis is clinically available for detecting mutations in the *PRNP* gene, found on 20p, that encodes major prion protein (PrP).

Peripheral Neuropathy

Broadly speaking, the structures involved in these conditions include any combination of lower motor nerves, sensory nerves, and autonomic nerves. The basic defect may be in the neuron, axon, or synapse. With regard to sensory and motor nerves, inherited peripheral neuropathies typically manifest as symmetric, predominantly distal, deficits.

Inherited peripheral neuropathies **T11.3** are numerous, and they are often classified according to the involved systems; thus those with predominantly sensory and motor deficits are considered hereditary motor and sensory neuropathies (HMSN), and those with mainly sensory and autonomic deficits are hereditary sensory and autonomic neuropathies (HSAN). Those whose effects are restricted to the lower motor neuron are the spinomuscular atrophies (SMA). The HMSNs are a group of disorders characterized by progressive muscular atrophy (initially affecting the feet, legs, and hands), with motor defects typically much more severe than sensory deficits, and onset in infancy or childhood. There are both demyelinating and axonal forms. The HSANs are a group of disorders that often result in acral injury because of marked sensory deficits (which are out of proportion to motor deficits, if any).

Charcot-Marie-Tooth (CMT) Disease

- CMT is an autosomal dominant group of inherited peripheral neuropathies, collectively termed HMSN. Type 1 CMT is most common, representing about 50% of cases, and type 2 accounts for about 30%. The neuropathy most often affects legs, hands, and feet, presenting with weakness, atrophy, and anesthesia.

T11.3
Neuropathies

	Syndrome	Gene (Locus)	Comment
HMSNs	CMT1a	PMP22 (17p)	Gene duplication
	HNPP	PMP22 (17p)	Gene deletion
	CMT1b, 1c, 1d	MPZ (1q), LITAF (16p), EGR2 (10q)	
	CMT2a	KIF1B (1p)	
	CMT2b, 2c, 2d	RAB7 (3q), 12q, GARS (7p)	
	CMT4a	GDAP1 (8q)	
	CMTX	GJB1(Xq)	
	HMN I - HMN VII	Unknown	
HSANs	HSAN I and HSAN III (Riley-Day)	SPTLC1 (9q) and IKBKAP (9q)	
Motor neuron disease	Amyotropic lateral sclerosis (ALS) type 1	SOD1 (21q)	Upper motor neuron + Lower motor neuron
	Amyotropic lateral sclerosis (ALS) type 3	Unknown (18q)	Upper motor neuron + Lower motor neuron
	SMA types I-III	SMN1 (5q)	Lower motor neuron
	Spinobulbar muscular atrophy	AR (Xq)	XLR

HMSN = hereditary motor and sensory neuropathies; HSAN = hereditary sensory and autonomic neuropathies; SMA = spinomuscular atrophy; XLR = X-linked recessive.

11: Neurolomuscular Diseases

Peripheral Neuropathy>Charcot-Marie-Tooth Disease; Familial Amyloidosis; Giant Axonal Neuropathy;
Hereditary Neuropathy with Liability to Pressure Palsies

- Type 1 CMT is associated with peripheral nerve demyelination. Biopsy of the nerve shows prominent onion bulb formation, and muscle biopsy findings are typical of denervation atrophy (angular atrophic fibers). The most common genetic basis for type 1 CMT is duplication of a 1.5-Mb region of DNA on 17p12 containing the *PMP22* gene. Incidentally, a 1.5-Mb deletion at this site causes hereditary neuropathy with pressure palsies (HNPP).

- Type 2 CMT is associated with axonal degeneration rather than demyelination. It is in many ways similar to CMT1, with distal muscle weakness, muscle atrophy, and impaired sensation; however, it tends to be less severe. Nerve biopsy shows axonal sprouting and atrophic axons. There are many genes which, when mutated, can give rise to CMT2. This makes genetic testing problematic. Sequence analyses are available for several of these, but a significant number of mutations are not detected.

Familial Amyloidosis (Transthyretin Amyloidosis, Familial Cardiac Amyloidosis, Familial Amyloid Polyneuropathy)

- Familial amyloidosis usually presents in the third or fourth decade. The diagnosis is suspected when there is a combination of peripheral neuropathy (dysautonomic and sensorimotor), cardiomyopathy, and/or a cardiac conduction block. Nephropathy, leptomeningeal amyloidosis, and vitreous opacities may also be seen. Some individuals have solely cardiac or leptomeningeal involvement, without any other features.

- The isolated cardiac variety is what has in the past been referred to as *senile cardiac amyloidosis*, and it has been associated with specific *TTR* gene mutations (D18N and others).

- Likewise, isolated leptomeningeal amyloidosis has been called *cerebral amyloid angiopathy*, and it has been linked to specific *TTR* mutations (L12P and others).

- In the past, tissue biopsy or immunometric techniques were used to detect transthyretin amyloid. Molecular assays are now available for mutations in the *TTR* gene, capable of detecting nearly 100% of disease-causing alleles. The *TTR* gene is located on 18q and encodes transthyretin. Targeted mutation analysis for the most common V30M mutation, can detect about 30% to 45% of affected persons. Direct sequence analysis can detect nearly 100%.

- Transthyretin amyloidosis displays autosomal dominant inheritance. Pockets of high prevalence exist in Portugal, Sweden, Japan, and parts of Africa. The frequency of TTR amyloidosis is about 1 in 500 in northern Portugal. In the United States, it is about 1 in 100,000 among Caucasians, but estimated to be much higher in African Americans.

Giant Axonal Neuropathy (GAN)

- GAN is an autosomal recessive disorder characterized by the histopathologic finding of axons enlarged by the presence of accumulated neurofilaments (an intermediate filament). Onion bulb formation (a sign of recurring demyelination-remyelination) is seen as well. Microscopic examination of hair shafts shows variation in shaft diameter and twisting (pili torti), similar to that seen in Menkes disease.

- The disease actually involves both the peripheral and central nervous system, presenting initially with peripheral motor and sensory neuropathy and progressing to ataxia and dementia.

- GAN is caused by mutations in the *GAN* gene, on 16q, that encodes gigaxonin. At this time, molecular testing is not clinically available.

Hereditary Neuropathy with Liability to Pressure Palsies (HNPP, Tomaculous Neuropathy)

- A tendency to develop pressure-related mononeuropathies is characteristic of this disorder. The onset is typically in the second to third decade, with abrupt sensory and motor deficits referable to a single peripheral nerve. The peroneal nerve, as it passes through the tarsal tunnel, is the most common site of involvement. This presents with sensory phenomena and foot drop. The median nerve may undergo compression, passing through the carpal tunnel (carpal tunnel syndrome), leading to numbness and tingling over the thumb and second digit, with thenar weakness. The radial nerve can be compressed at the elbow.

- A microdeletion is the cause of this syndrome. The affected gene locus, 17p11.2, is in fact the location of the *PMP22* gene (CMT types 1 and 4).

11: Neurolomuscular Diseases

Peripheral Neuropathy>Familial Dysautonomia; Dopamine β-Hydroxylase Deficiency; Spinomuscular Atrophy;
Amyotropic Lateral Sclerosis | Diseases of Skeletal Muscle>Dystrophin Muscular Dystrophies

Familial Dysautonomia (Riley-Day Syndrome, HSAN Type III)

- Familial dysautonomia displays autosomal recessive inheritance, is seen almost exclusively in Ashkenazi Jews, and manifests as autonomic, motor, and sensory deficits. The sensory findings include decreased pain sensation (tending to spare the hands and feet), abnormal temperature sensation, and decreased deep tendon reflexes. Autonomic dysfunction takes the form of hemodynamic instability, abnormal gastrointestinal motility, and insensitivity to hypercapnea. So-called autonomic crises can occur, manifesting as profuse sweating, hypertension, vomiting, drooling, and cutis marmorata. Some motor dysfunction (hypotonia) is also common.

- Histopathologic findings include a reduction in the size of dorsal root ganglia, and decreased numbers of neurons in sympathetic ganglia and parasympathetic ganglia.

- Molecular testing of the responsible *IKBKAP* gene, on 9q31, is clinically available. 2 mutations in this gene account for more than 99% of cases.

Dopamine β-Hydroxylase (DBH) Deficiency

- DBH catalyzes the conversion of dopamine to norepinephrine (noradrenaline). The enzyme's deficiency leads to absence of noradrenergic sympathetic outflow.

- While neonates with this disorder may be symptomatic (hypotension, hypothermia, hypoglycemia), and children have poor exercise tolerance, the diagnosis is usually not made until adulthood. Adults may present with sycope (resulting from orthostatic hypotension), reduced exercise tolerance, ptosis, and nasal congestion.

- Biochemical testing discloses low plasma norepinephrine, low plasma epinephrine, and markedly elevated plasma dopamine. Molecular testing of the *DBH* gene on 9q34 is not clinically available at this time.

Spinomuscular Atrophy (SMA)

- SMA is a disease of the lower motor neuron, located in the anterior horn of the spinal cord. It displays autosomal recessive inheritance. There are 3 clinicopathologic types.

- SMA type I (Werdnig-Hoffmann disease) is the most severe form of SMA. Affected infants are hypotonic, and the disease is fatal within 1 to 2 years.

- SMA type II has intermediate severity, with onset in early childhood or infancy and development of some gross motor skills such as sitting up. Still, death in childhood is the rule.

- SMA type III (Kugelberg-Welander disease) is the least severe form of SMA. It presents in childhood, but affected children are able to ambulate.

- All types of SMA are caused by mutations in the *SMN1* (survival motor neuron 1) gene. There are 2 SMN loci on each chromosome 5q—*SMN1* and *SMN2*. These differ in just a few nucleotides, such that *SMN2* is a less productive gene than *SMN1*. Most patients with SMA are homozygous for deletional mutations in *SMN1*.

- The molecular diagnosis of SMA is based on examination of exon 7. Exon 7 is deleted in nearly all patients with SMA, and exon 7 is the site of nucleotide differences between *SMN1* and *SMN2*; thus, the status of all 4 SMN loci can be simultaneously assessed with analysis of exon 7. Most patients with SMA, regardless of type, have homozygous absence of *SMN1* exon 7.

Amyotropic Lateral Sclerosis (ALS)

- ALS affects the upper and lower motor neurons, affecting about 1 in 20,000 people with onset at a mean age of 60 years. It can be difficult to distinguish ALS from SMA type III. However, ALS tends to have a later onset, and no definitive inherited basis has been established for most cases.

- About 10% of ALS cases, however, appear to be caused by a dominantly inherited trait. Most familial ALS cases are linked to an unknown locus on chromosome 18q; other cases have been associated with mutations in *SOD1* on chromosome 21.

Diseases of Skeletal Muscle T11.4

Dystrophin Muscular Dystrophies (Duchenne Muscular Dystrophy, Becker Muscular Dystrophy)

- Duchenne (DMD) and Becker (BMD) muscular dystrophy are X-linked recessive diseases that present in childhood with progressive skeletal muscle weakness. With sufficient longevity, both conditions eventually develop cardiomyopathy. Both DMD and BMD are caused by mutations in the *DMD* gene

Diseases of Skeletal Muscle>Dystrophin Muscular Dystrophies

T11.4
Muscular Dystrophies

Disease	Inheritance	Distribution	Gene (Locus)
Duchenne/Becker	X-linked recessive	Generalized	Dystrophin (Xp)
Myotonic	Autosomal dominant	Head, face, and neck, heart, smooth muscle	(19q)
Limb-girdle	Autosomal recessive	Pelvis, proximal lower extremities, scapulae, proximal upper extremity	Multiple (see below)
Facioscapulohumeral	Autosomal dominant	Shoulder girdle, face	4q
Emery-Dreifuss	X-linked recessive	Scapulae, proximal upper extremity	Xq

that is located at Xp21.2 and encodes the protein dystrophin. The Duchenne and Becker forms differ mainly in severity, with Becker having later onset and milder manifestations.

- The overall incidence of DMD is about 1 in 4000 live births. It is the most common form of inherited muscular dystrophy, followed by myotonic muscular dystrophy (MMD), facioscapulohumeral muscular dystrophy, and limb-girdle muscular dystrophies.

- DMD usually presents in early childhood (before 5 years of age) with delays in the development of gross motor skills such as sitting up and standing. Walking is delayed, often beyond 18 months, and comes with a characteristic waddling gait. Lumbar lordosis and calf enlargement are common physical findings. Weakness is symmetrical and proximal (typical of most primary myopathies), and it progresses to a state of wheelchair dependence by age 12 years and death by age 30 years. In those who survive beyond age 20 years, a dilated (congestive) cardiomyopathy invariably arises.

- In BMD affected individuals maintain ambulation well into their 20s, but cardiomyopathy becomes a major problem, causing death by the age of 50 years. Like DMD, the weakness is symmetrical and proximal. Often there is calf hypertrophy and muscle cramping with activity.

- Even female carriers of a DMD mutation are at increased risk for the DMD-related cardiomyopathy, and some affected males manifest only cardiomyopathy.

- All persons with a *DMD* mutation have elevated serum CPK. Males with DMD have CPK levels more than 10 times normal, males with BMD have CPK levels about 5 to 10 times normal, and smaller elevations are present in female carriers.

- Skeletal muscle biopsy findings are somewhat characteristic, showing variable fiber size and scattered hyper-eosinophilic small rounded fibers. Immunohistochemical staining (or Western blot) for dystrophin is negative. A mosaic pattern of staining is described in female carriers.

- The DMD gene is very large, composed of more than 2000 kilobases (kb) and 79 exons. It is expressed in skeletal muscle, myocardium, smooth muscle, and the brain. When skeletal muscle is stained by immunohistochemistry, dystrophin is found coating the inner aspect of the cell membrane; in DMD, dystrophin staining is absent. Most (about 65%) disease-causing mutations are large deletions that occur preferentially in a limited number of places in the gene. In particular, a 200-kB region spanning exon 45 (and the flanking introns 44 and 45) is the major site of DMD gene deletions. Another major group of deletions is found at the 5′ end. It is thought that mutations that alter the reading frame, leading to protein truncation, result in the more severe DMD phenotype, whereas those that do not alter the reading frame result in the BMD phenotype. About 10% of cases are the result of partial gene duplications. These are distributed in the same regions in which deletions are found. The remaining cases appear to be the result of randomly distributed point mutations.

- A small group of patients with DMD gene mutations manifest only dilated cardiomyopathy (X-linked dilated cardiomyopathy). It appears that this syndrome is caused by mutations in the dystrophin gene promoter region and that the isolated heart involvement results from so-called phenotypic rescue mediated by alternate promoters in skeletal muscle.

- To detect the majority of cases that are caused by deletions or duplications, various targeted Southern blot and multiplex PCR assays have been developed. In the Southern blot assay, endonuclease-digested patient DNA is subjected to electrophoresis, blotted, and then hybridized with several radiolabeled cDNA probes. Deletions (decreased hybridization) and duplications (increased hybridization) can thus be detected. The strength of hybridization signals are compared with those of a simultaneous normal male control. In the multiplex PCR assay, the major deletion/duplication sites are amplified using multiple primers. Amplicons are subjected to electrophoresis stained with ethidium bromide. A deletion will result in the absence of an expected amplicon band. While easier and faster than Southern blot and capable of detecting nearly 100% of deletions, the PCR assay is insensitive to the duplications. Both the multiplex PCR and Southern blot techniques are insensitive to point mutations. Direct sequence analysis would be required to detect the roughly 30% of cases that are caused by point mutations.

Myotonic Muscular Dystrophy (MMD; Steinert Disease)

- MMD is an autosomal dominant disease based on a trinucleotide repeat mechanism. As is common in trinucleotide repeat disorders, MMD displays anticipation (progressive severity with successive generations). Myotonic dystrophy is among the most common muscular dystrophies (just behind dystrophin muscular dystrophies) and is the most common muscular dystrophy presenting in adults. Its overall incidence is about 1 to 2 per 10,000. It can present in all age groups but usually comes to clinical attention in a young adult.

- In addition to skeletal muscle, it affects smooth muscle (bowel dysmotility), the cardiac conduction system, endocrine system, and central nervous system as well as having effects on the eyes (cataracts). In fact, cataracts may be the only manifestation in minimally affected patients, and those with the full syndrome often have ancestors with early-onset cataracts. The other unusual feature is that skeletal muscle, while weak, is persistently contracted (myotonic).

- The serum CPK is mildly elevated.

- Muscle biopsy findings are nonspecific but markedly abnormal, with rows of internalized nuclei, ring fibers, and type I fiber atrophy.

- The genetic causes of the MMD include a trinucleotide (CTG) expansion at the DMPK locus (19q) or a trinucleotide expansion in the CNBP locus (3q). The DMPK expansion causes MMD type 1 (DM1), and the CNBP expansion causes type 2 (DM2). Molecular testing in the form of targeted mutation analysis is clinically available to determine the number of repeats. Unaffected persons have up to 35 CTG repeats, and premutation alleles have up to 49. Disease-associated alleles have more than 50 repeats. Generally, the greater the number of repeats, the more severe the disease; for example, those with congenital-onset disease often have more than 2000 repeats.

Limb-Girdle Muscular Dystrophies (LGMD)

- LGMD refers to a large and heterogeneous group of muscular dystrophies that lack features of other distinctive forms of muscular dystrophy. The LGMDs show all the usual features of a myopathic process: (1) weakness that is symmetrical and proximal, (2) elevated serum CPK, and (3) a muscle biopsy showing myopathic changes (combined degeneration and regeneration). Cardiomyopathy is present in some cases.

- While the onset of symptoms may be in early childhood, it is more commonly in late childhood or early adulthood.

Diseases of Skeletal Muscle>Limb-Girdle Muscular Dystrophies; Facioscapulohumeral Muscular Dystrophy;
Inclusion Body Myositis

- In general, after dystrophin-related disease has been excluded, usually by means of genotyping studies, LGMD should be considered. Immunohistochemical staining of muscle biopsies can be useful in many of the LGMDs (sarcoglycanopathy, calpainopathy, and dysferlinopathy), but screening for genetic defects is sometimes required for definitive diagnosis.

Facioscapulohumeral Muscular Dystrophy (FSHD)

- Symptoms typically arise in late childhood or adolescence and consist of facial and scapular muscle weakness. This gives rise to a distinctive appearance, with gaping mouth, wide-open eyes, sloping shoulders, and scapular winging. The combination of winged scapulae and a normally developed deltoid muscle gives rise to a characteristic "double hump" when the arms are abducted.

- In addition to these features, patients often have cardiac conduction defects, retinal changes, and sensorineural hearing loss.

- FSHD shows an autosomal dominant pattern of inheritance. The genetic defect is located at 4q35,

in a region that normally contains a large number of repeats of a single DNA sequence (called D4Z4). Disease is associated with fewer than 11 D4Z4 repeats. Southern blot assays are capable of determining the size of this repeat region. The exact molecular effect of this anomaly is unknown.

Inclusion Body Myositis (IBM)

- IBM is a primary myopathic process that presents with distal muscle weakness. Other so-called distal myopathies include MMD. Many cases display autosomal recessive inheritance, and others occur as spontaneous new mutations.

- In classic cases, IBM presents in young adulthood with weakness of the anterior tibialis muscle, resulting in gait difficulties caused by foot drop, progressing to hand weakness and thigh muscle weakness. Characteristically, the quadriceps muscle is spared. Likewise, in the upper extremity, the triceps is usually spared.

- The CPK is modestly elevated, 2 to 4 times that of normal.

T11.5
Limb-Girdle Muscular Dystrophies (LGMDs)

Disease	Inheritance	Populations	Gene (Locus)	Gene Product
α-sarcoglycanopathy	AR	None	*SGCA* (17q)	α-sarcoglycan
β-sarcoglycanopathy	AR	Amish	*SGCB* (4q)	β-sarcoglycan
δ-sarcoglycanopathy	AR	Brazilians	*SGCD* (5q)	δ-sarcoglycan
γ-sarcoglycanopathy	AR	North Africans	*SGCG* (13q)	γ-sarcoglycan
Calpainopathy	AR	Amish, Basque	*CAPN3* (15q)	Calpain-3
Dysferlinopathy-Miyoshi distal myopathy (DYSF).	AR	Libyan Jews	*DYSF* (2p)	Dysferlin
Caveolinopathy	AD	None	*CAV3* (3p)	Caveolin
LGMD1a (myotilinopathy)	AD	None	*TTID* (5q31)	Myotilin
LGMD1b	AD	None	*LMNA* (1q)	Lamin A/C

- The muscle biopsy shows characteristic rimmed vacuoles and filamentous inclusions. The vacuoles are rimmed by basophilic granular material on hematoxylin-eosin (H&E)-stained sections and purple-red granular material on trichrome-stained sections. Note that rimmed vacuoles are seen only in frozen muscle biopsy tissue. Tissue fixed in glutaraldehyde or formalin does not show vacuoles. With electron microscopy, the vacuoles are found to be caused by whorls of membranous material.

- Inclusion body myositis is caused by mutations in the *GNE* gene, on 9p, that encodes the enzyme UDP-N-acetylglucosamine 2-epimerase/N-acetyl-mannosamine kinase. In persons of Middle-Eastern (especially Iranian) Jewish descent, the disease is almost exclusively the result of a single mutation for which targeted mutation analysis is clinically available.

Nemaline Rod Myopathy

- This term refers to a group of myopathies united by the finding of nemaline rods on muscle biopsy. Inheritance is autosomal dominant, autosomal recessive, or sporadic (simplex).

- The muscle biopsy shows rodlike inclusions (nemaline bodies) in the cytoplasm (sarcoplasm) of skeletal muscle fibers. The rods are easily visible in trichrome-stained sections but not seen in H&E-stained sections. The rods contain the same latticelike structure as the Z-discs, appear to be in continuity with them, and are composed of Z-disc proteins such as α-actinin. Rods are not specific for nemaline rod myopathy. They may sometimes be seen in other inherited and acquired myopathies, notably *RYR1* mutations.

- Several gene mutations may give rise to nemaline rod myopathy, including *ACTA1* (1q42: actin), *NEB* (2q22: nebulin), *TNNT1* (19q: troponin T), and *TPM3* (1q: tropomyosin).

Emery-Dreifuss Muscular Dystrophy (EDMD)

- EDMD presents with a typical triad of muscle weakness in a humeroperoneal distribution, joint contractures, and cardiac conduction defects.

- Several genetic defects produce this phenotype, associated with both X-linked and autosomal patterns

of inheritance. X-linked forms are caused by mutations in the *EMD* gene that encodes the emerin protein. Autosomal EDMD is most commonly caused by mutations in *LMNA*, which encodes the proteins lamin A and lamin C (by alternative mRNA splicing). Differing mutations in *LMNA* are associated with a type of LGMD.

Malignant Hyperthermia (MH)

- MH may be triggered by inhalational anesthesia (such as halothane or isoflurane) and succinylcholine. Without treatment, the mortality rate (70%) is very high. Since its recognition, the mortality rate has been reduced to about 5% with improved monitoring (particularly for hypercarbia during general anesthesia) and the use of dantrolene. The onset of MH is heralded by hypercarbia, a physiologic reaction to systemic lactic acidosis. Laboratory findings in MH include an increased $Paco_2$, metabolic (lactic) acidosis, hyperkalemia, increased creatine kinase, myoglobin in blood and urine, and abnormal coagulation test results. Untreated MH leads to rhabdomyolysis, hyperkalemia, myoglobinuria, disseminated intravascular coagulation, congestive heart failure, bowel ischemia, and compartment syndrome. Treatment includes discontinuation of the anesthetic agent and administration of dantrolene sodium, with supportive measures for hyperthermia, acidosis, hyperkalemia, and myoglobinuria.

- Patients with known susceptibility to MH can be safely administered regional anesthesia (spinal, epidural, or nerve block) or general anesthesia with nontriggering agents (barbiturates, benzodiazepines, opioids, propofol, ketamine, nitrous oxide, and nondepolarizing neuromuscular blockers).

- Underlying MH is an abnormally uncontrolled release of calcium from the sarcoplasmic reticulum of skeletal muscle, resulting in muscle contraction, adenosine triphosphate consumption, and increased anaerobic metabolism. The calcium channel, RYR1, located in the membrane of the sarcoplasmic reticulum is defective in MH, displaying prolonged channel opening when exposed to triggering agents and inhibition of this effect by dantrolene.

11: Neurolomuscular Diseases

Diseases of Skeletal Muscle>Malignant Hyperthermia; Hyperkalemic Periodic Paralysis; Mitochondrial Myopathy I
Hereditary Hearing Loss: Summary and Approach>Nonsyndromic Hearing Loss

- There are 2 main tests for MH susceptibility: a muscle contracture test and a genetic test. The caffeine-halothane contracture test has a sensitivity of more than 95%, with a specificity of only about 80%. This test involves removing a segment of skeletal muscle and, while the specimen is still fresh, determining its contractile properties when exposed to halothane and caffeine. Given the high sensitivity, a negative contracture test goes a long way toward excluding MH susceptibility, but the test is not widely available and some have questioned its reproducibility. Genetic testing for *RYR1* mutations has recently become available. The difficulty is that more than 60 mutations in *RYR1* have been found to be associated with MH susceptibility, most of which are private (confined to a particular kindred). Tests currently available are capable of screening for 17 of the most common mutations, but this permits for a sensitivity of only about 25%.

Hyperkalemic Periodic Paralysis (HPP)

- HPP is characterized by episodes of flaccid paralysis or weakness in association with hyperkalemia. The symptoms can be duplicated by the administration of oral potassium or vigorous exercise. These episodes begin in early childhood, increase in frequency over time, then drop off after the age of 50 years. They typically occur in the morning before a meal is taken. During an attack, serum potassium concentration is elevated by more than 1.5 mmol/L over normal. Cardiac arrhythmias seldom occur, but elevated T waves may be seen. The serum CPK is constitutively elevated.

- The disease is caused by mutations in the *SCN4A* gene, encoding the voltage-gated skeletal muscle transmembrane sodium channel. Targeted mutation analysis for the several most common mutations can detect 50% to 60% of mutations. Direct sequence analysis can detect nearly all mutations.

- This disease must be distinguished conceptually from *hypo*kalemic periodic paralysis, in which episodes of flaccid weakness are associated with decreased serum potassium. Hypokalemic periodic paralysis is caused by mutations in the *CACNA1S* or *SCN4A* genes. Those with hypokalemic periodic paralysis are at risk for malignant hyperthermia.

- Andersen-Tawil syndrome (potassium-sensitive cardiodysrhythmic periodic paralysis) is characterized by episodes of flaccid weakness, ventricular arrhythmias, a prolonged QT interval, and dysmorphic features (low-set ears, hypertelorism, small mandible, clinodactyly, and syndactyly). Mutations in the potassium channel gene *KCNJ2* are causative.

Mitochondrial Myopathy

- See chapter 10.

Hereditary Hearing Loss: Summary and Approach

There are numerous genetic defects related to hereditary hearing loss, either on the basis of a conductive defect or sensorineural defect, either syndromic or nonsyndromic, either prelingual (before language develops) or postlingual, and either congenital or progressive. Clinically, the cases are usually grouped as syndromic (present in association with a recognizable clinical syndrome) or nonsyndromic. Molecular genetic testing is available for many types of syndromic and nonsyndromic deafness, often only on a research basis and, for a more limited number, on a clinical basis.

The incidence of congenital hearing loss (prelingual deafness) is about 1 in 1000 births. Over 50% of such cases have a genetic basis, with the remaining cases arising from various causes, including toxin and infection (eg, TORCH agents). Of the genetic cases, about 70% are nonsyndromic and 30% syndromic. Furthermore, of the nonsyndromic cases, about 50% are caused by mutations in the *GJB2* gene (causing DFNB1).

Among noncongential hearing loss (which is most often postlingual), genetic causes remain important but proportionately less so than environmental factors. Still, genetics plays a major role; for example, aminoglycoside-associated ototoxicity appears to have a pharmacogenetic basis. Otosclerosis is an autosomal dominant trait, and chronic ear effusions may be the result of multifactorially encoded anatomic features.

Nonsyndromic Hearing Loss

- About 1 in 2000 newborns are affected by congenital nonsyndromic hearing loss, and more than half of these are caused by an autosomal recessive disorder known as DFNB1. DFNB1 is linked to the *GJB2* gene on 13q12 which encodes connexin 26 (Cx26). About 1 in 30 to 1 in 50 Americans are carriers for a mutated *GHB2* allele.

11: Neurolomuscular Diseases

Hereditary Hearing Loss: Summary and Approach>Nonsyndromic Hearing Loss; Syndromic Hearing Loss |
Mental Retardation and Developmental Delay: Summary and Approach

- Homozygosity for *GJB2* is responsible for about 1 in 2 cases of nonsyndromic hearing loss and about 1 in 3 cases of inherited hearing loss overall.

- The connexin defect results in sensorineural hearing loss that usually is congenital (present at birth).

- Mutation scanning assays are clinically available and designed to detect the most common several mutations. PCR-based assays are available to detect the most common *GJB2* mutation (35delG).

Syndromic Hearing Loss

- A multitude of genetic syndromes include hearing loss (syndromic hearing loss). Autosomal dominant forms of syndromic hearing loss include the Waardenburg syndrome, neurofibromatosis type 2, branchiootorenal syndrome, and Stickler syndrome. Autosomal recessive causes of syndromic hearing loss include the Usher syndrome, Jervell and Lange-Nielson syndrome, biotinidase deficiency, and Refsum disease. Alport syndrome is an example of X-linked syndromic hearing loss. Lastly, syndromic hearing loss with mitochondrial inheritance is seen in *MTTL1* gene mutations.

- Waardenburg syndrome is the most common type of autosomal dominant syndromic hearing loss. The syndrome consists of sensorineural hearing loss and pigmentary abnormalities of the skin, eyes (heterochromia iridis), and hair (white forelock). There are 4 types, distinguished by associated physical findings; Waardenburg syndrome type IV is associated with Hirschsprung disease and may be caused by mutations in the *EDNRB, EDN3,* or *SOX10* genes. Types I and III are caused by differing mutations in the *PAX3* gene. Type II is caused by mutations in the *MITF* gene.

- The second most common cause of autosomal dominant syndromic hearing loss is the branchiootorenal syndrome. Its features include hearing loss, branchial cleft cysts, preauricular pits, and renal anomalies. Mutations in the *EYA1* gene are found in about half of cases.

- Usher syndrome is the most common type of autosomal recessive syndromic hearing loss. It consists of sensorineural hearing loss and retinitis pigmentosa, ultimately leading to blindness. It is the most common cause of combined deafness and blindness. There are at present 3 forms of Usher syndrome (classified according to clinical severity) and 7 different loci associated with the most severe type 1 Usher syndrome, termed *USH1A* through *USH1G*.

- Pendred syndrome is the second most common cause of autosomal recessive syndromic hearing loss. Vaughan Pendred originally reported it in 1896 in a large family with deafness and goiters. The temporal anatomy is abnormal, described as having dilation of the endolymphatic sac and endolymphatic duct and enlargement of the vestibular aqueduct. So-called Mondini dysplasia (an abnormal cochlea in association with a dilated vestibular aqueduct) is present in most cases. These changes can be visualized by CT or MRI of the temporal bone. Goiter is almost always present, but the patients are euthyroid. The locus related to Pendred syndrome is found at 7q21-34. The causative gene is *PDS* (*SLC26A4*), in which several different mutations have been described. Most of these mutations are unique to single kindreds (private). Interestingly, 1 type of nonsyndromic deafness, DFNB4, is also connected to the *SLC26A4* gene.

- Jervell and Lange-Nielsen syndrome is the syndrome of prolonged QT interval with congenital deafness.

Mental Retardation and Developmental Delay: Summary and Approach

The terms m*ental retardation* and *global developmental delay* have essentially the same implication; however, mental retardation is generally assessed at an older age (over 5 years) and is based largely on IQ. In contrast, global developmental delay refers to delayed acquisition of a wide range of developmental skills, usually in a child under the age of 5.

Once developmental delay or mental retardation is identified, an etiologic explanation is often desired. The differential diagnosis is quite long, including several genetic causes, multifactorial conditions, and environmental causes (especially intrauterine infection, intrauterine exposure to alcohol or other toxins, and prematurity), and many cases are idiopathic. The likelihood of an identifiable genetic cause appears to increase as the degree of impairment increases; that is, a specific genetic cause is identified in around 30% of mild mental retardation and around 70% of severe mental retardation. In addition to the syndromes listed herein, several hundred genetic diseases, most of them rare, are associated with mental retardation and/or global developmental delay. Arriving at the underlying diagnosis may require, in addition to a history and physical examination, metabolic studies, cytogenetic studies, specific molecular studies, and/or neuroimaging.

A comprehensive metabolic study, it is estimated, can identify an etiologic diagnosis in up to 5% of cases. Such a study might involve screening for hyperammonemia, hyperlactic acidemia, thyroid function, lead level, amino acidurias, and organic acidurias. In the United States, however, many of the high-yield studies are performed as part of neonatal screening panels. Furthermore, the incidence of these diseases being as low as it is implies that false-positive findings are a major problem in such an approach. As a result, a directed metabolic assessment, based on history (especially consanguinity) and physical findings (including ophthalmologic examination) is recommended.

Cytogenetic and molecular studies may disclose an explanation, in this setting, in up to 10% of cases. Likely findings of conventional cytogenetics include trisomy 21 (Down syndrome) or trisomy 21 mosaicism, Turner syndrome, 47,XXY, fragile X syndrome, and a variety of translocations and deletions. Furthermore, specific testing for fragile X syndrome (as routine cytogenetic studies are relatively insensitive) should be considered, as it is an extremely common cause of global developmental delay and/or mental retardation. This test alone can explain around 5% of cases in males. Testing for Rett syndrome can identify roughly 5% of cases in females. Lastly, testing for so-called subtelomeric chromosomal rearrangements can explain up to another 5% of cases.

Down Syndrome (Chapter 2)

- This is probably the most common cause of global developmental delay and/or mental retardation overall.

Fragile X Syndrome (Chapter 2)

- Fragile X syndrome is second only to Down syndrome as a common cause of mental retardation, and it is the single most common cause of inherited mental retardation.

Rett Syndrome

- Rett syndrome is 1 of the most common causes of developmental delay and/or mental retardation in females and is very peculiar in its molecular pathogenesis. It is caused by anomalies in the DNA methylation mechanism of gene inactivation, resulting from mutations in the X-linked gene encoding methyl-CpG-binding protein 2 (MeCP2).

- There are several mechanisms by which methylation causes gene inactivation. 1 mechanism involves proteins that bind to methylated sequences, thus blocking transcription. Proteins that bind methylated DNA include MeCP2, MBD1, and others.

- The incidence of Rett syndrome is about 1 in 10,000 female births. Development is initially normal, but around 1 year of age there is a period of regression, with loss of recently acquired language and motor skills. Following this, the children continue to progress developmentally, though the rate is variable. Survival into adulthood is usually possible.

- The *MECP2* gene is found at Xq28. Rett syndrome is almost exclusively seen in females (males with the mutation die no later than infancy as a result of severe encephalopathy), and affected girls are heterozygous for the mutated allele. As a result of random X inactivation, half of somatic cells express the mutation. Thus, all affected girls are mosaics. While the vast majority of patients with Rett syndrome have *MECP2* mutations, not all *MECP2* mutations cause Rett syndrome (ie, some are benign polymorphisms).

Subtelomeric Rearrangements and Uniparental Disomy

- It has been reported that, in around 5% to 10% of children with developmental delay and/or mental retardation, small rearrangements involving the ends of chromosomes (subtelomeric rearrangements) can be found. In another 1% to 2% of such children, uniparental disomy (the inheritance of both copies of a chromosomal region from a single parent) can be found.

- These anomalies can only be detected using techniques more sensitive than conventional cytogenetics, ie, molecular cytogenetics or fluorescence in situ hybridization (FISH). FISH is generally used with subtelomeric probes to identify subtelomeric rearrangements and with microsatellite probes to find uniparental disomy.

- However, it is unclear whether these anomalies actually cause the observed phenotypic effects in all cases, because similar anomalies can be found in around 1% of phenotypically normal adults.

Craniosynostosis

- This is a condition in which 1 or more cranial sutures fuse prematurely. Without treatment, craniosynostosis can lead not only to an abnormality in the shape of the head, but more importantly, to inhibition of brain growth and increased intracranial pressure.

- Craniosynostosis should be distinguished from a common benign condition, having to do with sleep positioning, known as *deformational plagiocephaly*.

- The overall incidence is about 1 in 2000 live births. There are over 100 causes of craniosynostosis, with a variety of inheritance patterns, roughly divided into syndromic and nonsyndromic varieties. Nonetheless, the majority of cases are attributable to 1 of 2 entities: Crouzon disease and Apert syndrome.

  □ Crouzon disease is characterized by midfacial hypoplasia, mandibular prognathism, and marked proptosis (caused by increased intracranial pressure). The distal extremities are normal. Many cases are caused by new (spontaneous) mutations and are associated with advanced *paternal* age (older than 35 years). Crouzon disease is caused by mutations in the *FGFR2* gene on chromosome 10.

  □ The features of Apert syndrome include wide-set downslanting eyes and mitten-glove syndactyly. Radiographic examination discloses hypoplasia of the bones of the hand and extensive bony syndactyly. Apert syndrome is caused by mutations in the *FGFR2* gene.

References

Ackerman MJ, Clapham DE. Ion channels: basic science and clinical disease. *N Engl J Med* 1997; 336: 1575-1586.

Amberla K, Waljas M, Tuominen S, et al. Insidious cognitive decline in CADASIL. *Stroke* 2004; 35: 1598-1602.

Ando Y, Nakamura M, Araki S. Transthyretin-related familial amyloidotic polyneuropathy. *Arch Neurol* 2005; 62: 1057-1062.

Argov Z, Eisenberg I, Grabov-Nardini G, et al. Hereditary inclusion body myopathy: the Middle Eastern genetic cluster. *Neurology* 2003; 60: 1519-1523.

Axelrod FB, Goldberg JD, Ye XY, et al. Survival in familial dysautonomia: Impact of early intervention. *J Pediatr* 2002; 141: 518-523.

Aylward EH, Li Q, Stine OC, et al. Longitudinal change in basal ganglia volume in patients with Huntington's disease. *Neurology* 1997; 48: 394-399.

Aylward EH, Sparks BF, Field KM, et al. Onset and rate of striatal atrophy in preclinical Huntington disease. *Neurology* 2004; 63: 66-72.

Brandt J, Bylsma FW, Gross R, et al. Trinucleotide repeat length and clinical progression in Huntington's disease. *Neurology* 1996; 46: 527-531.

Benson MD. Leptomeningeal amyloid and variant transthyretins. *Am J Pathol* 1996; 148: 351-354.

Ben-Yosef T, Ness SL, Madeo AC, et al. A Mutation of PCDH15 among Ashkenazi Jews with the type 1 Usher syndrome. *N Engl J Med* 2003; 348: 1664-1670.

Berko BA, Swift M. X-linked dilated cardiomyopathy. *N Engl J Med* 1987; 316: 1186-1191.

Bertram L, Tanzi RE. Alzheimer's disease: one disorder, too many genes? *Hum Mol Genet* 2004; 13(review issue 1): R135-R141.

Biaggioni I, Goldstein DS, Atkinson T, et al. Dopamine-beta-hydroxylase deficiency in humans. *Neurology* 1990; 40: 370-373.

References

Bird TD. Genetic factors in Alzheimer's disease. *N Engl J Med* 2005; 352: 862-864.

Bird TD. Myotonic dystrophy type 1 (Steinert's disease). Available at www.GeneTests.org. Accessed November 22, 2005.

Boerkoel CF, Takashima H, Garcia CA, et al. Charcot-Marie-Tooth disease and related neuropathies: mutation distribution and genotype-phenotype correlation. *Ann Neurol* 2002; 51: 190-201.

Boeve BF, Tremont-Lukats IW, Waclawik AJ, et al. Longitudinal characterization of two siblings with frontotemporal dementia and parkinsonism linked to chromosome 17 associated with the S305N tau mutation. *Brain* 2005; 128: 752-772.

Boito CA, Melacini P, Vianello A, et al. Clinical and molecular characterization of patients with limb-girdle muscular dystrophy type 2I. *Arch Neurol* 2005; 62: 1894-1899.

Borm B, Moller LB, Hausser I, et al. Variable clinical expression of an identical mutation in the ATP7A gene for Menkes disease/occipital horn syndrome in three affected males in a single family. *J Pediatr* 2004; 145: 119-121.

Bradley WG, Taylor R, Rice DR, et al. Progressive myopathy in hyperkalemic periodic paralysis. *Arch Neurol* 1990; 47: 1013-1017.

Breitner JC. APOE genotyping and Alzheimer's disease. *Lancet* 1996; 347: 1184-1185.

Brett M, Persey MR, Reilly MM, et al. Transthyretin Leu12Pro is associated with systemic, neuropathic and leptomeningeal amyloidosis. *Brain* 1999; 122: 183-190.

Brugge KL, Nichols SL, Salmon DP, et al. Cognitive impairment in adults with Down's syndrome: similarities to early cognitive changes in Alzheimer's disease. *Neurology* 1994; 44: 232-238.

Bruno C, Bertini E, Federico A, et al. Clinical and molecular findings in patients with giant axonal neuropathy (GAN). *Neurology* 2004; 62: 13-16.

Bushby KM. Making sense of the limb-girdle muscular dystrophies. *Brain* 1999; 122: 1403-1420.

Bushby KM, Thambyayah M, Gardner-Medwin D. Prevalence and incidence of Becker muscular dystrophy. *Lancet* 1991; 337: 1022-1024.

Buxbaum JN, Tagoe CE. The genetics of the amyloidoses. *Annu Rev Med* 2000; 51: 543-569.

Chabriat H, Levy C, Taillia H, et al. Patterns of MRI lesions in CADASIL. *Neurology* 1998; 51: 452-457.

Chen L, Lee L, Kudlow BA, et al. LMNA mutations in atypical Werner's syndrome. *Lancet* 2003; 362: 440-445.

Chinnery PF, Walls TJ, Hanna MG, et al. Normokalemic periodic paralysis revisited: does it exist? *Ann Neurol* 2002; 52: 251-252.

Connors LH, Lim A, Prokaeva T, et al. Tabulation of human transthyretin (TTR) variants, 2003. *Amyloid* 2003; 10: 160-184.

Cox GF, Kunkel LM. Dystrophies and heart disease. *Curr Opin Cardiol* 1997; 12: 329-343.

Crawford DC, Meadows KL, Newman JL, et al. Prevalence of the fragile X syndrome in African-Americans. *Am J Med Genet* 2002; 110: 226-233.

Danek A, Rubio JP, Rampoldi L, et al. McLeod neuroacanthocytosis: genotype and phenotype. *Ann Neurol* 2001; 50: 755-764.

Danek A, Uttner I, Vogl T, et al. Cerebral involvement in McLeod syndrome. *Neurology* 1994; 44: 117-120.

Davies S, Ramsden DB. Huntington's disease. *J Clin Pathol: Mol Pathol* 2001; 54: 409-413.

DeDie-Smulders CE, Howeler CJ, Thijs C, et al. Age and causes of death in adult-onset myotonic dystrophy. *Brain* 1998; 121: 1557-1563.

DeJonghe P, Timmerman V, Ceuterick C, et al. The Thr124Met mutation in the peripheral myelin protein zero (MPZ) gene is associated with a clinically distinct Charcot-Marie-Tooth phenotype. *Brain* 1999; 122: 281-290.

Del Castillo I, Villamar M, Moreno-Pelayo MA, et al. A deletion involving the connexin 30 gene in nonsyndromic hearing impairment. *N Engl J Med* 2002; 346: 243-249.

References

Dias Da Silva MR, Cerutti JM, Arnaldi LA, et al. A mutation in the KCNE3 potassium channel gene is associated with susceptibility to thyrotoxic hypokalemic periodic paralysis. *J Clin Endocrinol Metab* 200; 87: 4881-4884.

Dichgans M, Mayer M, Uttner I, et al. The phenotypic spectrum of CADASIL: Clinical findings in 102 cases. *Ann Neurol* 1998; 44: 731-739.

DiFonzo A, Rohe CF, Ferreira J, et al. A frequent LRRK2 gene mutation associated with autosomal dominant Parkinson's disease. *Lancet* 2005; 365: 412-415.

Durr A, Cossee M, Agid Y, et al. Clinical and genetic abnormalities in patients with Friedreich's ataxia. *N Engl J Med* 1996; 335: 1169-1175.

Ebly EM, Parhad IM, Hogan DB, et al. Prevalence and types of dementia in the very old. *Neurology* 1994; 44: 1593-1600.

Estivill X, Fortina P, Surrey S, et al. Connexin-26 mutations in sporadic and inherited sensorineural deafness. *Lancet* 1998; 351: 394-398.

Fabrizi GM, Cavallaro T, Angiari C, et al. Giant axon and neurofilament accumulation in Charcot-Marie-Tooth disease type 2E. *Neurology* 2004; 62: 1429-1431.

Farrer M, Chan P, Chen R, et al. Lewy bodies and parkinsonism in families with parkin mutations. *Ann Neurol* 2001; 50: 293-300.

Filla A, De Michele G, Cavalcanti F, et al. The relationship between trinucleotide (GAA) repeat length and clinical features in Friedreich ataxia. *Am J Hum Genet* 1996; 59: 554-560.

Finckh U, Alberici A, Antoniazzi M, et al. Variable expression of familial Alzheimer disease associated with presenilin 2 mutation M239I. *Neurology* 2000; 54: 2006-2008.

Finsterer J, Stollberger C. The heart in human dystrophinopathies. *Cardiology* 2003; 99: 1-19.

Fox NC, Kennedy AM, Harvey RJ, et al. Clinicopathological features of familial Alzheimer's disease associated with the M139V mutation in the presenilin 1 gene. *Brain* 1997; 120: 491-501.

Frederick J. Pick disease: a brief overview. *Arch Pathol Lab Med* 2006; 130: 1063-1066.

Gabriel JM, Erne B, Pareyson D, et al. Gene dosage effects in hereditary peripheral neuropathy: expression of peripheral myelin protein 22 in Charcot-Marie-Tooth disease type 1A and hereditary neuropathy with liability to pressure palsies nerve biopsies. *Neurology* 1997; 49: 1635-1640.

Gouider R, LeGuern E, Gugenheim M, et al. Clinical, electro-physiologic, and molecular correlations in 13 families with hereditary neuropathy with liability to pressure palsies and a chromosome 17p11.2 deletion. *Neurology* 1995; 45: 2018-2023.

Greenberg DA. Calcium channels in neurological disease. *Ann Neurol* 1997; 42: 275-282.

Griggs RC, Askanas V, DiMauro S, et al. Inclusion body myositis and myopathies. *Ann Neurol* 1995; 38: 705-713.

Hagerman RJ, Leehey M, Heinrichs W, et al. Intention tremor, parkinsonism, and generalized brain atrophy in male carriers of fragile X. *Neurology* 2001; 57: 127-130.

Harding AE. Clinical features and classification of inherited ataxias. *Adv Neurol* 1993; 61: 1-14.

Hattori N, Yamamoto M, Yoshihara T, et al. Demyelinating and axonal features of Charcot-Marie-Tooth disease with mutations of myelin-related proteins (PMP22, MPZ and Cx32): a clinicopathological study of 205 Japanese patients. *Brain* 2003; 126: 134-151.

Hawley RJ, Milner MR, Gottdiener JS, et al. Myotonic heart disease: a clinical follow-up. *Neurology* 1991; 41: 259-262.

Hayflick SJ, Westaway SK, Levinson B, et al. Genetic, clinical, and radiographic delineation of Hallervorden-Spatz syndrome. *N Engl J Med* 2003; 348: 33-40.

Heckmann JM, Low WC, de Villiers C, et al. Novel presenilin 1 mutation with profound neurofibrillary pathology in an indigenous Southern African family with early-onset Alzheimer's disease. *Brain* 2004; 127: 133-142.

Hedera P, Turner RS. Inherited dementias. *Neurol Clin North Am* 2002; 20: 779-808.

References

Hoogerwaard EM, Bakker E, Ippel PF, et al. Signs and symptoms of Duchenne muscular dystrophy and Becker muscular dystrophy among carriers in The Netherlands: a cohort study. *Lancet* 1999; 353: 2116-2119.

Ikeda S. Cardiac amyloidosis: heterogenous pathogenic backgrounds. *Intern Med* 2004; 43: 1107-1114.

Ionasescu VV, Ionasescu R, Searby C, et al. Dejerine-Sottas disease with de novo dominant point mutation of the PMP22 gene. *Neurology* 1995; 45: 1766-1767.

Irobi J, De Jonghe P, Timmerman V. Molecular genetics of distal hereditary motor neuropathies. *Hum Mol Genet* 2004; 13(review issue 2): R195-R202.

Ishibashi-Ueda H, Imakita M, Yutani C, et al. Congenital nemaline myopathy with dilated cardiomyopathy: an autopsy study. *Hum Pathol* 1990; 21: 77-82.

Jacquemont S, Hagerman RJ, Leehey MA, et al. Penetrance of the fragile X-associated tremor/ataxia syndrome in a premutation carrier population. *JAMA* 2004; 291: 460-469.

Janssen JC, Beck JA, Campbell TA, et al. Early onset familial Alzheimer's disease: mutation frequency in 31 families. *Neurology* 2003; 60: 235-239.

Joutel A, Dodick DD, Parisi JE, et al. De novo mutation in the Notch3 gene causing CADASIL. *Ann Neurol* 2000; 47: 388-391.

Kabbani H, Raghuveer TS. Craniosynostosis. *Am Fam Physician* 2004; 69: 2863-2870.

Kamboh MI. Molecular genetics of late-onset Alzheimer's disease. *Ann Hum Genet* 2004; 68: 381-404.

Kanev PM. Congenital malformations of the skull and meninges. *Otolaryngol Clin North Am* 2007; 40: 9-26.

Krajewski KM, Lewis RA, Fuerst DR, et al. Neurological dysfunction and axonal degeneration in Charcot-Marie-Tooth disease type 1A. *Brain* 2000; 123: 1516-1527.

Kriaucionis S, Bird A. DNA methylation and Rett syndrome. *Hum Mol Genet* 2003; 12(review issue 2): R221-R227.

Kuhlenbaumer G, Young P, Oberwittler C, et al. Giant axonal neuropathy (GAN): case report and two novel mutations in the gigaxonin gene. *Neurology* 2002; 58: 1273-1276.

Labuda M, Labuda D, Miranda C, et al. Unique origin and specific ethnic distribution of the Friedreich ataxia GAA expansion. *Neurology* 2000; 54: 2322-2324.

Lamont PJ, Davis MB, Wood NW. Identification and sizing of the GAA trinucleotide repeat expansion of Friedreich's ataxia in 56 patients: clinical and genetic correlates. *Brain* 1997; 120: 673-680.

Lang AE, Lozano AM. Parkinson's disease: second of two parts. *N Engl J Med* 1998; 339: 1130-1143.

Lin SH, Lin YF, Chen DT, et al. Laboratory tests to determine the cause of hypokalemia and paralysis. *Arch Intern Med* 2004; 164: 1561-1566.

Lippa CF, Swearer JM, Kane KJ, et al. Familial Alzheimer's disease: site of mutation influences clinical phenotype. *Ann Neurol* 2000; 48: 376-379.

Litman RS, Rosenberg H. Malignant hyperthermia: update on susceptibility testing. *JAMA* 2005; 293: 2918-2924.

Loke J, MacLennan DH. Malignant hyperthermia and central core disease: disorders of calcium release channels. *Am J Med* 1998; 104: 470-486.

Lucking CB, Durr A, Bonifati V, et al. Association between early-onset Parkinson's disease and mutations in the parkin gene. *N Engl J Med* 2000; 342: 1560-1567.

Lupski JR, Chance PF, Garcia CA. Inherited primary peripheral neuropathies: molecular genetics and clinical implications of CMT1A and HNPP. *JAMA* 1993; 270: 2326-2330.

McCarthy TV, Quane KA, Lynch PJ. Ryanodine receptor mutations in malignant hyperthermia and central core disease. *Hum Mutat* 2000; 15: 410-417.

Manin't Veld AJ, Boomsma F, Moleman P, et al. Congenital dopamine-beta-hydroxylase deficiency: a novel orthostatic syndrome. *Lancet* 1987; 1: 183-188.

References

Markus HS, Martin RJ, Simpson MA, et al. Diagnostic strategies in CADASIL. *Neurology* 2002; 59: 1134-1138.

Margallo-Lana M, Morris CM, Gibson AM, et al. Influence of the amyloid precursor protein locus on dementia in Down syndrome. *Neurology* 2004; 62: 1996-1998.

Marrosu MG, Vaccargiu S, Marrosu G, et al. Charcot-Marie-Tooth disease type 2 associated with mutation of the myelin protein zero gene. *Neurology* 1998; 50: 1397-1401.

Mastrianni JA, Nixon R, Layzer R, et al. Prion protein conformation in a patient with sporadic fatal insomnia. *N Engl J Med* 1999; 340: 1630-1638.

Mastrianni JA, Roos RP. The prion diseases. *Semin Neurol* 2000; 20: 337-352.

Mateo I, Llorca J, Volpini V, et al. GAA expansion size and age at onset of Friedreich's ataxia. *Neurology* 2003; 2: 274-275.

Mayeux R, Saunders AM, Shea S, et al. Utility of the apolipoprotein E genotype in the diagnosis of Alzheimer's disease. *N Engl J Med* 1998; 338: 506-511.

Miller TM, Dias da Silva MR, Miller HA, et al. Correlating phenotype and genotype in the periodic paralyses. *Neurology* 2004; 63: 1647-1655.

Monnier N, Romero NB, Lerale J, et al. An autosomal dominant congenital myopathy with cores and rods is associated with a neomutation in the RYR1 gene encoding the skeletal muscle ryanodine receptor. *Hum Mol Genet* 2000; 9: 2599-2608.

Ng B, Connors LH, Davidoff R, et al. Senile systemic amyloidosis presenting with heart failure: a comparison with light chain-associated amyloidosis. *Arch Intern Med* 2005; 165: 1425-1429.

Nishino I, Noguchi S, Murayama K, et al. Distal myopathy with rimmed vacuoles is allelic to hereditary inclusion body myopathy. *Neurology* 2002; 59: 1689-1693.

Numakura C, Lin C, Oka N, et al. Hemizygous mutation of the peripheral myelin protein 22 gene associated with Charcot-Marie-Tooth disease type 1. *Ann Neurol* 2000; 47: 101-103.

Ogino S, Leonard DGB, Rennert H, et al. Spinal muscular atrophy genetic testing experience at an academic medical center. *J Mol Diagn* 2002; 4: 53-58.

Parman Y, Plante-Bordeneuve V, Guiochon-Mantel A, et al. Recessive inheritance of a new point mutation of the PMP22 gene in Dejerine-Sottas disease. *Ann Neurol* 1999; 45: 518-522.

Plante-Bordeneuve V, Said G. Transthyretin related familial amyloid polyneuropathy. *Curr Opin Neurol* 2000; 13: 569-573.

Prior TW, Bridgeman SJ. Duchenne muscular dystrophy. *J Mol Diagn* 2005; 7(3): 317-326.

Ravaglia G, Forti P, Maioli F, et al. Incidence and etiology of dementia in a large elderly Italian population. *Neurology* 2005; 64: 1525-1530.

Redman JB, Fenwick RG Jr, Fu YH, et al. Relationship between parental trinucleotide GCT repeat length and severity of myotonic dystrophy in offspring. *JAMA* 1993; 269: 1960-1965.

Rizzu P, Van Swieten JC, Joosse M, et al. High prevalence of mutations in the microtubule-associated protein tau in a population study of frontotemporal dementia in the Netherlands. *Am J Hum Genet* 1999; 64: 414-421.

Rosenblatt A, Liang KY, Zhou H, et al. The association of CAG repeat length with clinical progression in Huntington disease. *Neurology* 2006; 66: 1016-1020.

Rosenberg RN. The molecular and genetic basis of AD: the end of the beginning. *Neurology* 2000; 54: 2045-2054.

Rosenblatt A, Brinkman RR, Liang KY, et al. Familial influence on age of onset among siblings with Huntington disease. *Am J Med Genet* 2001; 105: 399-403.

Rosso SM, Kamphorst W, de Graaf B, et al. Familial frontotemporal dementia with ubiquitin-positive inclusions is linked to chromosome 17q21-22. *Brain* 2001; 124: 1948-1957.

Russo DC, Lee S, Reid ME, et al. Point mutations causing the McLeod phenotype. *Transfusion* 2002; 42: 287-293.

References

Ryan MM, Schnell C, Strickland CD, et al. Nemaline myopathy: a clinical study of 143 cases. *Ann Neurol* 2001; 50: 312-320.

Saito M, Kawai H, Akaike M, et al. Cardiac dysfunction with Becker muscular dystrophy. *Am Heart J* 1996; 132: 642-647.

Sambuughin N, de Bantel A, McWilliams S, et al. Deafness and CMT disease associated with a novel four amino acid deletion in the PMP22 gene. *Neurology* 2003; 60: 506-508.

Saunders AM, Hulette O, Welsh-Bohmer KA, et al. Specificity, sensitivity, and predictive value of apolipoprotein-E genotyping for sporadic Alzheimer's disease. *Lancet* 1996; 348: 90-93.

Sethi KD, Adams RJ, Loring DW, et al. Hallervorden-Spatz syndrome: clinical and magnetic resonance imaging correlations. *Ann Neurol* 1988; 24: 692-694.

Shaffer LG, Kennedy GM, Spikes AS, et al. Diagnosis of CMT1A duplications and HNPP deletions by interphase FISH: implications for testing in the cytogenetics laboratory. *Am J Med Genet* 1997; 69: 325-331.

Shaffer LG and the American College of Medical Genetics Professional Practice and Guidelines Committee. American College of Medical Genetics guideline on the cytogenetic evaluation of the individual with developmental delay or mental retardation. *Genet Med* 2005; 7: 650-654.

Shevell M. Hallervorden and history. *N Engl J Med* 2003; 348: 3-5.

Shevell M. Racial hygiene, active euthanasia, and Julius Hallervorden. *Neurology* 1992; 42: 2214-2219.

Shevell M, Ashwal S, Donley D, et al. Practice parameter: Evaluation of the child with global developmental delay. *Neurology* 2003; 60: 367-380.

Smith RJ, Hone S. Genetic screening for deafness. *Pediatr Clin North Am* 2003; 50: 315-329.

Spillantini MG, Crowther RA, Kamphorst W, et al. Tau pathology in two Dutch families with mutations in the microtubule-binding region of tau. *Am J Pathol* 1998; 153: 1359-1363.

Squitieri F, Gellera C, Cannella M, et al. Homozygosity for CAG mutation in Huntington disease is associated with a more severe clinical course. *Brain* 2003; 126: 946-955.

Stevens M, van Duijn CM, Kamphorst W, et al. Familial aggregation in frontotemporal dementia. *Neurology* 1998; 50: 1541-1545.

Tammaro A, Bracco A, Cozzolino S, et al. Scanning for mutations of the ryanodine receptor (RYR1) gene by denaturing HPLC: detection of three novel malignant hyperthermia alleles. *Clin Chem* 2003; 49: 761-768.

Taylor AM, Byrd PJ. Molecular pathology of ataxia telangiectasia. *J Clin Pathol* 2005; 58: 1009-1015.

Teunissen LL, Notermans NC, Franssen H, et al. Disease course of Charcot-Marie-Tooth disease type 2: a 5-year follow-up study. *Arch Neurol* 2003; 60: 823-828.

Tsujino A, Maertens C, Ohno K, et al. Myasthenic syndrome caused by mutation of the SCN4A sodium channel. *Proc Natl Acad Sci U S A* 2003; 100: 7377-7382.

Turner G, Webb T, Wake S, et al. Prevalence of fragile X syndrome. *Am J Med Genet* 1996; 64: 196-197.

Van der Kooi AJ, Barth PG, Busch HF, et al. The clinical spectrum of limb girdle muscular dystrophy: a survey in The Netherlands. *Brain* 1996; 119: 1471-1480.

Wagner KR. Genetic diseases of muscle. *Neurol Clin North Am* 2002; 20: 645-678.

Wijsman EM, Daw EW, Yu CE, et al. Evidence for a novel late-onset Alzheimer disease locus on chromosome 19p13.2. *Am J Hum Genet* 2004; 75: 398-409.

Wu WS, Holmans P, Wavrant-DeVrieze F, et al. Genetic studies on chromosome 12 in late-onset Alzheimer disease. *JAMA* 1998; 280: 619-622.

Chapter 12

Microbiology

Viral Hepatitis

Hepatitis B (HBV)

- The HBV virus is a DNA virus. The HBV genome has several major gene regions: pre-S, S, C, P, and X. The pre-S genes encode the hepatocyte receptor–binding site. The S gene encodes surface antigen (HBsAg), a component of the viral envelope. The C gene encodes core antigen (HBcAg) and e antigen (HBeAg). The P gene encodes a DNA polymerase.

- The diagnosis of HBV infection generally is based on clinical presentation and serologic findings. Important HBV-related serologic markers include:

  □ Hepatitis B surface antigen (HbsAg; Australia antigen), whose presence in serum indicates active disease; HBsAg would be expected to clear if infection is resolved and persist if infection is chronic.

  □ Hepatitis B e antigen (HBeAg) indicates active viral replication. In the hepatocyte, the genome of HBV can be present in 2 forms: (1) as replicating virus, or (2) integrated into the host genome as a nonreplicating form. HBeAg is only produced when the virus is in replicating form; thus, it has for some time been used as a marker of HBV replication. HBV DNA in serum is a more sensitive indicator of viral replication, however, and is now replacing HBeAg for this purpose.

  □ Antibody against hepatitis B core antigen (IgM and IgG anti-HBc) is present throughout the lifetime of somebody who has been infected with HBV. Its presence cannot be used to classify a patient's condition as acute, resolved, or chronic. While IgM anti-HBc usually disappears after acute infection, it may persist for over a year; furthermore, in patients with chronic infection, IgM anti-HBc may reappear in acute flares. IgM anti-HBc emerges shortly after HBsAg and persists for many months. It is eventually replaced by IgG anti-HBc, sometimes 18 to 24 months after infection. Thus, IgG anti-HBc indicates past infection, either resolved (anti-HBsAb+) or in the chronic phase (HBsAg+).

  □ Antibody against hepatitis B e antigen (anti-HBe) is found when HBe becomes negative. The presence of anti-HBe does not imply resolved infection or immunity.

  □ Antibody against surface antigen (HBsAb) indicates resistance to infection. It is found in immunized persons and those who have successfully cleared HBV infection. With older less sensitive assays, there was a brief interval between disappearance of HBsAg and appearance of HBsAb, termed the "window" period. The possibility of a false-negative serologicdiagnosis of HBV infection existed during this period, unless IgM anti-HBc was measured. With current more sensitive assays,this window has narrowed considerably.

- Serologic markers become detectable between 2 and 10 weeks following exposure, with HBsAg emerging first. HBV DNA is detectable in serum before HBsAg, and both are detectable before clinical symptoms appear. The development of antibodies (anti-HBs, anti-HBc) roughly coincides with the development of clinical symptoms.

- Most patients experience complete resolution of acute HBV infection. This is heralded by the emergence of anti-HBe and anti-HBs. Usually the latter developments somewhat following the disappearance of HBsAg and HBeAg from serum. Anti-HBs therefore is indicative of resolved HBV hepatitis and implies life-long immunity.

- It is in those patients whose infection does not resolve that molecular methods are most important. Chronic hepatitis B infection is defined by persistence of HBsAg after the acute phase (for more than 6 months). Persistent HBsAg without clinical hepatitis is called the chronic "carrier" state. Chronicity develops in around 5% of healthy infected adults, 10% of immunocompromised adults, and up to 90% of neonates who have become infected transplacentally. Hepatitis D virus (HDV) is capable of infecting hepatocytes with HBV DNA but not uninfected hepatocytes.

- The HBV genome frequently undergoes mutation. Some mutations can significantly alter the clinical features.

  □ 1 such mutation takes the form of so-called HBeAg-negative chronic hepatitis B. This is characterized by circulating HBV DNA, fluctuating aminotransferases, and a tendency toward fulminant hepatitis with liver failure.

This form of hepatitis B results from mutations in the C or pre-C region, the most common mutation being an adenosine (A) for guanine (G) substitution at nucleotide position 1896 (G1896A), leading to a premature stop codon that impairs synthesis of HBeAg.

☐ Mutations in the DNA polymerase gene often arise during treatment with lamivudine, resulting in decreased binding of lamivudine. These mutations may lead to abrupt progression of chronic hepatitis B in patients previously stable on treatment.

☐ A mutation in the S gene, a glycine to arginine substitution at codon 145 (G145R), causes a type of HBsAg that binds poorly to anti-HBs antibody. Thus, a productive HBV infection can take place in somebody "adequately" immunized against HBV.

■ There are 3 major applications of molecular assays in HBV infection: making the initial diagnosis, particularly when serologic findings are equivocal; distinguishing replicative from nonreplicative chronic HBV infection; and monitoring therapy.

☐ With regard to diagnosis, HBV DNA can be detected approximately 3 weeks before HBsAg becomes detectable in serum. This lead-time is particularly useful to evaluate patients after an exposure (eg, a needle stick).

☐ The HBe antigen status is the traditional way to distinguish carriers who are replicative from those who are not. Certain limitations in this approach, such as a tendency of HBe antigen to be undetectable in reactivation disease or to never appear in precore mutations, have made HBV DNA a more attractive analyte for this purpose. Currently, those with more than 10^5 copies of HBV DNA per mL are considered replicative.

☐ The response to therapy is monitored in several ways: (1) in the liver biopsy, a decrease in the histologic activity index (HAI) of more than or equal to 2 is considered a histologic response, (2) normalization of serum alanine aminotransferase (ALT) is definitive of a biochemical response, and (3) either a negative HBeAg or an undetectable HBV DNA level (<10^5 copies/mL) is considered a virologic response.

■ Note that HBsAg status continues to define chronic HBV. Circulating HBV DNA can be found by means of polymerase chain reaction (PCR) in a high percentage of patients with negative HBsAg and positive anti-HBs, anti-HBe, and anti-HBc. The significance of this is unclear at this time.

Hepatitis C Virus (HCV)

■ HCV is an RNA virus from the *Flavivirus* family. It causes the vast majority of transfusion-associated viral hepatitis and the vast majority of what was previously called non-A, non-B hepatitis. About 55% to 85% of those infected with HCV will develop chronic HCV infection. About 10% to 15% of those with chronic HCV will develop cirrhosis, usually after an illness of about 20 years. Those with cirrhosis caused by HCV have a roughly 5% chance of developing hepatocellular carcinoma. The most powerful predictor of progression to cirrhosis is the finding of more-than-portal fibrosis (Ishak 3) on a liver biopsy.

■ HCV infection has traditionally been diagnosed with enzyme immunoassay (EIA)–based assays for anti-HCV antibodies, their presence indicative of infection. It is important to note that IgM and IgG anti-HCV cannot be reliably used to distinguish acute from chronic HCV infection; in fact, there is no reliable way to distinguish acute from chronic HCV infection and, for that matter, no compelling reason to do so. Most patients diagnosed with HCV, it is believed, are diagnosed with HCV in the chronic phase.

■ Both qualitative and quantitative tests are available for detecting HCV RNA. Qualitative assays for HCV RNA are based on conventional PCR or transcription-mediated amplification (TMA) platforms. The presence of HCV RNA in serum is the earliest marker of HCV infection. It is usually detectable within 1 to 2 weeks of exposure and precedes both the appearance of anti-HCV antibody and the elevation of ALT. For making the initial diagnosis of HCV infection, the anti-HCV antibody test is now augmented by molecular assays for HCV RNA. While either a qualitative or a quantitative HCR RNA test will suffice for this purpose, many clinicians request the quantitative test. Based on combined serologic and molecular assays, 4 sets of results are possible **T12.1**.

T12.1

Possible Results of Hepatitis C Virus (HCV) Testing

Anti-HCV	HCV RNA	Interpretation
–	–	No infection
+	–	Probably not HCV infection; may represent recovery from acute HCV; retest for HCV RNA in several weeks
–	+	Probable early HCV infection; may also be seen rarely in chronic HCV infection, when patient is profoundly immunosuppressed, agammaglobulinemic, or on hemodialysis; retest for anti-HCV in several weeks
+	+	Infection

- HCV RNA is particularly helpful for diagnosing transplacentally (vertically) transmitted HCV from mother to fetus. Since the neonate has circulating maternal antibody, the anti-HCV antibody test cannot be used.

- Donor blood can now be screened using qualitative HCV RNA tests. This can reduce the window period from about 70 days to about 40 days.

- Chronic HCV develops in over 60% of infections. In some patients, the decision is made to treat, and the standard treatment presently is a combination of peginterferon alpha with ribavirin (PEGIFNa/RBV). The most significant pretreatment predictor of treatment response is the viral genotype: genotypes 2 and 3 have a high (70%) rate of response; genotype 1 has a low (40%) rate of response. Furthermore, the nature and duration of treatment is influenced by the genotype. The other genotypes—4 through 9—have not been sufficiently studied because of low prevalence. Other pretreatment predictors of treatment response include viral load (<2 × 10^6 copies per mL portends a favorable response), biopsy assessment of fibrosis (less than cirrhosis is favorable), younger age, and female sex.

- HCV genotyping may be performed on the basis of either molecular or serologic assays. The molecular assays involve direct sequencing of portions of the HCV genome (eg, the 5V noncoding region), hybridization with genotype-specific sequences, or restriction fragment length polymorphism (RFLP) analysis. Serologic assays detect serum antibodies against genotype-specific antigens. In the United States, the most common HCV genotype is 1 (about 80% of patients). Genotype 1 is further subdivided

into 1a (about 60%) and 1b (about 20%), but to date, no clinical significance has been attributed to differing genotypes. Genotype 2 represents about 20% of all infections, and genotype 3 about 5%.

- Quantitative assays for HCV RNA can be performed by real-time reverse transcriptase PCR (RT-PCR), transcription-mediated amplification (TMA), or branched DNA (bDNA). These techniques must be capable of detecting levels as low as 50 IU/mL, because this is the definition of a sustained virologic response. Furthermore, they must be equally sensitive to RNA from the different genotypes. The same testing platform should be used throughout treatment, because quantitative results of the different methods are not directly comparable. The desired endpoint of treatment is a sustained virologic response (SVR), defined as undetectable HCV RNA for a period of 24 weeks (6 months) after the end of treatment. Early clearance (undetectable) or rapid decline (>2 logs) of HCV RNA is predictive of a sustained virologic response.

- The liver biopsy remains important, particularly in making treatment decisions in patients infected with HCV genotype 1 or 4 to 9. Furthermore, the quantitative HCV RNA reflects neither the degree (grade) of hepatic inflammation nor the extent (stage) of hepatic fibrosis. And while HCV RNA is a good predictor of treatment response, it does not correlate, as histology does, with the likelihood of progressing to cirrhosis. Serial ALT measurements are only slightly better at predicting histologic findings in the liver. Most clinicians, therefore, continue to rely on the liver biopsy for assessing severity of liver disease, predicting prognosis, and deciding whether to treat.

Human Immunodeficiency Virus (HIV)

HIV-1

- HIV-1 is the major cause of acquired immunodeficiency syndrome (AIDS) in the world. HIV-2 is found predominantly in parts of West Africa. In most ways similar to HIV-1, HIV-2 is considered somewhat less virulent.

- For classification purposes, HIV-1 is divided into major (M) and outlier (O) groups, with M group viruses further segregated into subtypes (clades) A through H. These distinctions are based on genetic diversity present in the *gag* and *env* genes. Subtype C viruses account for half of all HIV-1 infections worldwide, because of its predominance among the large number of cases in sub-Saharan Africa, followed by subtype A (12%), subtype B (10%), subtype G (6%), and subtype D (3%). In the United States and Europe, subtype B predominates.

Diagnosis

- Enzyme-linked immunosorbent assay (ELISA) is the principal method for HIV screening. The sensitivity of current HIV ELISA tests is more than 99%. Anti-HIV antibodies are usually detectable within 6 to 8 weeks of infection; however, some patients experience seroconversion only after many months. So it is in these first weeks to months that most false-negative ELISA findings occur (the window period). Because of passive transfer of maternal antibodies, the serologic diagnosis of neonatal HIV infection is not reliable. ELISA has suffered from insensitivity to HIV-2 and HIV-1 subtype O; however with recent improvements most, but not all, cases of HIV-2 and subtype O can be detected with current ELISA assays.

- Confirmatory testing is based generally on the Western blot. In this assay, a sample containing known HIV proteins is subjected to gel electrophoresis. The gel is then transferred (blotted) onto nitrocellulose paper, to which patient serum is added. After staining, visible bands reflect antibodies in the patient's serum. The Centers for Disease Control and Prevention (CDC) has defined a positive HIV-1 Western blot as the presence of any 2 of the following bands: p24, gp41, gp120/160. If no bands are present, the test result is considered negative. If 1 or more bands are present but not in a combination that meets criteria for positivity, then the test result is considered indeterminate. The specificity of Western blot, when these criteria are rigorously applied, approaches 100%. Conventional Western blot results can give a false-negative result in subtype O, and false-positive Western blots have been reported in hyperbilirubinemia, patients with HLA antibodies, autoantibodies, and polyclonal hypergammaglobulinemia. Patients who test as indeterminate should have a repeat test within 6 months. Those who are repeatedly indeterminate over 6 months and who have no risk factors can be considered negative. If there are risk factors and repeatedly indeterminate results, a nucleic acid–based test is advised.

- Detection of proviral DNA can be used to confirm the diagnosis of HIV infection. Proviral DNA is the result of HIV RNA reverse transcription into cDNA which then integrates into the host-cell genome. Its presence can be detected with PCR; the sensitivity of this assay is about 95% and the specificity 98%.

- The p24 protein is expressed very early in HIV infection, capable of reducing the width of the serologic window by more than half. Serum p24 assays are based on an antigen-capture ELISA platform, in which a solid substrate with attached anti-p24 antibody is washed over with patient sample (thus capturing the p24). Enzyme-linked IgG is then added, and the reaction is measured colorimetrically. While the p24 assay has been used to diagnose pre-seroconversion HIV infection, the quantitative p24 level has been used for predicting prognosis (this has been supplanted by viral load testing).

- Detection of HIV infection shortly after a presumed exposure may be very important, because there appears to be significant merit in the early administration of highly-active antiretroviral therapy (HAART). Serology (ELISA and Western blot) is not useful in this setting, because antibodies do not reliably appear for many weeks. The p24 antigen seems to wane at various times during acute infection, leading to a suboptimal sensitivity of 89%. The best test in this setting may be HIV RNA quantification. HIV proviral DNA detection may be just as good but has not been studied in the acute stage. The sensitivity of HIV RNA in acute infection is essentially 100%. However, the specificity is not 100%, and some false positives occur; as soon as feasible, a positive HIV RNA should be confirmed with ELISA and Western blot.

■ Detection of HIV infection in neonates and infants is sometimes difficult. ELISA and Western blot are not useful because of the persistence of transplacentally acquired maternal antibodies. Furthermore, p24 antigen has a poor sensitivity in neonates and young infants, as low as 20% in the first month of life. PCR testing for HIV proviral DNA is the recommended test in this setting, but HIV RNA may be equally good. Umbilical cord blood should not be tested.

Monitoring

■ The CD4 count has been used for some time to monitor disease progression. The count is determined by means of flow cytometry. Counts are monitored approximately every 6 months while the disease is stable and more frequently when treatment is being altered or there is illness. While CD4 counts are still instrumental in making treatment decisions (eg, the decision to instigate *Pneumocystis carinii* [PCP] prophylaxis) and to define AIDS, the quantitative HIV RNA (viral load) is the preferred means of assessing response to antiretroviral therapy.

■ Quantification of circulating HIV RNA (viral load) has become a mainstay in HIV management.

 □ Long-term outcome correlates extremely well with the viral load (quantity of HIV RNA). The viral load has been found to be superior to the CD4 count for predicting disease progression; however, it appears that the combination of the 2 is superior to either in isolation. Furthermore, while viral load correlates very well with long-term (>10 years) prognosis, the CD4 count correlates better with short-term (6 months) prognosis and susceptibility to infection.

 □ Transient increases in the quantitative viral load may occur following immune provocation; eg, following immunization. Up to a 0.3-log change can be attributed to nonspecific alteration in the quantitative HIV RNA; changes greater than 0.5 log are considered significant.

 □ The viral load is the primary variable used to determine when to initiate HAART, and it is the viral load that determines the efficacy of this treatment. The anticipated duration of viral suppression relates to both the rate of decline in viral load and the magnitude of the nadir.

 □ 3 methods are currently available for measuring the HIV RNA (viral load): real-time RT-PCR,

branched DNA (bDNA), and nucleic acid sequence–based amplification (NASBA). These methods have comparable analytic sensitivity and precision, but the quantities cannot be directly compared between methods. An individual patient should be followed with a single method. In the RT-PCR assay, HIV-1 RNA and known standard RNA (a control of known copy number) compete for amplification in the same reaction chamber. First, the RNA is converted to cDNA by adding reverse transcriptase. Then a specific portion of the cDNA—within the *gag* gene—is amplified by PCR. Enzyme-linked oligonucleotide probes are added, 1 complementary for the HIV gag sequence and 1 for the RNA standard, and reaction product is measured. The ratio of reaction products determines the quantity of HIV RNA that is present. In the bDNA assay, complementary oligonucleotide is fixed to a solid substrate (microplate). The patient sample is added, capturing any HIV RNA present. Then chemiluminescent enzyme-linked probes are added, which are complementary to additional sequences of HIV RNA. The chemiluminescent signal is measured and compared with a known standard. The NASBA method is similar in concept to RT-PCR, with the exception that RNA is amplified instead of DNA.

 □ The goal of therapy is to reach a viral load below the lower limit of detection.

Detection of Drug Resistance

■ As in bacteriology, viral drug resistance can be measured as the ability of the organism to replicate in the presence of drug (phenotypic testing); alternatively, drug resistance can be evaluated by looking for genetic aberrations known to be associated with drug resistance (genotypic testing).

■ Genotypic testing can be performed by direct sequencing, with comparison to known sequences, or by hybridization assays. In either case, interpretation of the findings is complex, as (1) there are many mutations that do not display a binary relationship between mutation and drug resistance, (2) new mutations are always emerging, and (3) treatment nearly always involves a combination of drugs, for which the effect of a mutation is significantly more difficult to predict.

12: Microbiology

Human Immunodeficiency Virus (HIV)>Detection of Drug Resistance | Bacterial Infection>Primary Diagnosis; Detection of Antimicrobial Resistance

- Despite these challenges, there is evidence that treatment in combination with genotypic drug resistance information is more effective than treatment without. At this time, drug resistance testing is recommended for those who do not respond (failed viral load reduction) to first-line treatment.

Bacterial Infection

Primary Diagnosis

- For most bacterial infections, conventional culture methods provide adequate rapidity, sensitivity, and specificity. Molecular diagnosis is principally of interest for those bacteria that are slow-growing, fastidious, or cannot be cultured. Examples include the detection of *Bordetella pertussis* (whooping cough), *Borrelia burgdorferi* (Lyme disease), *Rickettsia rickettsii* (Rocky Mountain spotted fever), *Bartonella henselae* (bacillary angiomatosis), and *Ehrlichia chaffeensis* (human monocytic Ehrlichiosis). Furthermore, some organisms that are readily isolated may be growth-impaired by delayed transport, inappropriate collection systems, or preculture administration of antibiotics.

- While a small number of assays are commercially available at this time, there is now a mass of literature on the successful identification of bacteria through amplification of genus- or species-specific DNA sequences. In addition, panels have been developed that, depending on the clinical presentation, are capable of detecting several of the most common isolates. For example, assays are presently commercially available for detection of slow-growing causes of sexually transmitted diseases (eg, *C trachomatis N gonorrhoeae*, and herpes simplex virus), causes of atypical pneumonia (eg, *Chlamydia pneumoniae, Mycobacterium tuberculosis, Mycoplasma pneumoniae*), and causes of septic arthritis (culture has only 50% sensitivity for gonococcal arthritis).

Detection of Antimicrobial Resistance

- Antimicrobial-resistant bacteria have caused great difficulty in hospitalized patients and are now emerging in community-acquired infections. Principal concerns are methicillin (oxacillin)–resistant *Staphylococcus aureus* (MRSA), some of which are now vancomycin resistant, and vancomycin-resistant enterococci.

- While identifying most bacteria with conventional culture-based procedures may take 24 to 48 hours, detecting antimicrobial resistance with conventional methods may take an additional 24 to 72 hours. Molecular methods can detect antimicrobial resistance in laboratory isolates or directly from clinical specimens within hours.

- Staphylococci
  - Staphylococci are common colonizers, being present on the skin and nares of uninfected patients and hospital staff. Between 30% and 60% of healthy adults are colonized with *S aureus*, primarily in the nares. About 10% are colonized with MRSA.
  - Methicillin acts by binding to and inactivating proteins involved in cell wall synthesis called penicillin-binding proteins (PBPs). Low-level methicillin resistance results either from production of a large quantity of β-lactamase or by mutations in bacterial-encoded PBP such that they bind less avidly. The major mechanism by which *S aureus* acquires high-level methicillin resistance is the production of a foreign (acquired) PBP, called PBP2a. The *mecA* gene, which is found outside the normal bacterial genome on a mobile element called the staphylococcal cassette chromosome mec (SCCmec), encodes PBP2a.
  - MRSA strains are usually resistant not only to methicillin but (based on other mechanisms it is thought) are multidrug resistant. Resistance in MRSA includes fluoroquinolones (eg, ciprofloxacin), macrolides (erythromycin), aminoglycosides (gentamicin), and others. Fluoroquinolones were initially considered a useful drug class in MRSA, especially because they can be taken by mouth, but this is no longer the case as an increasing proportion of MRSA is also ciprofloxacin-resistant.
  - Vancomycin continues to be effective in most MRSA strains, but it must be administered intravenously. Furthermore, in recent years vancomycin resistance has emerged in a growing number of cases. Vancomycin resistance is thought to be caused by 2 mechanisms: cell wall thickening (which causes a moderate degree of resistance) and acquisition of a gene called *vanA* (which is associated with marked resistance).

12: Microbiology

Bacterial Infection>Detection of Antimicrobial Resistance | Mycobacteria>Diagnosis; Molecular Species Identification; Molecular Typing

□ Detecting strains that are methicillin resistant by virtue of mecA by traditional methods is difficult, because these strains exhibit so-called heteroresistance (a mixture of resistant and sensitive bacteria). Traditional (agar-based) susceptibility tests may appear falsely sensitive.

□ The detection of the *mecA* gene by PCR has become the gold standard for detection of MRSA strains. One problem with PCR is that inhibitors may be present, requiring the co-amplification of a constitutive bacterial gene as an internal positive control. For example, 1 assay uses a multiplex PCR that co-amplifies *mecA* and bacterial *gyrA* gene as the internal control; another amplifies *mecA* with the *femA* gene. Several non-PCR genotype-based screening assays are available with comparable performance, including a fluorescein-labeled *mecA* gene probe, a latex agglutination test that uses beads coated with anti-PBP2 antibodies, and others. The advantages of these screening assays include rapid (2-hour) turnaround time and avoidance of establishing the infrastructure for PCR.

Mycobacteria

Diagnosis

■ Traditionally, the diagnosis of tuberculosis has been made based on a positive culture with or without a positive smear (eg, of sputum) for acid fast bacilli (AFB). This approach suffers from several limitations, including (1) the lengthy incubation period required for mycobacteria, (2) the low sensitivity of direct smears for AFB, and (3) the species nonspecificity of a positive AFB smear. The reported sensitivity of AFB smear microscopy using the traditional Ziehl-Neelsen staining varies from 20% to 70%.

■ At this time, molecular methods have been approved for direct detection of mycobacteria, collectively referred to as nucleic acid amplification tests (NAAT). These are based on amplification of either *M tuberculosis* species–specific mRNA or *Mycobacterium* genus–specific rRNA.

■ In the diagnosis of *M tuberculosis*, the CDC now recommends that AFB smear and NAAT be performed on the first sputum sample collected. If both are positive, then the diagnosis of pulmonary tuberculosis is made. If the smear is positive and the NAAT is negative, the CDC recommends testing the sputum sample for inhibitors (by adding lysed *M tuberculosis* to the sample and repeating the NAAT assay. If inhibitors are not detected, then testing is repeated on additional samples. If the sputum is repeatedly AFB positive with negative NAAT, then the diagnosis of non-TB mycobacterial infection is made. When the AFB stain is negative but the sputum is NAAT positive, additional samples should be tested. If the sputum is repeatedly NAAT positive but AFB negative, then a diagnosis of pulmonary tuberculosis is made.

Molecular Species Identification

■ The current microbiologic approach to tuberculosis involves (1) detection of growth in culture and (2) species identification. Initial detection has been made faster using broth methods in which growth is detected within 1 to 2 weeks by automated methods. For species identification, however, a number of growth characteristics and biochemical test reactions must be noted in a process that can take 6 weeks or longer.

■ NAAT probes can be used for the rapid identification of organisms growing on solid or broth media which can distinguish *M tuberculosis, Mycobacterium avium complex, Mycobacterium kansasii,* and *Mycobacterium gordonae.*

Molecular Typing (Strain Identification)

■ Strain identification is relevant primarily for epidemiologic purposes, particularly for identifying the source of an outbreak.

■ The most widely used technique is RFLP analysis of a sequence called IS6110. IS6110 is a sequence repeated throughout the genome in copy numbers ranging from 0 to 30. Endonuclease digestion will yield strain-specific patterns after gel electrophoresis. Isolates with matching bands can be considered related (clonal), indicating that that are derived from a common source.

■ Another approach is based on a separate sequence known as IS1081, a GC-rich sequence with polymorphism throughout the *M tuberculosis* population.

Detection of Antimicrobial Resistance

- The current recommendation is for testing isolates against isoniazid (at 2 concentrations), rifampin, ethambutol, and pyrazinamide.

- Traditional testing for drug resistance is a slow process and depends on the ability of the isolate to grow in an uninhibited fashion in the presence of antibiotics. It has been known for some time that organisms acquire resistance through the acquisition of genetic changes—through such mechanisms as spontaneous mutation and bacteriophage transfer. Instead of traditional assays, one can simply look for these changes in the bacterial genome. For example, the anti-tuberculosis agent pyrazinamide must be activated by a bacterial enzyme which converts it to its active form, pyrazinoic acid. The *pncA* (pyrazinamidase) gene product carries out this conversion, and mutations in the *pncA* gene can result in reduced activation of pyrazinamide and therefore resistance. Because these mutations can be spread throughout the coding sequence, the entire gene must be sequenced to locate these mutations. The *katG* gene mutations are the cause of isoniazid resistance. Mutations in codon 315 of the *katG* gene are responsible for most instances of isoniazid resistance. *RIF* gene mutations are the basis for rifampin resistance. Like mutations in the *katG* gene, these occur in a limited "hotspot" region of the gene.

- DNA sequencing is considered the definitive way to identify resistance-associated mutations, but there are several limitations. For 1, this approach is labor-intensive and expensive. Several more rapid identification kits have been developed to screen for mutant alleles after DNA amplification with PCR.

References

Aires de Sousa M, de Lencastre H. Evolution of sporadic isolates of methicillin-resistant *Staphylococcus aureus* (MRSA) in hospitals and their similarities to isolates of community acquired MRSA. *J Clin Microbiol* 2003; 41: 3806-3815.

Bangham CR. HTLV-1 infections. *J Clin Pathol* 2000; 53: 581-586.

Barlow K, Tosswill J, Clewley J. Analysis and genotyping of PCR products of the amplicor HIV-1 kit. *J Virol Methods* 1995; 52: 65-74.

Chevaliez S, Pawlotsky J-M. Use of virologic assays in the diagnosis and management of hepatitis C virus infection. *Clin Liver Dis* 2005; 9: 371-382.

Chinen J, Shearer WT. Molecular virology and immunology of HIV infection. *J Allergy Clin Immunol* 2002; 110: 189-198.

Cooksey RC. Recent advances in laboratory procedures for pathogenic mycobacteria. *Clin Lab Med* 2003; 23: 801-821.

Daar E, Little S, Pitt J. Diagnosis of primary HIV-1 infection. *Ann Intern Med* 2001; 134: 25-29.

Daley CL. Molecular epidemiology: a tool for understanding control of tuberculosis transmission. *Clin Chest Med* 2005; 26: 217-231.

Dickson DW, Rademakers R, Hutton ML. Progressive supranuclear palsy: pathology and genetics. *Brain Pathol* 2007; 17: 74-82.

Dumler JS. Molecular methods for Ehrlichiosis and Lyme disease. *Clin Lab Med* 2003; 23: 867-884.

Fish DN, Ohlinger MJ. Antimicrobial resistance: factors and outcomes. *Crit Care Clin* 2006; 22: 291-311.

Fluit AC, Visser MR, Schmitz FJ. Molecular detection of antimicrobial resistance. *Clin Microbiol Rev* 2001; 14: 836-871.

Glenn JS. Molecular virology of the hepatitis C virus: implication for novel therapies. *Infect Dis Clin North Am* 2006; 20: 81-98.

References

Harris KR, Dighe AS. Laboratory testing for viral hepatitis. *Am J Clin Pathol* 2002; 118: S18-S25.

Hiramatsu K. Vancomycin-resistant *Staphylococcus aureus*: a new model of antibiotic resistance. *Lancet Infect Dis* 2001; 1: 147-155.

Hirsch MS, Brun F, Clotet B, et al. Antiretroviral drug resistance testing in adults infected with human immunodeficiency virus type 1: 2003 recommendations of an International AIDS Society. *Clin Infect Dis* 2003; 37: 113-128.

Houpikian P, Raoult D. Diagnostic methods current best practices and guidelines for identification of difficult-to-culture pathogens in infective endocarditis. *Infect Dis Clin North Am* 2002; 16: 377-392.

Karim SSA, Abdool Karim Q, Gouws E, et al. Global epidemiology of HIV-AIDS. *Infect Dis Clin North Am* 2007; 21: 1-17.

Lauer GM, Walker BD. Medical progress: hepatitis C infection. *N Engl J Med* 2001; 345: 41-52.

Louie M, Cockerill FR III. Susceptibility testing: phenotypic and genotypic gests for bacteria and mycobacteria. *Infect Dis Clin North Am* 2001; 15: 1205-1226.

Nagai M, Usuku K, Matsumoto W. Analysis of HTLV-I proviral load in 202 HAM/TSP patients and 243 asymptomatic HTLV-I carriers: high proviral load strongly predisposes to HAM/TSP. *J Neurovirol* 1998; 4: 586-593.

Nolte FS. Impact of viral load testing on patient care. *Arch Pathol Lab Med* 1999; 123: 1011-1014.

Pawlotsky JM. Use and interpretation of virological tests for hepatitis C. *Hepatology* 2002; 36(suppl 1): S65-S73.

Picken MM, Picken RN, Han D, et al. A two year prospective study to compare culture and polymerase chain reaction amplification for the detection and diagnosis of lyme borreliosis. *Mol Pathol* 1997; 50: 186-193.

Rebucci C, Cerino A, Cividini A, et al. Monitoring response to antiviral therapy for patients with chronic hepatitis C virus infection by a core-antigen assay. *J Clin Microbiol* 2003; 41: 3881-3884.

Rice LB. Antimicrobial resistance in Gram-positive bacteria. *Am J Med* 2006; 119(6A): S11-S19.

Sakoulas G, Gold HS, Venkataraman L, et al. Methicillin-resistant *Staphylococcus aureus*: comparison of susceptibility testing methods and analysis of mecA-positive susceptible strains. *J Clin Microbiol* 2001; 39: 3946-3951.

Steketee RW, Abrams EJ, Thea DM, et al. Early detection of perinatal human immunodeficiency virus type 1 infection using HIV RNA amplification and detection. *J Infect Dis* 1997; 175: 707-711.

Sterling TR, Vlahov D, Astermborski J, et al. Initial plasma HIV-1 RNA levels and progression to AIDS in women and men. *N Engl J Med* 2001; 344: 720-725.

Swenson JM, Williams PP, Killgore G, et al. Performance of eight methods, including two new rapid methods, for detection of oxacillin resistance in a challenge set of *Staphylococcus aureus* organisms. *J Clin Microbiol* 2001; 39: 3785-3788.

Van Swieten J, Spillantini MG. Hereditary frontotemporal dementia caused by *Tau* gene mutations. *Brain Pathol* 2007; 17: 63-73.

Thomson MM, Parez-Alvarez L, Naijera R. Molecular epidemiology of HIV-1 genetic forms and its significance for vaccine development and therapy. *Lancet Infect Dis* 2002; 2: 461-471.

Whiley DM, Tapsall JW, Sloots TP. Nucleic acid amplification testing for *Neisseria gonorrhoeae*. *J Mol Diagn* 2006; 8: 3-15.

Wolk D, Mitchell S, Patel R. Principles of molecular microbiology testing methods. *Infect Dis Clin North Am* 2001; 15: 1157-1204.

Woods GL. Molecular methods in the detection and identification of mycobacterial infections. *Arch Pathol Lab Med* 1999; 123: 1002-1006.

Woods GL. The mycobacteriology laboratory and new diagnostic techniques. *Infect Dis Clin North Am* 2002: 127-144.

Yang S, Rothman RE. PCR-based diagnostics for infectious diseases: uses, limitations, and future applications in acute-care settings. *Lancet Infect Dis* 2004; 4: 337-348.

Chapter 13

Inherited Tumor Syndromes

13: Inherited Tumor Syndromes

Gastrointestinal Tumor Syndromes>General Features; APC-Associated Syndromes: Familial Adenomatous Polyposis, Gardner Syndrome, and Turcot Syndrome

Gastrointestinal Tumor Syndromes

General Features

- About 5% to 10% of colorectal carcinomas arise in association with an inherited germline mutation. Furthermore, the very same genes that underlie inherited colorectal carcinoma syndromes are commonly found to be mutated in sporadic tumors (somatic mutations). While these syndromes are transmitted in classic Mendelian patterns, there are undoubtedly numerous less-well-defined predisposition genes. This assertion arises from numerous observations regarding apparently sporadic colorectal carcinomas: that first-degree relatives of patients with sporadic tumors are themselves at increased risk; that this risk is enhanced by having more than 1 affected relative or 1 affected while young; and that the concordance risk for identical twins is over 30%.

- There are 2 major types of inherited colorectal carcinoma: (1) the adenomatous polyposis coli (*APC*) gene-associated conditions such as FAP, and (2) the mismatch-repair (MMR)-related conditions, such as hereditary nonpolyposis colorectal cancer (HNPCC), which are caused by mutations in 1 of several mismatch repair genes.

- APC-related tumors generally are located more distally (left colon and rectum). They have the histologic features of usual-type colonic adenocarcinoma (formation of abortive glands, dirty necrosis, infiltrative tumor margin), DNA aneuploidy, additional somatically acquired mutations in k-ras and p53, and a more aggressive biology. In contrast, MMR-related tumors tend to be proximally located (right colon), and to express a characteristic mucinous or medullary carcinomalike appearance. Their DNA is more likely to be diploid, and they behave indolently.

APC-Associated Syndromes: Familial Adenomatous Polyposis (FAP), Gardner Syndrome, and Turcot Syndrome

- The common feature in the APC group of disorders, in addition to *APC* gene mutations, is the presence of a large number of adenomatous polyps, predominantly in the colon. The adenomatous polyp in FAP is histologically indistinguishable from other adenomas, characterized as a discrete, raised (sessile or pedunculated) lesion composed of dysplastic colonic epithelium. The dysplasia is usually of low grade, distinguished by abnormal but not overly complex crypt branching, paucity of goblet cells, nuclear enlargement, and stratification. Just as in sporadic adenomas, these usually have tubular architecture but may occasionally be villous or tubulovillous, and, over time, may demonstrate high-grade dysplasia.

- The APC-related group of disorders is caused by mutations in the *APC* gene, located on 5q. Several hundred different mutations have been described, but a few generalizations are worth noting:

  - Nearly all mutations that result in the full FAP syndrome are mutations that result in *premature truncation* of the APC protein and occur between codons 169 and 1393. Marked polyposis, with several thousand polyps, is associated with mutations between 1250 and 1393. The most common of these is a 5–base pair deletion at codon 1309.

  - The attenuated form of FAP (as described later in this section) is associated with mutations at the extreme 5′ and 3′ ends of the *APC* gene (before 169 or after 1393).

  - A mutation at codon 1307, the I1307K mutation, is present in about 6% of Ashkenazi Jews and produces a partial FAP phenotype, with only a moderately increased risk of carcinoma. It does this by a somewhat unique mechanism, the production of an adenine-poor region (oligoadenine tract) that results in slippage of DNA polymerase.

  - Mutations between codons 460 and 1440 are associated with congenital hypertrophy of the pigmented retinal epithelium (CHPRE).

  - Mutations between codons 1440 and 1578 are associated with desmoid tumors.

- Because of the large number of potential mutations, definitive molecular diagnosis of FAP requires direct DNA sequencing of the entire *APC* gene. This can be costly, so several screening assays may be employed, including a protein truncation assay, conformation-sensitive gel electrophoresis (CSGE), and denaturing gradient gel electrophoresis (DGGE). Because the overwhelming majority of mutations causing FAP cause truncation of the *APC* gene product, truncation testing is capable of effectively screening nearly all clinically significant cases. An in vitro system is used which is capable of transcribing and translating the APC gene. The recovered protein product is then subjected to electrophoresis to determine its size.

- The normal APC gene product acts as a tumor suppressor protein that appears to be involved in maintaining a normal level of apoptosis, regulating cell entry into the cell cycle, and maintaining chromosomal positioning during mitosis through anchoring mechanisms. The APC protein exerts many of its effects through interaction with a second protein, β-catenin.

- Familial adenomatous polyposis.

  □ Without colectomy, colorectal carcinoma is an inevitability in FAP. By the age of 20 years, most patients have at least 1 adenomatous polyp. By the age of 35 years, the colon is carpeted with 100 polyps. By the age of 50 years (average age 39 years), most have developed adenocarcinoma. Overall, FAP is estimated to cause about 1% of all cases of colorectal carcinoma. In addition, there is an increased incidence of gastric polyps (fundic gland polyps, especially) and small intestinal polyps (adenomas) with a slightly increased risk of small bowel adenocarcinoma, ampullary adenocarcinoma, thyroid cancer, and fibromatosis (desmoids). The recommended treatment for FAP is prophylactic colectomy in young adulthood.

  □ A somewhat lower risk for colon cancer and fewer adenomatous polyps (less than 100, with an average of 30) characterize a variant form of FAP, so-called attenuated FAP. These polyps tend to be located more proximally, and colon cancer develops at a somewhat older age.

  □ While most cases are inherited in an autosomal dominant manner because of transmission of a mutation in the *APC* gene as many as 30% represent a new mutation (a simplex case).

  □ FAP may be considered the prototypical hereditary tumor syndrome. It demonstrates features that should lead the physician to suspect such a syndrome in any given patient: a malignancy presenting at an unusually young age and the development of multiple (synchronous or metachronous) such tumors. Other clues, not seen in FAP, include a characteristic histologic appearance (eg, Lynch syndrome tumors and *BRCA*-associated breast tumors) and tumor types that are uncommon (eg, medullary thyroid carcinoma). Hereditary cancer syndromes can be identified through the demonstration of specific germline mutations. That is, the disease-causing mutation is found in all somatic cells, not just the tumor cells. A germline mutation is one that is present in all cells in the body (all somatic cells), whereas a somatic mutation is found only in the lesional cells.

- Gardner syndrome is an autosomal dominant disorder combining the features of FAP with epidermal cysts, osteomas, and fibromatosis (desmoids). The epidermal cysts are found in more than 50% of patients and tend to appear on the lower extremities, face, and scalp. Osteomas, located most frequently in the mandible or maxilla, occur in at least 75% of patients. Desmoid tumors may be of either the visceral or the nonvisceral type. Additional features may include pilomatricomas, dental abnormalities, and pigmented ocular lesions of the ocular fundus termed *congenital hypertrophy of the retinal epithelium.*

- Turcot syndrome is the association of adenomatous polyposis and central nervous system (CNS) tumors, most commonly medulloblastoma and glioblastoma multiforme. While this association has been recognized for a long time, the availability of molecular testing has permitted distinction of 2 types of Turcot syndrome. Most (70%) of cases are caused by germline mutations in the APC gene; the CNS tumors seen in this type of Turcot syndrome are mainly medulloblastomas and, less commonly, low-grade astrocytomas or ependymomas. Around 30% have a normal APC gene and instead have mutations in 1 of the mismatch repair (MMR) genes associated with HNPCC (see following subsection). Glioblastoma multiforme is a feature of this variant of Turcot syndrome.

MMR-Associated Syndromes: Hereditary Nonpolyposis Colorectal Carcinoma (Lynch Syndrome) and Muir-Torre Syndrome

- Hereditary non-polyposis colorectal carcinoma (HNPCC) is an autosomal dominant condition associated with a 60% to 80% lifetime risk of colorectal carcinoma. It is caused by germline mutations that result in defective mismatch repair (MMR), which in turn results in microsatellite instability (MSI).

- There are 2 main types of HNPCC: Lynch syndrome I (colon cancer), and Lynch syndrome II (colon, endometrial, and ovarian cancer).

- Additional tumors found with increased incidence in HNPCC include small intestinal adenocarcinoma,

Gastrointestinal Tumor Syndromes>MMR-Associated Syndromes: Hereditary Nonpolyposis Colorectal Carcinoma and Muir-Torre Syndrome

pancreaticobiliary adenocarcinoma, gastric adenocarcinoma, and urothelial carcinoma.

- HNPCC is caused by a germline (present in all somatic cells) mutation in 1 of the DNA mismatch repair (MMR) genes: *MLH1*, *MSH2*, *MSH6*, *PMS2*, *MSH3*, *PMS1*, and *MLH3*. Taken together, *MLH1* (40%), *MSH2* (40%), and *MSH6* (10%) account for more than 90% of cases. Mutations are of several types, most often resulting in premature truncation. In addition, an unusual mechanism involving germline hypermethylation (germline epimutation) has been described some cases of HNPCC (and is the most common mechanism in sporadic MSI tumors).

- Approximately 15% of sporadic colorectal carcinomas display MSI, caused by somatic cell inactivation of the MMR genes by hypermethylation. Most commonly inactivated in these sporadic cases is the *MLH1* gene. Thus, the mere demonstration of MSI in a tumor is not diagnostic of HNPCC. MSI tumors in HNPCC tend to arise at a younger age than sporadic MSI-high tumors. Furthermore, HNPCC tumors are more likely to be tubular adenoma-associated; while sporadic MSI-high tumors are more often serrated adenoma-associated.

- Nonetheless, MSI tumors, with or without HNPCC, have unique biologic features. They tend to be located in the right colon, and they are often large at presentation (probably a reflection of their location rather than their genetics). Histologically, they may display trabecular, mucinous (colloid), or signet-ring growth. They tend to have prominent tumor-infiltrating lymphocytes (TIL) and a peritumoral "Crohn-like" nodular lymphoid infiltrate. A "pushing" rather than infiltrative tumor margin is characteristic. Because of this circumscribed appearance, high nuclear grade, and infiltrating lymphocytes, the tumors have been described as medullary-like (referring to medullary breast carcinoma). Despite their high-grade appearance and large size, MSI tumors have a relatively favorable clinical course, with a lower incidence of metastasis, and longer overall survival compared with MSI-stable tumors. Furthermore, MSI tumors do not benefit from adjuvant chemotherapy. Again, these generalities apply whether the tumor is a product of HNPCC or is a sporadic MSI tumor.

- Like colonic tumors, HNPCC-related endometrial carcinomas appear to have a medullary-like appearance. They have been described as having high nuclear grade, a Crohn-like lymphoid reaction, tumor-infiltrating lymphocytes, and a pushing margin. Further, there is an increased rate of angiolymphatic invasion.

- While the gold standard for mutation detection is direct DNA sequencing of the suspected gene, this process would be extremely difficult in the case of HNPCC, because there are not only multiple genes involved but also multiple possible mutations in each. Thus, the approach to molecular diagnosis in HNPCC involves 2 tiers of screening: first, clinicopathologic criteria are applied to determine which patients should be studied, and second, indirect assays are applied to determine which patients should be genotyped. Even in patients qualifying on both counts, sequencing is often confined only to *MLH1* and *MSH2*, the location of the vast majority of HNPCC-causing mutations.

- With regard to clinicopathologic criteria, the Amsterdam criteria were the first established, later to be modified (Amsterdam II). While identifying a great number of cases, the iterations of the Amsterdam criteria proved too exclusive. Slightly more liberal (and thereby more sensitive) Bethesda guidelines were then published and themselves modified. The modified Bethesda criteria are as follows: (1) colorectal carcinoma in a patient younger than 50 years; (2) patient of any age with 2 synchronous or metachronous HNPCC-related tumors (colonic carcinoma, small bowel carcinoma, gastric carcinoma, urothelial carcinoma, biliary carcinoma, glioblastoma multiforme, sebaceous adenomas, keratoacanthomas); (3) colorectal carcinoma with morphologic findings suggestive of MSI in a patient younger than 60 years (tumor-infiltrating lymphocytes, Crohn-like lymphocytic reaction, mucinous or signet-ring cell differentiation, medullary growth pattern); (4) colorectal carcinoma in a patient whose first-degree relative had an HNPCC-related tumor before the age of 50 years or adenomas before the age of 40 years; (5) colorectal carcinoma in a patient with 2 first-degree relatives having HNPCC-related tumors at any age.

- For the second tier of screening, in those patients fulfilling the above criteria or in whom testing is otherwise desired, 2 types of tests are often employed: MSI testing or immunohistochemistry (IHC).

  □ MSI testing is performed on neoplastic and nonneoplastic tissue. A microsatellite is a DNA sequence, normally present in the genome, which consists of nucleotide repeats; eg, a stretch

Gastrointestinal Tumor Syndromes>MMR-Associated Syndromes: Hereditary Nonpolyposis Colorectal Carcinoma and Muir-Torre Syndrome; Juvenile Polyposis

of several CA dinucleotides. The number of repeats is normally stable; that is, from 1 cell to the next the number is the same. MSI refers to a gain or loss in the number of repeats in tumor DNA compared with the number of repeats in the DNA of nontumor tissue. MSI testing is performed by extracting DNA from paraffin-embedded nonneoplastic and neoplastic tissue (either a carcinoma or an adenoma). Polymerase chain reaction (PCR), using a set of primers, is used to amplify 5 specific microsatellite regions—BAT25, BAT26 (both of which are regions of mononucleotide repeats), D2S123, D5S346, and D17S250 (regions of dinucleotide repeats). These regions from the tumor are compared with those from adjacent nonneoplastic tissue to assess for differences in length, indicative of MSI. Note that while a person with HNPCC has the responsible gene mutation in all cells of the body (a germline mutation), MSI will be confined to tumor tissue. That is, the gene causing MSI is present in tumor tissue and adjacent normal tissue, but MSI, while present in DNA, is a phenotypic, not a genotypic, feature. Tumors are classified as MSI-High (MSI-H) when differences are present in 2 or more markers, MSI-Low (MSI-L) when present in 1 marker, and microsatellite stable (MSS) when all markers are unchanged.

☐ IHC testing is performed on neoplastic and nonneoplastic tissue for expression of the proteins encoded by MMR genes: MLH1, PMS2, MSH2, and MSH6. While the analysis may be performed on either a carcinoma or an adenoma, sensitivity in adenomas is only about 60%. Dim or absent staining is indicative of gene mutation/inactivation. IHC appears to have good sensitivity (>90%) and specificity (nearly 100%) for MSI.

☐ If a tumor is deemed to have MSI by 1 of these studies, this implies that the patient may have HNPCC, and testing for mutations is indicated. Because there are several genes and no mutational hot-spots, DNA sequencing for mutation detection is a daunting prospect. The results of the screening tests (eg, immunohistochemistry) may point to a particular gene to study. Furthermore, several molecular laboratories employ a molecular screening assay (mutation scanning), which involves the amplification of large segments to detect physicochemical evidence of sequence changes;

sequencing is then restricted to those segments in which alterations are detected. These scanning techniques include denaturing high pressure liquid chromatography (DHPLC), conformation-sensitive gel electrophroreis (CSGE), denaturing gradient gel electrophoresis (DGGE), and others. All operate on the principal that a small genetic alteration (e.g., substitution or deletion) will produce a change in the properties (e.g., electrophoretic) of the oligonucleotide segment. Overall, these screening assays have less than 100% sensitivity (80%–90% is considered pretty good); even direct sequencing of the entire gene, however, lacks 100% sensitivity, because structural rearrangements (duplications or large deletions) can be missed by this technique.

■ Muir-Torre syndrome is a related condition. In 1967, Muir and Torre independently noted the association of cutaneous sebaceous adenomas and colorectal carcinoma. This tendency has been attributed to a DNA MM R gene mutation. Colonic polyps are present in only about half of the cases, but colonic adenocarcinoma develops in well over half of the cases. Other sites of malignancy include the larynx, duodenum, ileum, stomach, uterus, ovary, and urothelium.

■ Unlike FAP, colectomy is not currently recommended in HNPCC. The current recommendation is for annual colonoscopy, beginning at age 20 to 25 years. Once a malignancy is detected, however, colectomy may be recommended. Women with HNPCC should also undergo screening for tumors of the gynecologic tract. The current recommendation is for annual transvaginal ultrasound.

Juvenile Polyposis

■ Juvenile polyposis is associated with a moderately increased risk of colorectal cancer, but its foremost expression is the juvenile polyp. A number of juvenile polyps form in the stomach, small intestine, and large intestine. The juvenile polyp is a particular histologic type of polyp (the name does not refer to age of onset) with a smooth outer contour, cystically dilated mucus-filled glands lined by nonadenomatous epithelium, and a dense nonmuscular collagenous stroma permeated by inflammatory cells. Most affected individuals have some polyps by the age of 20 years, but the number of polyps developed over a lifetime is highly variable, ranging from 1 to over 100.

- The lifetime risk of malignancy ranges from 9% to 50%, and most of these are colorectal adenocarcinomas.

- Juvenile polyposis is inherited as an autosomal dominant trait. 2 genes have thus far been implicated: *BMPR1A* (10q22.3) and *MADH4/SMAD4* (18q21.1). However, these combined account for slightly fewer than half of all cases. A small subset of patients has mutations in the *PTEN* gene (causative of Cowden and Bannayan-Riley-Ruvalcaba syndromes) and in fact has juvenile polyps as part of 1 of those syndromes.

Peutz-Jeghers Syndrome (PJS)

- PJS is an autosomal dominant condition manifesting with mucocutaneous pigmentation and a particular type of hamartomatous polyp. There is a more than 90% lifetime risk of malignancy, with a risk of 50% by age 65 years, especially of the gastrointestinal tract and breast.

- Peutz-Jeghers polyps arise in greatest number in the small intestine, especially the jejunum, but also crop up in the stomach and colon. They begin to arise around the age of 10 years. Lined by mucinous epithelium, the distinguishing feature of the Peutz-Jeghers polyp is stroma built of thin complexly branching muscle bundles with an arborizing appearance.

- Mucocutaneous hyperpigmentation begins in early childhood with dark blue or brown macules which form around the mouth, eyes, nostrils, perianal area, and sometimes the fingers.

- The sex cord tumor with annular tubules (SCTAT) of the ovary and adenoma malignum (minimal deviation adenocarcinoma) of the cervix are largely restricted to Peutz-Jeghers syndrome; likewise, the calcifying Sertoli cell tumors of the testes are rarely encountered outside this syndrome.

- There is a high incidence of nasal polyposis in some patients with PJS, and PJS should be considered along with cystic fibrosis in pediatric patients presenting with nasal polyps. Compared with allergic-type sinonasal polyps, PJS polyps contain a paucity of eosinophils.

- Mutations in the *STK11* gene (chromosome 19p) underlie about 75% of cases. *STK11* encodes a serine/threonine kinase. The genetic cause of the remaining 25% has yet to be uncovered, but some cases have been linked to a locus on 19q13.

Hereditary Diffuse Gastric Cancer

- 2 main types of gastric adenocarcinoma are routinely recognized: intestinal type and diffuse (signet ring) type. The intestinal type is more common, affects older patients, and is strongly associated with atrophic gastritis. The diffuse type affects younger patients (mean age around 40 years), and aside from heredity, no major risk factors have been identified.

- Decreased expression of E-cadherin is identified in diffuse gastric cancer, whether inherited or sporadic. E-cadherin, a protein involved in cell-to-cell adhesion, is encoded by the *CDH1* gene found on 16q. Germline mutations in the CDH1 gene are the cause of hereditary diffuse gastric cancer. This appears to follow a classic "2-hit" model, in which 1 copy of a mutated gene is inherited, and the second mutation takes place somatically.

Cronkhite-Canada Syndrome

- While Cronkhite-Canada is a syndrome of multiple GI polyps, it has not yet been demonstrated to be inherited. Some authors have demonstrated MSI in a subset of cases, but this has not been confirmed. It is an extremely rare syndrome, so far arising mostly in Japanese patients, that presents with the tetrad of diffuse macular hyperpigmentation, alopecia, nail atrophy, and gastrointestinal polyposis. An additional crucial feature of the disease, since it is a common cause of death, is a chronic refractory malabsorptive diarrhea; thus, it appears that even the nonpolypoid intestinal mucosa is constitutively abnormal.

- Most of the intestinal polyps are juvenile polyp–like hamartomatous polyps; nonetheless, adenomatous polyps occur with increased frequency in this syndrome. The intervening nonpolypoid mucosa also appears histologically abnormal, displaying inflammation, mucosal edema, and crypts that are cystically dilated and tortuous.

Inherited Pancreatic Cancer

- Familial pancreatic cancer (FPC) is an inherited condition in which 2 or more family members have pancreatic adenocarcinoma. The *BRCA2* gene, known for its association with familial breast cancer, is also the culprit in FPC. A particular mutation, 6174delT, appears to cause most cases, and is found predominantly in Ashkenazi Jews. Families with this mutation do not have a high incidence of breast or ovarian cancer.

- Other inherited syndromes associated with an increased risk of pancreatic carcinoma include *BRCA2*-associated breast cancer, HNPCC, FAP, PJS, hereditary pancreatitis, ataxia-telangiectasia, and the familial atypical multiple mole and melanoma (FAMMM) syndrome.

Breast Tumor Syndromes

BRCA Gene Mutations

- In families harboring germline *BRCA* gene mutations, there are often 2 or more generations of women with premenopausal breast cancer, sometimes arising bilaterally. Many such kindreds display an increased incidence of epithelial ovarian malignancies, as well as carcinomas of the pancreas, colon, uterus, and prostate. In fact, it appears that a variant mutation in *BRCA2* (6174delT) is the cause of familial pancreatic cancer.

- A mutated BRCA gene (*BRCA1* or *BRCA2*) is expressed in an autosomal dominant fashion. The lifetime risk of breast cancer in those with BRCA mutations is over 80% (compared with an overall 10% lifetime incidence in all women), and the risk of ovarian cancer is about 50%. *BRCA1* mutations carry a higher ovarian cancer risk (60%) than does *BRCA2* (20%). Furthermore, cancers associated with BRCA mutations often present at a young age, with many diagnosed in 20- to 30-year-old women. The risk of breast cancer in a male who carries a BRCA mutation is about 6%; *BRCA2* carries a higher male risk than does *BRCA1*.

- About 5% of all women with breast cancer and 25% of Ashkenazi Jewish women with breast cancer have a BRCA mutation **T13.1**. Additionally, in a woman with breast cancer who is found to harbor a BRCA mutation, the risk of cancer developing in the contralateral breast is 25%.

- About 50% of familial breast cancer is linked to *BRCA1*, about 30% to *BRCA2*, and perhaps 10% to an as-yet poorly characterized *BRCA3*. Families with *BRCA1* are more likely to show a high incidence of associated ovarian malignancies, while families with *BRCA2* have breast carcinoma in both male and female members.

- The BRCA genes

  □ *BRCA1* (chromosome 17q21) and *BRCA2* (13q12-13) are tumor suppressor genes that encode proteins involved in the DNA repair process.

  □ The genes are large, each spanning several kilobases, and each with over 20 exons. Several thousand different mutations have been identified among the 2 genes.

  □ 3 mutations appear with high frequency in persons of Ashkenazi Jewish descent (so-called founder mutations), together accounting for over 90% of the BRCA mutations in this population: (1) a 2–base pair deletion in codon 23 (185delAG) of *BRCA1*, (2) a 5385insC mutation in *BRCA1*, and (3) a 6174delT mutation of *BRCA2*. About 2% of the Ashkenazim harbor 1 of these mutations.

T13.1
Contribution of Inherited Syndromes to Breast Cancer Incidence

Syndrome	Approximate Proportion of Cases, %	Gene
BRCA1	3	*BRCA1*
BRCA2	2	*BRCA2*
Cowden's	1	*PTEN*
Li-Fraumeni	1	*TP53*
Muir-Torre and hereditary nonpolyposis colorectal carcinoma	<1	*MLH1/MSH2*
Peutz-Jeghers	<1	*STK11*
Sporadic	90	

13: Inherited Tumor Syndromes

Breast Tumor Syndromes>BRCA Gene Mutations; Other Breast Cancer-Associated Mutations |
Renal Cell Carcinoma Syndromes>Von Hippel-Lindau Disease

□ Outside the Ashkenazi Jewish population, disease-causing mutations are dispersed widely throughout the *BRCA* genes, precluding targeted mutation analysis. Thus, entire gene sequencing is required to detect a mutation in a never-before-evaluated family. Given the size of the BRCA genes, this is a highly labor-intensive and expensive process. Nonetheless, 3 results are possible from this analysis: a mutation may be found that is known to be associated with high cancer risk (deleterious mutation); a mutation may be found that is of unknown significance; or no mutation may be found. In this latter scenario, several possibilities still exist: no mutation, a mutation in a noncoding region (promoter), a gene duplication or balanced translocation, or familial breast cancer on the basis of some other gene.

□ While direct gene sequencing is the gold standard technique for detecting BRCA mutations, several mutation scanning strategies exist which trade cost for sensitivity. These include DHPLC (denaturing high-performance liquid chromatography), single strand conformational polymorphism (SSCP) analysis, CSGE (conformation-sensitive gel electrophoresis), and others. DHPLC appears capable of sensitivity of up to 99% compared with direct sequencing and seems most promising at this time.

■ The histologic appearance of some BRCA-associated breast tumors is somewhat distinctive, a fact that can aid in directing DNA-based testing. The morphologic features are not sufficiently sensitive, however, to warrant restricting molecular testing to cases having distinctive features.

□ *BRCA1*-linked cases often have medullary histology, including a high nuclear grade, pushing margins, tumor-infiltrating lymphocytes, and lack of estrogen receptor (ER) or progesterone receptor (PR) expression. Only about 10% of *BRCA1*-associated tumors express ER or PR (compared with 70% of sporadic tumors). In 1 study, a lack of hormone receptor expression was the strongest predictor of *BRCA1* mutation status. Furthermore, these *BRCA1*-associated tumors have been shown to express a basal-type phenotype, with immunohistochemical expression of cytokeratins 5/14 (in contrast to the usual-type ductal carcinoma, having a luminal-type phenotype that is CK 5/14 negative, CK 8/18 positive). Reports of the rate of Her2

expression have been variable, but overall it appears that there is a *lower* rate of Her2 expression in these tumors. Lastly, *BRCA1*-associated tumors are less likely to be found in association with ductal carcinoma in situ (DCIS).

□ Tumors associated with *BRCA2* germline mutations are much more likely to appear as usual-type ductal carcinomas; however, a tendency for pushing margins and higher grade has been demonstrated. There is no difference in the rate of associated DCIS or in ER/PR expression.

■ Currently it is recommended that women in breast cancer kindreds undergo close clinical monitoring for the development of breast carcinoma. In some cases, prophylactic mastectomy is recommended. Likewise, these women must undergo close scrutiny for the development of ovarian malignancy. Prophylactic oophorectomy is sometimes considered.

Other Breast Cancer-Associated Mutations

■ An increased risk of breast cancer has been associated with germline mutations in *TP53* (Li-Fraumeni syndrome), *PTEN* (Cowden syndrome), *MLH1/MSH2* (Muir-Torre and HNPCC syndromes), and *STK11* (PJS).

■ A mutation in the *CHEK2* (cell-cycle–checkpoint kinase 2) gene has been strongly associated with familial breast cancer, so far predominantly in European kindreds.

Renal Cell Carcinoma Syndromes

Von Hippel-Lindau (VHL) Disease

■ VHL disease is an autosomal dominant disease in which patients are at high risk for hemangioblastoma (cerebellar, cerebral, or retinal), pheochromocytoma, renal cell carcinoma, pancreatic cysts, islet cell tumors, epidymal/broad ligament cystadenomas, and tumors of the endolymphatic sac of the inner ear.

■ Renal cell carcinoma develops in about 70% of those with VHL. They tend to present at a young age (mean 37 years) and to be multifocal and bilateral. They have exclusively clear cell histology, but they are somewhat more indolent than sporadic clear cell tumors (metastasize only when quite large).

■ Deletion or other alteration of 3p, where the *VHL* tumor suppressor gene is found, is extremely common

13: Inherited Tumor Syndromes

Renal Cell Carcinoma Syndromes>VHL Disease; Birt-Hogg-Dubé Syndrome; Familial Clear Cell Renal Cell Carcinoma; Hereditary Papillary Renal Cell Carcinoma | Other Tumor Syndromes>Tuberous Sclerosis; Multiple Endocrine Neoplasia Type 1

in sporadic clear cell renal cell carcinoma. VHL disease is caused by inheritance of a germline mutation in 1 *VHL* gene, and tumorigenesis in VHL is caused when a "second hit" is acquired in the other *VHL* gene (loss-of-heterozygosity).

- Based on genotypic and phenotypic features, VHL is further divisible into 2 major types. A form of the syndrome having all the usual features except pheochromocytoma is known as type 1 VHL. Type 1 is associated with major loss-of-function mutations, such as a gene deletion or missense mutation. Forms of the syndrome with a high risk of pheochromocytoma are known as type 2 VHL, and these are associated with minor loss-of-function mutations, such as missense mutations.

Birt-Hogg-Dubé Syndrome

- This is an autosomal dominant disorder characterized by 3 cardinal features: multiple skin lesions, spontaneous pneumothorax, and renal tumors.

- Skin lesions include fibrofolliculomas, trichodiscomas, and acrochordons, especially affecting the head, neck, and upper trunk.

- Renal tumors actually develop in only about 15% to 20% of cases, but they tend to be multifocal, bilateral, and have features of combined oncocytoma and chromphobe carcinoma.

- The lung contains numerous cystic parenchymal spaces in addition to blebs and bullae, causing recurrent spontaneous pneumothorax. The differential diagnosis of spontaneous pneumothorax, particularly in a young patient, includes several other inherited and acquired conditions: alpha-1 antitrypsin deficiency–associated emphysema, lymphangiomyomatosis (often associated with tuberous sclerosis), Langerhans cell histiocytosis (eosinophilic granuloma), Ehlers-Danlos syndrome, and Marfan syndrome. 1 unique feature of Birt-Hogg-Dubé is its tendency to involve the lower lobes. In contrast, spontaneous pneumothoraces in other conditions usually involve the upper lobes.

- Birt-Hogg-Dubé is caused by mutations in the *BHD* gene (chromosome 17p11.2) encoding the protein folliculin.

Familial Clear Cell Renal Cell Carcinoma

- A non-VHL form of familial clear cell renal cell carcinoma, caused by inherited translocations involving 3p, has been described in rare kindreds. Translocation partners have included chromosomes 4, 6, and 8.

- Additional families with clear cell renal cell carcinoma, lacking VHL mutations and 3p translocations, have been described. The genetic basis for these kindreds in unknown.

Hereditary Papillary Renal Cell Carcinoma

- Tumors in this syndrome have features typical of papillary renal cell carcinoma, but they are multiple and bilateral.

- The syndrome is caused by gain-of-function mutations or duplications in the *C-MET* gene on chromosome 7q31. C-MET functions in a manner similar to C-KIT, with mutation resulting in a constitutively activated tyrosine kinase.

Other Tumor Syndromes

Tuberous Sclerosis (Bourneville Disease)

- Tuberous sclerosis is an autosomal-dominant syndrome characterized by numerous, mostly benign, tumors: angiofibromas (adenoma sebaceum) of the skin, periungual fibromas, shagreen patches, hypopigmented macules, cardiac rhabdomyomas, pulmonary lymphangioleiomyomatosis (LAM), subependymal giant cell astrocytomas (SEGA), and renal angiomyolipomas. Subependymal nodules form, most commonly along the sulcus terminalis associated with the caudate nucleus, and these have been called "candle drippings." There is an increased risk of renal neoplasms, including clear cell carcinoma and oncocytomas.

- 2 genes have been implicated in tuberous sclerosis. Most (80%) cases are caused by mutations in the *TSC1* gene, located on chromosome 9q34, which encodes the protein hamartin. The remaining cases are the result of mutations in the *TSC2* gene, located on chromosome 16p13, which encodes the protein tuberin. Approximately 60% of tuberous sclerosis cases arise sporadically, reflecting the high rate of de novo mutations.

Multiple Endocrine Neoplasia Type 1 (MEN1, Wermer Syndrome)

- The cardinal manifestations of MEN1 syndrome **T13.2** include parathyroid adenomas, pituitary adenomas, and pancreatic islet cell tumors. Endocrine tumors may also develop in the adrenal cortex, bronchus, thymus, and GI tract. The most common and earliest manifestation is usually primary hyperparathyroidism. Most of the pituitary tumors are

T13.2
Multiple Endocrine Neoplasia Syndromes

Syndrome	Tumors	Gene (Chromosome)
MEN I (Wermer)	Parathyroid adenoma Pituitary adenoma (especially prolactinoma) Pancreatic islet cell tumor (especially gastrinoma)	*MEN1* (11q)
MEN II/IIa (Sipple's)	Parathyroid adenoma Adrenal pheochromocytoma Thyroid medullary carcinoma	*RET* (10q)
MEN IIb/III	Features of MEN IIa Mucosal ganglioneuromas Marfanoid body habitus	*RET* (10q)

prolactinomas. Pancreatic and other GI tumors often produce gastrin (gastrinomas) or insulin (insulinomas).

- Nonendocrine lesions associated with MEN1 include facial angiofibromas, collagenomas, lipomas, and meningiomas.

- The *MEN1* gene is found on chromosome 11q13 where it encodes the protein menin. Direct sequence analysis is capable of identifying germline *MEN1* gene mutations in about 90% of families with MEN1. Persons with so-called simplex cases (MEN1 syndrome developing sporadically in a single person, without apparent inheritance) have the mutation about 60% of the time. Among those with a single, sporadic, MEN1-associated tumor, it is rare to find a germline mutation; however somatic *MEN1* mutations are found in 15% to 20% of sporadic parathyroid adenomas, islet cell tumors, and gastrinomas.

- Specific germline mutations in the *MEN1* gene can give rise to familial isolated hyperparathyroidism.

RET-Associated Diseases: MEN2A (Sipple Syndrome), MEN2B, and Familial Medullary Thyroid Carcinoma (FMTC)

- The *RET* gene is found on 10q. MEN2A is caused by mutations affecting exons 10-11 of the *RET* gene, most often affecting a particular cysteine residue (634 Cys). FMTC is caused by *RET* mutations affecting other cysteine residues, particularly 609, 611, 618, and 620 Cys. MEN2B is most often caused by a *RET* mutation affecting exon 16, encoding the tyrosine kinase domain.

- Interestingly, about 20% of cases of Hirschsprung disease are caused by germline or sporadic mutations in *RET*.

- In addition, about 40% of sporadic papillary thyroid carcinomas have somatic mutations in *RET*.

- The 3 syndromes—MEN2A, MEN2B, and FMTC—have some things in common: all imparting a high risk for medullary thyroid carcinoma, all autosomal dominant, and all due to a *RET* gene mutation. These features alone comprise FMTC. These features plus pheochromocytoma and parathyroid adenoma make up the MEN2A syndrome; and these plus pheochromocytoma, ganglioneuromatous intestinal polyps, and Marfanoid body habitus comprise MEN2B.

- While the histologic appearance of medullary thyroid carcinomas is not particularly distinctive in these syndromes, the appearance of the background thyroid is: C-cell hyperplasia and numerous microscopic foci of medullary carcinoma.

Carney Complex (LAMB Syndrome, NAME Syndrome)

- Carney complex is characterized by the formation of multiple tumors, most of them benign. Cutaneous lentigines (simple lentigos) are the most common presenting finding, located on the face (particularly the oral and conjunctival mucosa), vagina, and penis. Blue nevi are common, particularly the cellular blue nevus. Cardiac myxomas occur frequently, at a young age, and may affect any chamber. Myxomas arise at other sites as well, including the breast, female genital tract, and skin (especially on the eyelid and external ear). Endocrine tumors form, particularly follicular adenomas of the thyroid, pituitary adenomas (growth hormone–secreting), and the so-called primary pigmented nodular adrenocortical disease (PPNAD) of the adrenal gland.

13: Inherited Tumor Syndromes

Other Tumor Syndromes>Carney Complex; Cowden Syndrome and Other PTEN-Related Disorders; Gorlin Syndrome; Neurofibromatosis Type 1

The latter is a form of multinodular hyperplasia of the adrenal cortex and causes Cushing syndrome. Large-cell calcifying Sertoli cell tumors arise in most affected males. Note that this unusual tumor is also seen in PJS; however, the SCTAT of PJS is not seen in females with Carney complex. Psammomatous melanotic schwannoma, rare as a sporadic tumor, is common in the Carney complex.

- Note that, though similarly named, the Carney triad is an entirely different syndrome (triad of gastric gastrointestinal stromal tumor, pulmonary chondroma, and extraadrenal paraganglioma).

- About half of all cases are the result of mutations in the *PRKAR1A* gene, located on 17q24, which encodes a regulatory subunit of cyclic adenosine monophosphate–dependent protein kinase. In the remaining cases, a specific gene has not been implicated, but a locus at 2p16 appears promising. Direct sequence analysis for the *PRKAR1A* gene is clinically available.

Cowden Syndrome and Other PTEN-Related Disorders

- The *PTEN* gene is located at 10q23 and encodes the phosphatidylinositol-3,4,5-trisphosphate 3-phosphatase (PTEN). Disorders associated with mutations in the *PTEN* gene share a tendency to develop hamartomatous lesions and include Cowden syndrome, Bannayan-Riley-Ruvalcaba syndrome, and Proteus syndrome.

- Hamartomatous intestinal polyps, multiple lipomas, fibromas, genitourinary malformations, and multiple mucocutaneous lesions (facial trichilemmomas, papillomas, palmoplantar keratoses, and palmoplantar hyperkeratotic pits) characterize Cowden syndrome. Microcephaly and mental retardation are common, and it is strongly associated with cerebellar dysplastic gangliocytoma (Lhermitte-Duclos), which is considered pathognomonic. There is an increased risk of malignancy, especially of the breast, thyroid (follicular carcinoma), colon, and endometrium.

- Bannayan-Riley-Ruvalcaba syndrome is characterized by high birth weight with macrocephaly, mental retardation, myopathy, joint hypermobility, pectus excavatum, scoliosis, hamartomatous intestinal polyps, lipomas, and pigmented macules of the glans penis.

- Proteus syndrome has highly variable manifestations and appears to affect individuals in a mosaic distribution; ie, some organs or tissues heavily affected, others entirely spared. Some examples include connective tissue nevi (considered pathognomonic), asymmetric limb growth, skull hyperostosis, megaspondylodysplasia of the vertebrae, or visceral overgrowth (especially spleen and thymus).

Gorlin Syndrome (Nevoid Basal Cell Carcinoma Syndrome)

- Gorlin syndrome manifests as multiple basal cell carcinomas presenting at a young age, odontogenic keratocysts, calcification of the falx cerebri, palmoplantar pits, and skeletal anomalies. In addition, there is a high incidence of medulloblastoma, often presenting before the age of 2 years.

- The skin is hypersensitive to ionizing radiation.

Neurofibromatosis Type 1 (NF1, Von Recklinghausen Disease)

- When inherited, NF1 is an autosomal dominant trait, but about half of all cases are caused by new mutations. NF1 has an incidence of about 1 in 2500 live births.

- Specific criteria for the diagnosis of NF1 were published by the National Institutes of Health in 1988. In childhood, NF1 initially presents with multiple café au lait spots and intertriginous (groin, axilla) freckling. Neurofibromas typically begin to emerge in adolescence or early adulthood (diagnosis is often delayed into the second decade as a result), and the less common plexiform neurofibroma is considered pathognomonic. Many women with NF1 experience a rapid increase in the number and size of neurofibromas during pregnancy. Ocular Lisch nodules are fairly common but innocuous. Inconsistent features include vertebral dysplasia, scoliosis, bone cortical thinning, pseudoarthrosis, mental retardation, pulmonic stenosis, and NF1 vasculopathy with associated hypertension.

- Tumors arising with increased incidence in NF1 include neurofibromas and malignant peripheral nerve sheath tumors (MPNST). The latter arise either de novo or in association with a plexiform neurofibroma, but rarely (if ever) in association with a typical neurofibromas. Other tumors with high incidence in NF1 include optic gliomas, leukemia, medulloblastoma, pheochromocytoma, adenocarcinoma of the ampulla of Vater, and breast cancer.

- Hyperintense lesions, seen on magnetic resonance imaging and often called "unidentified bright objects," may be seen in the optic tracts, basal ganglia, brainstem, cerebellum, or cortex. They are usually inconsequential clinically and seen primarily in childhood, disappearing in adulthood.

- An appearance resembling Noonan syndrome (see chapter 2) is seen in about 12% of individuals with NF1.

- NF1 is caused by mutations in the *NF1* gene (17q11.2), encoding the protein neurofibromin. Half of affected individuals have NF1 as the result of a de novo *NF1* mutation. Neurofibromin appears to act as an inhibitor of the *RAS* proto-oncogene; thus neurofibromin is a tumor suppressor protein. Most clinically significant NF1 mutations are nonsense mutations, missense mutations, or microdeletions that, while distributed throughout the gene, cause protein truncation. Discrete point mutations are responsible for only about 10% of cases. Thus, while there are an enormous variety of mutations, the laboratory can screen for about 80% of them with protein truncation tests. Fluorescence in situ hybridization (FISH) can detect the 5% to 10% of cases that are caused by microdeletions (conventional cytogenetic testing is not sensitive enough). When there is a strong clinical suspicion and negative protein truncation and/or FISH, then direct DNA sequencing of the entire gene must be considered.

Neurofibromatosis Type 2 (NF2, Bilateral Acoustic Neuromas)

- NF2 is an autosomal dominant condition, but about 1 in 3 cases are caused by new mutations (simplex cases). Much about the nomenclature of this syndrome is confusing: NF2 is characterized by bilateral vestibular nerve (not acoustic nerve) schwannomas (neither neurofibromas nor neuromas occur), and it has almost no relationship to NF1.

- The disease first manifests around the age of 20 years, and nearly all affected individuals have bilateral vestibular schwannomas by the age of 30 years. Schwannomas may arise in association with other nerves as well, and there is a tendency to develop meningiomas, ependymomas, and astrocytomas.

- Mutations in the *NF2* gene (22q), which encodes merlin, are the cause of NF2.

Osteochondromatosis (Hereditary Multiple Exostoses)

- This is an autosomal dominant condition in which there are multiple osteochondromas, differing from solitary sporadic osteochondromas in their location and malignant potential.

- Affected individuals have additional skeletal anomalies such as short stature, premature osteoarthritis, and bone deformities.

- Osteochondromas develop on the femur in 70% of cases. While this site is typical for sporadic osteochondromas, the lesions tend to be bilateral and symmetrical in osteochondromatosis.

- Furthermore, osteochondromas are found in uncommon sites such as the forearm, scapula, pelvis, vertebrae, phalanges, wrist, and ankle.

- Sarcomatous change occurs in about 1% of cases.

- 2 genes have been implicated: *EXT1* (70%) and *EXT2* (30%). These are found on 8q and 11p and encode exostosin-1 and exostosin-2, respectively.

Li Fraumeni Syndrome

- Mutations in the tumor suppressor gene *TP53* (p53) are found in about 50% of malignancies, regardless of type, and are the most common genetic anomaly found in malignant tumors. An inherited (germline) mutation in *TP53* causes Li Fraumeni syndrome; as might be predicted, Li Fraumeni is associated with a tendency to develop numerous widespread malignancies,

- Early reports focused on the association with a number of tumors, including osteosarcoma, soft tissue sarcomas, breast cancer, adrenal cortical carcinoma, and acute leukemia. It seems now that there is no limit to the variety of tumors, however, with an increased risk for gastric adenocarcinoma, colorectal carcinoma, pancreatic carcinoma, esophageal carcinoma, germ cell tumors, melanoma, Wilms tumor, and CNS malignancy. Perhaps the only characteristic features of Li Fraumeni are (1) that any given tumor type arises at a younger age than would be expected for a sporadic tumor of the same type, and (2) that multiple disparate tumors may arise in the same person. About 40% of those with Li Fraumeni syndrome have developed a malignancy by the age of 20 years, 60% by the age 40 years, and 90% by age 60 years.

- Adrenocortical carcinoma is rare overall, and they often occur in children with Li Fraumeni syndrome. The likelihood of Li Fraumeni syndrome in a young patient with adrenocortical carcinoma is high (>50%). Thus, the occurrence of an adrenocortical carcinoma in a child or young adult is sufficient indication for Li Fraumeni syndrome testing.

- About 85% of cases are caused by *TP53* mutations (chromosome 17p); mutations in the *CHEK2* gene (whose product is 1 of the intracellular targets of p53) has been identified in a minority of cases. While there are a variety of *TP53* mutations, most arise between exons 4 through 9 (or amino acids 91 through 309). This permits good (95%) sensitivity for sequencing analyses confined to this portion of the gene. The limited sequencing assay does not detect the small percentage of cases are caused by duplications, deletions, inversions, and mutations outside exons 4 through 9.

- IHC can be performed for p53 expression. Most mutated forms of p53, though nonfunctional as tumor suppressor proteins, have a prolonged half-life in the cell (the mutated forms are able to avoid protein degradation). Thus, tumors with *TP53* mutations (and decreased p53 activity) have overexpression of p53.

Aniridia/WAGR Syndrome

- Aniridia may be a sporadic or inherited trait, usually occurring as an isolated finding; however, in some it occurs as part of a mendelian syndrome that includes Wilms tumor, aniridia, genitourinary anomalies, and mental retardation (WAGR syndrome).

- The WAGR syndrome is a contiguous gene syndrome in which a microdeletion spanning 11p13 affects several genes.

- In approximately 20% to 30% of cases, the deletion is detectable by high-resolution chromosome studies. FISH studies, utilizing several probes that span the affected band, can also be diagnostically useful.

Beckwith-Wiedemann Syndrome

- Embryonal tumors (Wilms tumor and hepatoblastoma, in particular) occur with a high rate in Beckwith-Wiedemann syndrome. The syndrome may become apparent in utero, with a fetus that is large for gestational age and has polyhydramnios. At birth, the placenta is large, and the umbilical cord is abnormally long. Additional features that may be identified at birth include macrosomia, macroglossia, hemihypertrophy (asymmetric growth), omphalocele (exomphalos), and anterior ear creases or pits. A peculiar adrenocortical cytomegaly has been described in patients with Beckwith-Wiedemann syndrome, and renal anomalies (renal medullary dysplasia, nephrocalcinosis, medullary sponge kidney, and nephromegaly) are very common.

- About 80% of cases are inherited, and the remaining are sporadic (simplex).

- Beckwith-Weidemann syndrome can be caused by any 1 of several defects, the common thread being abnormal transcription of genes in the 11p15.5 band. 11p normally is an imprinted domain (expression depends on whether inherited from the mother or from the father), 1 in which maternally derived alleles are preferentially expressed. Several genes are located in 11p, including: (1) *KCNQ1*, encoding a potassium channel, and the same gene implicated in Romano-Ward and Jervell Lange-Nielsen syndromes (see chapter 6), (2) *IGF2*, encoding an insulinlike growth factor, (3) *H19*, encoding a nontranslated mRNA, (4) CDKN1C, encoding a cyclin-dependent kinase inhibitor.

- This is primarily a clinical diagnosis. The molecular diagnosis of Beckwith-Wiedemann syndrome is problematic, because no single finding defines it. Conventional cytogenetics can identify an anomaly at 11p15 in only about 1% of cases. FISH can identify another 1% to 2%. Methylation assays are capable of finding abnormalities in over half of patients (either gain or loss of methylation). Uniparental disomy studies can identify abnormalities in about 15% of cases. Lastly, a single gene defect in *CDKN1C* appears to underlie around 10% of simplex cases and up to 40% of familial cases.

Chromosomal Breakage Syndromes: Ataxia-Telangiectasia, Bloom Syndrome, Fanconi Anemia, Xeroderma Pigmentosum, and Nijmegen Syndrome

- This is a group of genetic disorders, usually transmitted in an autosomal recessive fashion, whose unifying feature is a tendency, in cell culture, to exhibit elevated rates of chromosomal breakage or instability. Underlying this tendency are defects in DNA repair mechanisms, and the clinical effect is a predisposition to cancer (see chapter 9).

13: Inherited Tumor Syndromes

Other Tumor Syndromes>Chromosomal Breakage Syndromes: Ataxia-Telangiectasia, Bloom Syndrome, Fanconi Anemia, Xeroderma Pigmentosum, and Nijmegen Syndrome; Immunodeficiency Syndromes | References

■ This group of disorders should be conceptually distinguished from the trinucleotide repeat disorders associated with the presence of "fragile sites." These do not cause a cancer predisposition (see chapter 2).

Immunodeficiency Syndromes

■ As a group, the inherited immunodeficiencies are associated with a higher than normal rate of malignancy, especially hematolymphoid neoplasms (see chapter 9).

References

Aaltonen LA, Salovaara R, Kristo P, et al. Incidence of hereditary nonpolyposis colorectal cancer and the feasibility of molecular screening for the disease. *N Engl J Med* 1998; 338: 1481-1487.

Aarnio M, Mecklin JP, Aaltonen LA, et al. Life-time risk of different cancers in hereditary non-polyposis colorectal cancer (HNPCC) syndrome. *Int J Cancer* 1995; 64: 430-433.

Algar E, Brickell S, Deeble G, et al. Analysis of CDKN1C in Beckwith Wiedemann syndrome. *Hum Mutat* 2000; 15: 497-508.

Allinen M, Huusko P, Mantyniemi S, et al. Mutation analysis of the CHK2 gene in families with hereditary breast cancer. *Br J Cancer* 2001; 85: 209-212.

Andersson J, Sihto H, Meis-Kindblom JM, et al. NF1-associated gastrointestinal stromal tumors have unique clinical, phenotypic, and genotypic characteristics. *Am J Surg Pathol* 2005; 29: 1170-1176.

Ars E, Kruyer H, Morell M, et al. Recurrent mutations in the NF1 gene are common among neurofibromatosis type 1 patients. *J Med Genet* 2003; 40: e82.

Bane AL, Beck JC, Bleiweiss I, et al. BRCA2 mutation-associated breast cancers exhibit a distinguishing phenotype ba)sed on morphology and molecular profiles from tissue microarrays. *Am J Surg Pathol* 2007; 31: 121-128.

Baser ME, Friedman JM, Evans DG. Increasing the specificity of diagnostic criteria for schwannomatosis. *Neurology* 2006; 66: 730-732.

Baser ME, Kuramoto L, Joe H, et al. Genotype-phenotype correlations for nervous system tumors in neurofibromatosis 2: a population-based study. *Am J Hum Genet* 2004; 75: 231-239.

Beckwith JB. Nephrogenic rests and the pathogenesis of Wilms tumor: developmental and clinical considerations. *Am J Med Genet* 1998; 79: 268-273.

Biesecker LG, Happle R, Mulliken JB, et al. Proteus syndrome: diagnostic criteria, differential diagnosis, and patient evaluation. *Am J Med Genet* 1999; 84: 389-395.

References

Birch JM, Alston RD, McNally RJ, et al. Relative frequency and morphology of cancers in carriers of germline TP53 mutations. *Oncogene* 2001; 20: 4621-4628.

Birt AR, Hogg GR, Dube WJ. Hereditary multiple fibrofolliculomas with trichodiscomas and acrochordons. *Arch Dermatol* 1977; 113: 1674-1677.

Boardman LA, Couch FJ, Burgart LJ, et al. Genetic heterogeneity in Peutz-Jeghers syndrome. *Hum Mutat* 2000; 16: 23-30.

Boardman LA, Thibodeau SN, Schaid DJ, et al. Increased risk for cancer in patients with the Peutz-Jeghers syndrome. *Ann Intern Med* 1998; 128: 896-899.

Bonneau D, Longy M. Mutations of the human PTEN gene. *Hum Mutat* 2000; 16: 109-122.

Brandi ML, Gagel RF, Angeli A, et al. Guidelines for diagnosis and therapy of MEN type 1 and type 2. *J Clin Endocrinol Metab* 2001; 86: 5658-5671.

Brauckhoff M, Gimm O, Hinze R, et al. Papillary thyroid carcinoma in patients with RET proto-oncogene germline mutation. *Thyroid* 2002; 12: 557-561.

Brown GJ, St John DJ, Macrae FA, et al. Cancer risk in young women at risk of hereditary nonpolyposis colorectal cancer: implications for gynecologic surveillance. *Gynecol Oncol* 2001; 80: 346-349.

Burger B, Uhlhaas S, Mangold E, et al. Novel de novo mutation of MADH4/SMAD4 in a patient with juvenile polyposis. *Am J Med Genet* 2002; 110: 289-291.

Butnor KJ, Guinee DG. Pleuropulmonary pathology of Birt-Hogg-Dubé syndrome. *Am J Surg Pathol* 2006; 30: 395-399.

Carney JA. Familial multiple endocrine neoplasia: the first 100 years. *Am J Surg Pathol* 2005; 29: 254-274.

Carney JA, Hruska LS, Beauchamp GD, et al. Dominant inheritance of the complex of myxomas, spotty pigmentation, and endocrine overactivity. *Mayo Clin Proc* 1986; 61: 165-172.

Casey M, Mah C, Merliss AD, et al. Identification of a novel genetic locus for familial cardiac myxomas and Carney complex. *Circulation* 1998; 98: 2560-2566.

Cheadle JP, Reeve MP, Sampson JR, et al. Molecular genetic advances in tuberous sclerosis. *Hum Genet* 2000; 107: 97-114.

Cheung PK, McCormick C, Crawford BE, et al. Etiological point mutations in the hereditary multiple exostoses gene EXT1: a functional analysis of heparan sulfate polymerase activity. *Am J Hum Genet* 2001; 69: 55-66.

Church J, Simmang C. Practice parameters for the treatment of patients with dominantly inherited colorectal cancer (familial adenomatous polyposis and hereditary nonpolyposis colorectal cancer). *Dis Colon Rectum* 2003; 46: 1001-1012.

Cohen MS, Moley JF. Surgical treatment of medullary thyroid carcinoma. *J Intern Med* 2003; 253: 616-626.

Cunningham JM, Kim CY, Christensen ER, et al. The frequency of hereditary defective mismatch repair in a prospective series of unselected colorectal carcinomas. *Am J Hum Genet* 2001; 69: 780-790.

Curless RG. Use of "unidentified bright objects" on MRI for diagnosis of neurofibromatosis 1 in children. *Neurology* 2001; 55: 1067-1068.

Czene K, Hemminki K. Familial papillary renal cell tumors and subsequent cancers: a nationwide epidemiological study from Sweden. *J Urol* 2003; 169: 1271-1275.

DeBella K, Poskitt K, Szudek J, Friedman JM. Use of "unidentified bright objects" on MRI for diagnosis of neurofibromatosis 1 in children. *Neurology* 2000; 54: 1646-1651.

DeBella K, Szudek J, Friedman JM. Use of the National Institutes of Health criteria for diagnosis of neurofibromatosis 1 in children. *Pediatrics* 2000; 105: 608-614.

Delahunt B, Eble JN. Papillary renal cell carcinoma: a clinicopathologic and immunohistochemical study of 105 tumors. *Mod Pathol* 1997; 10: 537-544.

DeLeeuw WJ, Dierssen J, Vasen HF, et al. Prediction of a mismatch repair gene defect by microsatellite instability and immunohistochemical analysis in endometrial tumours from HNPCC patients. *J Pathol* 2001; 192: 328-335.

References

DeLeng WW, Westerman AM, Weterman MA, et al. Nasal polyposis in Peutz-Jeghers syndrome: a distinct histopathological and molecular genetic entity. *J Clin Pathol* 2007; 60: 392-396.

Du M, Zhou W, Beatty LG, et al. The KCNQ1OT1 promoter, a key regulator of genomic imprinting in human chromosome 11p15.5. *Genomics* 2004; 84: 288-300.

Eng C, Brody LC, Wagner TM, et al. Interpreting epidemiological research: blinded comparison of methods used to estimate the prevalence of inherited mutations in BRCA1. *J Med Genet* 2001; 38: 824-833.

Eng C, Hampel H, de la Chapelle A. Genetic testing for cancer predisposition. *Annu Rev Med* 2001; 52: 371-400.

Evans DG, Sainio M, Baser ME. Neurofibromatosis type 2. *J Med Genet* 2000; 37: 897-904.

Farshid G, Balleine RL, Cummings M, et al. Morphology of breast cancer as a means of triage of patients for BRCA1 genetic testing. *Am J Surg Pathol* 2006; 30: 1357-1366.

Ferner RE. Neurofibromatosis 1 and neurofibromatosis 2: a twenty first century perspective. *Lancet Neurol* 2007; 6: 340-351.

Forster LF, Defres S, Goudie DR, et al. An investigation of the Peutz-Jeghers gene (LKB1) in sporadic breast and colon cancers. *J Clin Pathol* 2000; 53: 791-793.

Francannet C, Cohen-Tanugi A, Le Merrer M, et al. Genotytpe-phenotype correlation in hereditary multiple exostoses. *J Med Genet* 2001; 38: 430-434.

Frank TS. Laboratory determination of hereditary susceptibility to breast and ovarian cancer. *Arch Pathol Lab Med* 1999; 123: 1023-1026.

Frank-Raue K, Hoppner W, Frilling A, et al. Mutatins of the ret protooncogene in German multiple endocrine neoplasia families: Relation between genotype and phenotype. *J Clin Endocrinol Metab* 1996; 81: 1780-1783.

Friedman JM. Neurofibromatosis 1. Available at www.genetests.org. Accessed 7 November, 2007.

Friedman JM, Birch PH. Type 1 neurofibromatosis: a descriptive analysis of the disorder in 1,728 patients. *Am J Med Genet* 1997; 70: 138-143.

Giardiello FM, Brensinger JD, Tersmette AC, et al. Very high risk of cancer in familial Peutz-Jeghers syndrome. *Gastroenterology* 2000; 119: 1447-1453.

Gologan A, Krasinskas A, Hunt J, et al. Performance of the revised Bethesda guidelines for identification of colorectal carcinomas with a high level of microsatellite instability. *Arch Pathol Lab Med* 2005; 129: 1390-1397.

Gosden R, Trasler J, Lucifero D, et al. Rare congenital disorders, imprinted genes, and assisted reproductive technology. *Lancet* 2003; 361: 1975-1977.

Gryfe R, Kim H, Hsieh ET, et al. Tumor microsatellite instability and clinical outcome in young patients with colorectal cancer. *N Engl J Med* 2000; 342: 69-77.

Guilford PJ, Hopkins JB, Grady WM, et al. E-cadherin germline mutations define an inherited cancer syndrome dominated by diffuse gastric cancer. *Hum Mutat* 1999; 14: 249-255.

Gutmann DH. Recent insights into neurofibromatosis type 1: clear genetic progress. *Arch Neurol* 1998; 55: 778-780.

Gutmann DH, Aylsworth A, Carey JC, et al. The diagnostic evaluation and multidisciplinary management of neurofibromatosis 1 and neurofibromatosis 2. *JAMA* 1997; 278: 51-57.

Hahn SA, Bartsch DK. Genetics of hereditary pancreatic carcinoma. *Clin Lab Med* 2005; 25: 117-133.

Halvarsson B, Lindblom A, Johansson L, et al. Loss of mismatch repair protein immunostaining in colorectal adenomas from patients with hereditary nonpolyposis colorectal cancer. *Mod Pathol* 2005; 18: 1095-1101.

Hamilton SR, Liu B, Parsons RE, et al. The molecular basis of Turcot's syndrome. *N Engl J Med* 1995; 332: 839-847.

Hampel H, Frankel WL, Martin E, et al. Screening for the Lynch syndrome (hereditary nonpolyposis colorectal cancer). *N Engl J Med* 2005; 352: 1851-1860.

References

Hartmann LC, Schaid DJ, Woods JE, et al. Efficacy of bilateral prophylactic mastectomy in women with a family history of breast cancer. *N Engl J Med* 1999; 340: 77-84.

Hedenfalk I, Duggan D, Chen Y, et al. Gene-expression profiles in hereditary breast cancer. *N Engl J Med* 2001; 344: 539-548.

Hisada M, Garber JE, Fung CY, et al. Multiple primary cancers in families with Li-Fraumeni syndrome. *J Natl Cancer Inst* 1998; 90: 606-611.

Hitchins MP, Wong JJL, Suthers G, et al. Inheritance of a cancer-associated MLH1 germline epimutation. *N Engl J Med* 2007; 356: 697-705.

Howe JR, Mitros FA, Summers RW. The risk of gastrointestinal carcinoma in familial juvenile polyposis. *Ann Surg Oncol* 1998; 5: 751-756.

Hoyme HE, Seaver LH, Jones KL, et al. Isolated hemihyperplasia (hemihypertrophy): report of a prospective multicenter study of the incidence of neoplasia and review. *Am J Med Genet* 1998; 79: 274-278.

Iino H, Simms L, Young J, et al. DNA microsatellite instability and mismatch repair protein loss in adenomas presenting in hereditary non-polyposis colorectal cancer. *Gut* 2000; 47: 37-42.

Inabnet WB, Caragliano P, Pertsemlidis D. Pheochromocytoma: inherited associations, bilaterality, and cortex presentation. *Surgery* 2000; 128: 1007-1011.

Inoue K, Shimotake T, Inoue K, et al. Mutational analysis of the RET proto-oncogene in a kindred with multiple endocrine neoplasia type 2A and Hirschsprung's disease. *J Pediatr Surg* 1999; 34: 1552-1554.

Jarvinen HJ, Aarnio M, Mustonen H, et al. Controlled 15-year trial on screening for colorectal cancer in families with hereditary nonpolyposis colorectal cancer. *Gastroenterology* 2000; 118: 829-834.

Kauff ND, Satagopan JM, Robson ME, et al. Risk-reducing salpingo-oophorectomy in women with a BRCA1 or BRCA2 mutation. *N Engl J Med* 2002; 346: 1609-1615.

Kruse R, Rutten A, Lamberti C, et al. Muir-Torre phenotype has a frequency of DNA mismatch-repair-gene mutations similar to that in hereditary nonpolyposis colorectal cancer families defined by the Amsterdam criteria. *Am J Hum Genet* 1998; 63: 63-70.

Laakso M, Loman N, Borg A, et al. Cytokeratin 5/14-positive breast cancer: true basal phenotype confined to BRCA1 tumors. *Modern Pathology* 2005; 18: 1321-1328.

Legoix P, Sarkissian HD, Cazes L, et al. Molecular characterization of germline NF2 gene rearrangements. *Genomics* 2000; 65: 62-66.

Li FP, Fraumeni JF Jr. Soft-tissue sarcomas, breast cancer, and other neoplasms. a familial syndrome? *Ann Intern Med* 1969; 71: 747-752.

Li M, Squire J, Shuman C, et al. Imprinting status of 11p15 genes in Beckwith-Wiedemann syndrome patients with CDKN1C mutations. *Genomics* 2001; 74: 370-376.

Li M, Squire JA, Weksberg R. Molecular genetics of Wiedemann-Beckwith syndrome. *Am J Med Genet* 1998; 79: 253-259.

Lonser RR, Kim J, Butman JA, et al. Tumors of the endolymphatic sac in von Hippel–Lindau disease. *N Engl J Med* 2004; 350: 2481-2486.

Loukola A, Salovaara R, Kristo P, et al. Microsatellite instability in adenomas as a marker for hereditary nonpolyposis colorectal cancer. *Am J Pathol* 1999; 155: 1849-1853.

MacCollin M, Chiocca EA, Evans DG, et al. Diagnostic criteria for schwannomatosis. *Neurology* 2005; 64: 1838-1845.

McGarrity TJ, Kulin HE, Zaino RJ. Peutz-Jeghers syndrome. *Am J Gastroenterol* 2000; 95: 596-604.

Machens A, Ukkat J, Brauckhoff M, et al. Advances in the management of hereditary medullary thyroid cancer. *J Intern Med* 2005; 257: 50-59.

Machin P, Catasus L, Pons C, et al. Microsatellite instability and immunostaining for MSH-2 and MLH-1 in cutaneous and internal tumors from patients with the Muir-Torre syndrome. *J Cutan Pathol* 2002; 29: 415-420.

Maher ER, Webster AR, Richards FM, et al. Phenotypic expression in von Hippel-Lindau disease: correlations with germline VHL gene mutations. *J Med Genet* 1996; 33: 328-332.

References

Massoll N, Mazzaferri EL. Diagnosis and management of medullary thyroid carcinoma. *Clin Lab Med* 2004; 24: 49-83.

Misago N, Narisawa Y. Sebaceous neoplasms in Muir-Torre syndrome. *Am J Dermatopathol* 2000; 22: 155-161.

Moers AM, Landsvater RM, Schaap C, et al. Familial medullary thyroid carcinoma: not a distinct entity? *Am J Med* 1996; 101: 635-641.

National Institutes of Health Consensus Conference Statement. Neurofibromatosis. *Arch Neurol* 1988; 45: 575-578.

Neumann HP, Bausch B, McWhinney SR, et al. Germ-line mutations in nonsyndromic pheochromocytoma. *N Engl J Med* 2002; 346: 1459-1466.

Neumann HP, Eng C, Mulligan LM, et al. Consequences of direct genetic testing for germline mutations in the clinical management of families with multiple endocrine neoplasia, type II. *JAMA* 1995; 274: 1149-1151.

Newman EA, Mulholland MW. Prophylactic gastrectomy for hereditary diffuse gastric cancer syndrome. *J Am Coll Surg* 2006; 202: 612-617.

Nilsson O, Tisell LE, Jansson S, et al. Adrenal and extra-adrenal pheochromocytomas in a family with germline RET V804L mutation. *JAMA* 1999; 281: 1587-1588.

Oncel M, Church JM, Remzi FH, et al. Colonic surgery in patients with juvenile polyposis syndrome: a case series. *Dis Colon and Rectum* 2005; 48: 49-56.

Peltomaki P. Role of DNA mismatch repair defects in the pathogenesis of human cancer. *J Clin Oncol* 2003; 21: 1174-1179.

Pharoah PD, Guilford P, Caldas C. Incidence of gastric cancer and breast cancer in CDH1 (E-cadherin) mutation carriers from hereditary diffuse gastric cancer families. *Gastroenterology* 2001; 121: 1348-1353.

Pyatt RE, Pilarski R, Prior TW. Mutation screening in juvenile polyposis syndrome. *J Mol Diagn* 2006; 8: 84-88.

Raue F, Frank-Raue K, Grauer A. Multiple endocrine neoplasia type 2: clinical features and screening. *Endocrinol Metab Clin North Am* 1994; 23: 137-136.

Rijcken FEM, Hollema H, Kleibeuker JH. Proximal adenomas in hereditary non-polyposis colorectal cancer are prone to rapid malignant transformation. *Gut* 2002; 50: 382-386.

Romeo G, Ceccherini I, Celli J, et al. Association of multiple endocrine neoplasia type 2 and Hirschsprung disease. *J Intern Med* 1998; 243: 515-520.

Rowley PT. Inherited susceptibility to colorectal cancer. *Annu Rev Med* 2005; 56: 539-554.

Rustgi AK. Hereditary gastrointestinal polyposis and nonpolyposis syndromes. *N Engl J Med* 1994; 331: 1694-1702.

Santoro M, Melillo RM, Carlomagno F, et al. RET: normal and abnormal functions. *Endocrinology* 2004; 145: 5448-5451.

Schrager CA, Schneider D, Gruener AC, et al. Clinical and pathological features of breast disease in Cowden's syndrome: an underrecognized syndrome with an increased risk of breast cancer. *Hum Pathol* 1998; 29: 47-53.

Sieber OM, Lipton L, Crabtree M, et al. Multiple colorectal adenomas, classic adenomatous polyposis, and germline mutations in MYH. *N Engl J Med* 2003; 348: 791-799.

Simon S, Pavel M, Hensen J, et al. Multiple endocrine neoplasia 2A syndrome: surgical management. *J Pediatr Surg* 2002; 37: 897-900.

Sipple JH. The association of pheochromocytoma with carcinoma of the thyroid gland. *Am J Med* 1961; 31: 163-166.

Skinner MA, Moley JA, Dilley WG, et al. Prophylactic thyroidectomy in multiple endocrine neoplasia type 2A. *N Engl J Med* 2005; 353: 1105-1113.

Smith JM, Kirk EP, Theodosopoulos G, et al. Germline mutations of the tumour suppressor PTEN in Proteus syndrome. *J Med Genet* 2002; 39: 937-940.

Szinnai G, Meier C, Komminoth P, et al. Review of multiple endocrine neoplasia type 2A in children: therapeutic results of early thyroidectomy and prognostic value of codon analysis. *Pediatrics* 2003; 111: E132-139.

References

Takahashi M, Asai N, Iwashita T, et al. Molecular mechanisms of development of multiple endocrine neoplasia 2 by RET mutations. *J Intern Med* 1998; 243: 509-513.

Thull DL, Vogel VG. Recognition and management of hereditary breast cancer syndromes. *Oncologist* 2004; 9: 13-24.

Valentini AM, Armentano R, Pirrelli M, et al. Immunohistochemical mismatch repair proteins expression in colorectal cancer. *Appl Immunohistochem Mol Morphol* 2006; 14: 42-45.

Van den Bos M, Van den Hoven M, et al. More differences between HNPCC-related and sporadic carcinomas from the endometrium as compared to the colon. *Am J Surg Pathol* 2004; 28: 706-711.

Van Kessel AG, Wijnhoven H, Bodmer D, et al. Renal cell cancer: chromosome 3 translocations as risk factors. *J Natl Cancer Inst* 1999; 91: 1159-1160.

Varley JM, Evans DG, Birch JM. Li-Fraumeni syndrome: a molecular and clinical review. *Br J Cancer* 1997; 76: 1-14.

Vasen HF, Watson P, Mecklin JP, et al. New clinical criteria for hereditary nonpolyposis colorectal cancer (HNPCC, Lynch syndrome) proposed by the International Collaborative group on HNPCC. *Gastroenterology* 1999; 116: 1453-1456.

Veugelers M, Bressan M, McDermott DA, et al. Mutation of perinatal myosin heavy chain associated with a Carney complex variant. *N Engl J Med 2004*; 351: 460-469.

Watanabe T, Wu TT, Catalano PJ, et al. Molecular predictors of survival after adjuvant chemotherapy for colon cancer. *N Engl J Med* 2001; 344: 1196-1206.

Watson JC, Stratakis CA, Bryant-Greenwood PK, et al. Neurosurgical implications of Carney complex. *J Neurosurg* 2000; 92: 413-418.

Watson P, Lin KM, Rodriguez-Bigas MA, et al. Colorectal carcinoma survival among hereditary nonpolyosis colorectal carcinoma family members. *Cancer* 1998; 83: 259-266.

Weksberg R, Nishikawa J, Caluseriu O, et al. Tumor development in the Beckwith-Wiedemann syndrome is associated with a variety of constitutional molecular 11p15 alterations including imprinting defects of KCNQ1OT1. *Hum Mol Genet* 2001; 10: 2989-3000.

Wicklund CL, Pauli RM, Johnston D, et al. Natural history study of hereditary multiple exostoses. *Am J Med Genet* 1995; 55: 43-46.

Wuyts W, Van Hul W. Molecular basis of multiple exostoses: mutations in the EXT1 and EXT2 genes. *Hum Mutat* 2001; 15: 220-227.

Yip L, Cote GJ, Shapiro SE, et al. Multiple endocrine neoplasia type 2: evaluation of the genotype-phenotype relationship. *Arch Surg* 2003; 138: 409-416.

Young S, Gooneratne S, Straus FH, et al. Feminizing Sertoli cell tumors in boys with Peutz-Jeghers syndrome. *Am J Surg Pathol* 1995; 19: 50-58.

Zhou X, Hampel H, Thiele H, et al. Association of germline mutation in the PTEN tumour suppressor gene and Proteus and Proteus-like syndromes. *Lancet* 2001; 358: 210-211.

Chapter 14

Solid Tumors

Genitourinary Tumors

Renal Cell Carcinoma (RCC)

- Most renal tumors can be classified, based on morphology alone, in accordance with the 2004 World Health Organization **T14.1** nomenclature. Correct classification is important, because the tumors manifest clinically significant differences in behavior that influence both prognosis and treatment. In fact, one may be asked to make these distinctions intraoperatively, particularly to identify 1 of the benign lesions—oncocytoma and angiomyolipoma. However, an occasional tumor is difficult to classify, and immunohistochemistry (IHC) is only marginally helpful. For example, histochemical staining for Hale colloidal iron and immunohistochemical expression of CD117 have been well described in chromophobe carcinoma, but results are often disappointing in practice. In these instances, one occasionally must appeal to the molecular laboratory for assistance.

- Conventional clear cell renal cell carcinoma

  - This is the most common variant encountered in routine practice. Clear cell histology is often predictable macroscopically, because areas of degeneration, hemorrhage, and necrosis give these tumors a highly variegated gross appearance. Microscopically, a clear cell carcinoma is composed of cells with clear cytoplasm, arranged in small packets surrounded by a rich network of uniform, thin-walled vessels.

  - Portions of the short arm of chromosome 3 are deleted in most cases. 3 particular loci are disproportionately affected: 3p14, 3p25.3 (the location of the *VHL* gene), and 3p21.3.

  - Del (3p) is the sole abnormality in only about 15% of cases, however. Additional anomalies at 14q, 9p, 8p, and 6q are common; in fact, it appears that 3p is necessary for initial tumorigenesis, but the additional anomalies contribute to tumor progression. Furthermore, del(3p) by itself has no impact on prognosis, while loss of 14q, 9p, and 8p each correlates with higher stage and a worse prognosis.

- Papillary (chromophil) renal cell carcinoma

  - About 15% of RCCs are of the papillary type. The likelihood increases in connection with end-stage renal disease–associated polycystic kidneys. Like many of the nonclear variants,

T14.1
2004 World Health Organization Classification of Renal Tumors (Modified)

Tumor	Immunophenotype	Chromosomes	Behavior
Clear cell renal cell carcinoma	CD10+, Vimentin+	del (3p)	Aggressive
Papillary renal cell carcinoma	CD10+, Vimentin+, AMACR+	Loss of Y, gains of 7 & 17	Indolent
Chromophobe renal cell carcinoma	CD10−/+, Vimentin −, CD117+	Loss of Y, 1, 2, 6, 10, 13, 17, and 21	Indolent
Collecting (Bellini) duct carcinoma	CD10−, Vimentin −, high MW keratin+	del (1q)	Aggressive
Renal medullary carcinoma	CD10−, Vimentin −, CEA+	Unknown	Aggressive
Xp11.2 translocation carcinoma	TFE3+ (nuclear)CD10+	Xp11.2 translocation	Indolent
Oncocytoma	CD10−/+, Vimentin +/−, CD117+	Highly variable: loss of 1, 14. t(5;11).	Benign
Mucinous, tubular, and spindle cell carcinoma	CD10−, Vimentin+	Loss of 1, 4, 6, 8, 13, 14	Indolent
Angiomyolipoma	HMB45+	LOH at *TSC2* on 16p	Benign

the gross appearance is that of a uniform brown tumor; however, papillary carcinomas are often multifocal. Microscopically the tumor may grow in either tubular or papillary formations, on the surface of which the tumor cells grow as either a bland cuboidal monolayer (type 1 papillary RCC) or a pseudostratified proliferation of larger cells (type 2 papillary RCC). A highly consistent feature is packets of foamy interstitial macrophages.

☐ Papillary carcinoma is associated with loss of the Y chromosome (in males) and gains of (trisomy or tetrasomy of) 7 and 17. The only consistent cytogenetic difference between the papillary types is that type 2 tumors have a greater number of anomalies than type 1. In the very rare familial form of papillary RCC, the responsible gene has been mapped to 7q.

☐ The mucinous tubular and spindle cell carcinoma of the kidney, which is easily mistaken for papillary renal cell carcinoma, lacks the gains and losses that characterize papillary RCC.

■ Chromophobe renal cell carcinoma

☐ Chromophobe renal cell carcinoma may be difficult to distinguish from both clear cell carcinoma and oncocytoma. The clinical behavior is intermediate between these 2 look-alikes. The gross appearance is typically a uniform brown tumor. Microscopically, key features are the sharp "plantlike" cell borders and irregular "human papillomavirus (HPV)–like" nuclei. Hale colloidal iron is reported to stain chromophobe carcinomas preferentially, as is the immunohistochemical marker CD117 (c-kit).

☐ With multiple chromosomal losses, especially of Y, 1, 2, 6, 10, 13, 17, and 21, chromophobe carcinomas often achieve hypodiploidy. Oncocytomas show similar, though far fewer, chromosomal losses; they especially show a high incidence of 1p1 deletion.

■ Renal carcinoma with Xp11.2 translocation (TFE3-associated carcinoma)

☐ This tumor most often arises in children and young adults. The tumor has a distinctive appearance with alveolar (nested) and papillary architecture, clear cells, and psammoma bodies. Based on the foregoing, therefore, TFE3-associated carcinoma should be thought of whenever (1) a diagnosis of an RCC with a mixed histologic pattern is entertained, or (2) any RCC is seen

in a child. A thick, calcified capsule is seen in some cases. The tumor is characteristically negative for epithelial membrane antigen (a marker uniformly positive in conventional clear cell carcinoma) but positive for CD10.

☐ Several Xp11.2 abnormalities have been described in connection with these tumors, including t(X;1)(p11.2;q21), producing the TFE3-PRCC fusion gene, t(X;17)(p11.2;q25), producing TFE3-ASPL, and t(X;1)(p11.2;p34), producing TFE3-PSF. The TFE3-ASPL gene fusion of t(X;17) is also seen in alveolar soft part sarcoma (ASPS); however, a key difference is that the translocation in ASPS is an unbalanced one, while that in renal carcinoma is balanced.

☐ The TFE-ASPL renal tumors character-istically present at advanced stage but, like ASPS, follow an indolent course marked by very late relapses/metastases.

☐ RCCs with t(6:11)(p11.2;q12) involves the TFEB gene which is closely related in function to the TFE3 gene. The resulting tumor is essentially identical to Xp11.2 tumors.

Prostate Cancer

■ By far, the most common form of prostate cancer is adenocarcinoma derived from acinar cells (acinar adenocarcinoma). Presently, there is little role for molecular techniques in routine diagnostic prostate pathology, but the role of such techniques in prostate cancer screening is increasing.

■ When studied by conventional cytogenetics, most prostatic adenocarcinomas have a normal karyotype. However, numerous small abnormalities are demonstrable by fluorescence in situ hybridization (FISH) or comparative genomic hybridization, the most common of which may be loss of 8p. Several oncogenes are overexpressed in prostatic adenocarcinoma, MYC and BCL2 especially. Furthermore, mutations in PTEN and/or P53 are present in a proportion of tumors, particularly in advanced disease.

■ About 5% of cases are associated with a strong family history. The proportion may be as high as 40% in cases diagnosed before age 55 years. Presently, most cases are thought to be linked to a locus on chromosome 1q24-25 (the HPC1 locus), and the responsible gene at this locus is believed to be the RNASEL gene (encoding ribonuclease L).

In addition, families with germline mutations of the *BRCA1* or *BRCA2* genes have a higher rate of prostatic adenocarcinoma.

- From a practical standpoint, the most exciting development has to do with the availability of a molecular marker for the detection of prostatic adenocarcinoma. The effectiveness of the serum assay for prostate specific antigen (PSA) is limited by significant overlap between those with benign and malignant disease; a significant number of cancers are found in men with a "normal" PSA value of less than 4 ng/dL. Nucleic acid tests are now available that can be performed on urine, obtained after prostatic massage, to detect RNA transcripts of genes overexpressed in prostate cancer. 1 example is the assay for PCA3 (prostate cancer 3). PCA3 (uPM3) encodes a nontranslated mRNA known as DDT (differential display 3). PCA3 (DDT) is overexpressed in more than 95% of prostate cancers, at an average of 66 times the rate of expression in benign glands. By contrast, the KLK3 gene, which encodes PSA, is not overexpressed in prostate cancer (the increased concentration of PSA in the serum of some patients with prostate cancer seems to be related to an increase in leakage into the extracellular matrix rather than increased expression). Using quantitative reverse transcriptase polymerase chain reaction (PCR), the quantity of the PCA3 transcript can be measured and compared with the urine PSA (to correct for the number of prostatic cells obtained). Sensitivity of about 70% and a specificity approaching 90% has been demonstrated through the use of this assay.

- Specimen identity testing is occasionally required in the practice of prostate and other types of biopsy pathology. Specimen identity testing refers to the use of molecular techniques to ensure that a specimen belongs to a particular patient. Most pathologists are familiar with the uniquely alarming circumstance in which cancer cannot be found in a prostatectomy after a positive biopsy. Often the issue can be resolved with thorough sectioning, but there are rare cases in which even after exhaustive efforts one is left with the predicament of an unequivocally positive biopsy specimen and a negative prostate gland. This situation has been called the "vanishing cancer" phenomenon. While there are a number of possible explanations, 1 that must occasionally be entertained is a specimen mix-up. 1 approach to this problem is the comparison of DNA microsatellites, either between biopsy and patient or between biopsy and prostatectomy. Microsatellites are regions of the genome composed of a short repetitive sequence; eg, a run of adenine bases or a run of alternating cytosine-adenine (CA) couplets. They are usually found in noncoding segments of DNA, and each person inherits, for every microsatellite locus, 1 maternal and 1 paternal allele. The parental alleles are usually of differing length (heterozygous), but they are occasionally the same (homozygous); within a particular person, every cell in the body has microsatellites of equal length. From person-to-person, microsatellites are usually of different lengths, and, particularly if several microsatellite loci are looked at simultaneously, they can be used to very reliably distinguish 1 person from another. This analysis can be performed on formalin-fixed, paraffin-embedded tissue from which DNA is extracted. The recovered DNA is subjected to multiplex (multiple primers) PCR designed to amplify several microsatellite markers. The amplified products can be subjected to electrophoresis on a gel and analyzed visually. The pattern derived from a prostate biopsy should match exactly that obtained from the prostatectomy.

Urothelial (Transitional Cell) Carcinoma

- There appear to be at least 2 distinct biologic types of urothelial carcinoma, arrived at by way of 2 separate pathways. The first is the common low-grade papillary urothelial carcinoma which has the capacity to recur but has almost no metastatic potential. Clinically, it serves mainly as a marker of risk for developing a high-grade urothelial carcinoma, for which the low-grade tumor may be a precursor. High-grade tumors may arise from low-grade tumors or from flat carcinoma in situ. High-grade tumors readily invade the bladder wall and may then disseminate.

- Thus, grading is a critical part of bladder biopsy interpretation. Low-grade papillary urothelial carcinomas are distinctive mainly for their architectural findings: the formation of papillae. There must be a mild degree of cytologic change as well, to distinguish them from the rare papilloma. These changes may include an increase in nuclear size, irregularities of nuclear shape, and coarsened chromatin, but mitotic figures are rare and confined to parabasal cells. In contrast, high-grade lesions may be papillary (high-grade papillary urothelial carcinoma) or flat (urothelial carcinoma in situ). In either case, the defining features are loss of polarity, marked nuclear enlargement (at least 6 times the size of a stromal lymphocyte), inky chromatin, and readily identifiable mitoses. In cases that present a grading difficulty, adjunctive IHC (using CK20, Ki-67, and/or p53) can be very helpful. Thus far, however, molecular methods have not shown much practical merit in the biopsy setting.

- Urothelial carcinomas have been extensively studied on the molecular level, with results that support this bimodal concept. Low-grade tumors generally display a limited variety of genetic anomalies, including deletion of the *P16* tumor suppressor gene and mutations in the *FGFR3* (fibroblast growth factor receptor 3) gene. Low-grade tumors usually have either a normal karyotype or a single anomaly: the loss of 9p (the consequence of which is thought to be loss of the tumor suppressor gene *P16*, found at 9p21). In contrast, high-grade tumors usually lack *FGFR3* mutations but do have *P16* inactivation; in addition, they commonly display *TP53* inactivation, chromosomal instability, and a complex karyotype including, in addition to del 9p, multiple aneuploidies. In particular, gains or losses of 6p, 7, 9, and 17 are associated with aggressive behavior. Gain of 6p is a common theme in multiple tumor types—urothelial carcinoma, colon cancer, melanomas, several lymphoma types, and several sarcoma types—and is especially associated with tumor progression (increasing grade or stromal invasion). Gain in 6p genetic material may occur via the formation of an isochromosome, a translocation, or amplification (with the appearance of double minutes or homogeneously staining regions).

- FISH assays are now available which can be applied to urothelial cells exfoliated in urine. The available assays include a "cocktail" of several probes, which are fluorescein-tagged single-stranded DNA segments, designed to hybridize with specific chromosome regions that are often aneuploid in urothelial carcinoma. Each probe produces a unique color, and each normal nucleus would be expected to produce 2 signals in each color. For example, the UroVysion probe cocktail includes 3 chromosome enumeration probes (CEP) probes—CEP 3, CEP 7, and CEP17—and 1 locus-specific indicator (LSI) probe. The 4-probe set was approved initially for detection of tumor recurrence but is now also approved for evaluation of microhematuria. After incubation with these probes, the slide is examined for cytologically abnormal cells, and the number of probe signals within each abnormal nucleus is noted. A predetermined number of cells must be examined, after which specific

criteria are applied to categorize the study as positive or negative. This method has demonstrated high sensitivity and specificity for urothelial carcinoma, particularly for high-grade tumors. As would be expected, sensitivity for the normally diploid low-grade tumors is not high (or necessarily desired). An interesting phenomenon, noted even in early clinical trials, is that in some cases a positive FISH study is not initially associated with a cystoscopically confirmed tumor; however, in nearly all such cases a tumor later developed, usually within a few months. The identification of such "anticipatory positives" reflects the impressive sensitivity of these methods.

Wilms Tumor

- *WT1* is a tumor suppressor gene located at 11p13. The WAGR syndrome (Wilms tumor, aniridia, genitourinary anomalies, retardation) is caused by a large germline 11p13 deletion that encompasses the *PAX6* gene (causing aniridia) and the *WT1* gene. Germline mutations in *WT1* are also present in the Denys-Drash syndrome. Sporadic Wilms tumors have *WT1* mutations, but in almost all such cases, these are present only in tumor tissue (somatic mutations).

- *WT2* is a gene located at 11p15. The Beckwith-Wiedemann syndrome is caused by germline mutations in *WT2*.

Central Nervous System Tumors

Gliomas

- In adults, gliomas are the most common form of central nervous system tumor, and astrocytomas and oligodendrogliomas represent the most common forms of glioma. Because gliomas usually cannot be fully removed surgically, radiotherapy and chemotherapy are frequently entertained as therapeutic modalities. It has been known for some time that *oligodendrogliomas respond much better to radiation and chemotherapy, and have an overall better prognosis.* Distinguishing oligodendrogliomas from astrocytomas T14.2, and thus predicting tumor response and overall prognosis, has traditionally been based on tumor morphology. Several immunohistochemical markers—GFAP, Leu7, p53—have failed to demonstrate sufficient discrimination. While routine histology can reliably classify a large proportion of cases, there remains a considerable number with indeterminate morphologic features.

Central Nervous System Tumors>Gliomas

T14.2
Oligodendroglioma vs Astrocytoma

Diagnostic Method	Oligodendroglioma	Astrocytoma
Imaging	Peripheral (cortical), well-demarcated, calcified	Central (subcortical), infiltrative
Histology	Round, regular nuclei Paucity of glial processes Perineural satellitosis Microcysts filled with mucin	Elongated, irregular nuclei Abundant glial processes
WHO types	Grade II (oligodendroglioma) Grade III (anaplastic oligodendroglioma)	Grade II (low-grade astrocytoma) Grade III (anaplastic astrocytoma) Grade IV (GBM)
IHC	Not generally useful, although astrocytomas are more likely to express strong GFAP and p53, with considerable overlap.	
Genetics (by LOH or FISH)	Loss of 1p in 80% Loss of 19q in 80% Loss of 1p and 19q in 60-80% Losses in 9p and 10q increase with grade No EGFR amplification	Loss of 1p in 30%-40% Loss of 19q in 10%-15% Loss of 1p and 19q in 5% Losses in 9p and 10q increase with grade EGFR amplification in high grade astros (esp GBM)
Prognosis	Better, with combined loss of 1p and 19q associated with chemosensitivity	Worse, with unclear significance of combined loss of 1p and 19q cases

EGFR = epidermal growth factor receptor; FISH = fluorescence in situ hybridization; GFAP = glial fibrillary acidic protein; IHC = immunohistochemistry; LOH = loss of heterozygosity; WHO = World Health Organization.

■ Genetic markers have shown the greatest potential, to date, in this crucial distinction. There are genetic alterations that occur with equal frequency in astrocytomas and oligodendrogliomas, usually with devolution to a higher grade, including loss of 9p21 (*p16/CDKN2A*) and losses involving chromosome 10 (*PTEN/DMBT1*). These markers may provide prognostic information but do not aid in the distinction of oligodendrogliomas from astrocytomas. The genetic markers with the greatest power in this regard are the *combined loss of genetic material from chromosomes 1p and 19q*. The loss of either of these is more common in oligodendrogliomas, and their combined loss is highly specific (but only about 60%–80% sensitive). Furthermore, other tumors often confused with oligodendrogliomas, such as the dysembryoblastic neuroectodermal tumor (DNET), protoplasmic astrocytoma, and central neurocytoma, lack 1p/19q losses.

■ Perhaps distinct from and more important than the question of oligodendrogliomas versus astrocytoma, the combined loss of 1p and 19q identifies a set of tumors with enhanced chemosensitivity and prolonged survival. Deletions of 1p and 19q can be detected in formalin-fixed, paraffin-embedded tissue by means of PCR or FISH. The strategy for PCR in this setting is to detect loss-of-heterozygosity (LOH) for particular markers on 1p or 19q. Microsatellites (multiple repeats of a single nucleotide or dinucleotide) occur throughout the genome, usually in noncoding segments of DNA. Because of polymorphism in the population, the maternally derived and paternally derived microsatellite at a particular locus are likely to be of somewhat different length. From cell-to-cell, these lengths are constant, however, and variability is the marker of microsatellite instability (see section on colorectal carcinoma). Thus, when a segment of DNA that contains a microsatellite is amplified, there will be 2 products, usually of differing lengths. In the context of glioma diagnosis, primers are applied that will amplify specific microsatellites on 1p and 19q. The retrieval of product on only a single length is indicative of LOH and suggests a deletion. Simultaneous amplification of nontumor DNA can confirm this, if products of 2 different lengths are obtained. FISH is much more straightforward, employing probes for specific 1p or 19q sequences. A positive centromere marker probe must also be included.

- *TP53* (17p) mutations are present in about 30% of diffuse astrocytomas of any grade (II, III, or IV), but they are not very common in oligodendrogliomas. Immunohistochemical staining for p53 correlates well with, and is a useful substitute for, molecular testing. It appears that the subset of p53 expressing grade II/III astrocytomas are *no more likely* than p53 negative tumors to progress to grade IV (glioblastoma multiforme). However, among GBMs, p53 expression is more likely in a tumor that arose out of a preexisting low-grade glioma; as de novo GBMs are usually p53 negative (epidermal growth factor receptor [EGFR] positive).

- *EGFR* mutations are common in high-grade (III-IV) gliomas; interestingly, EGFR and TP53 are overexpressed rarely in the same tumor. EGFR overexpression by IHC, like p53, correlates well with mutational status, and is indicative of an aggressive tumor. Importantly, it may also be indicative of sensitivity to EGFR inhibitors. Amplification of the *EGFR* gene is found in about half of glioblastomas and rarely in lower grade astrocytomas or oligodendrogliomas; thus, it may be useful in correctly categorizing small cell astrocytomas.

- Chromosome 10q LOH is among the most common molecular anomalies found in GBM. 10q is the site of the *PTEN* gene, and its loss indicates an unfavorable prognosis.

- In summary, poor prognostic molecular factors in gliomas include retention of 1p and 19q, LOH 10q, and EGFR amplification. TP53 mutation or p53 overexpression does not seem to impact prognosis.

Retinoblastoma

- The *RB1* gene is critical in the development of retinoblastoma. About 70% of *RB1* mutations are in the form of point mutations, detectable only by direct sequence analysis. Larger deletions of all or part of the *RB1* gene may be identified by FISH in about 15% of cases. Hypermethylation, particularly within the promoter region, is found in about 10% of cases.

- Most cases (85%) are sporadic. About 5% of children with retinoblastoma harbor a germline chromosome deletion, detectable by cytogenetics, involving chromosome 13q14. The incidence is higher in children with bilateral retinoblastoma. About another 10% have no detectable deletion but have a family history of retinoblastoma. Inheritance of a germline *RB1* mutation markedly increases the risk of several extraocular tumors as well: pineal gland tumors, peripheral neuroectodermal tumors (PNETs), and *osteosarcomas*. These secondary tumors usually present in late childhood or adulthood.

Meningioma

- Monosomy of chromosome 22 is the most common abnormality found in meningiomas. The key region appears to be 22q12.2 where the *NF2* gene is located. Recall that meningioma is 1 of the features of the NF2 syndrome (caused by germline *NF2* mutations).

- Merlin is the protein encoded by the *NF2* gene. Merlin is found in the cell membrane where its function is to mediate cell-cell contact and cell contact inhibition. It is thought that CD44, 1 of the merlin ligands, is a signal for the cessation of growth.

- Certain histologic features have shown moderate correlation with aggressive behavior (recurrence and progression). The term *anaplastic meningioma* has been applied to such tumors. The mitotic rate is perhaps the strongest single predictive feature. Others, in combination, portend a high rate of recurrence: the presence of true cerebral invasion, high cellularity, small cell growth, prominent nucleoli, sheet-like growth, and necrosis. In addition, particular histologic subtypes are felt to have a higher rate of progression: clear cell, chordoid, rhabdoid, and papillary. Lastly, a high proportion of cells with MIB-1 (Ki-67) immunohistochemical staining is associated with recurrence.

- While 22q12.2 deletion is thought to be a key early step in development of meningiomas, tumor progression seems to involve other alterations. Anaplastic meningiomas show frequent losses (eg, 1p, 9p, 14, and others) as well as gains (eg, 1q, 9q, and others). In fact, del 1p is the second most common chromosomal abnormality found in meningiomas. Deletion of 14 (monosomy 14) and/or deletion of 9p21 have been associated with shortened survival.

Soft Tissue Tumors T14.3

Ewing/PNET (Ewing Family of Tumors)

- The Ewing tumor family encompasses several entities previously considered distinct, including Ewing sarcoma, peripheral neuroectodermal tumor (PNET), Askin tumor, and others. In addition to common histologic and immunohistochemical traits, this group of tumors has various molecular rearrangements all of which result in the formation of a *EWS* fusion gene and the production of *EWS* fusion transcripts.

- The most common structural rearrangement is t(11;22)(q24;q12), involving the *EWS* gene on 22q12 and the *FLI1* gene on 11q24, forming an *FLI1/EWS* fusion gene. The precise location of fusion differs from case to case, but most commonly it is formed between exon 7 of *EWS* and exon 6 of *FLI1* (termed the *type 1 fusion*). The type 1 fusion is associated with a relatively favorable prognosis. Some cases have instead a t(21;22) translocation, involving *EWS* and *ERG*, or rarely a t(7;22) or t(17;22).

- Intraabdominal desmoplastic small round cell tumor (IADSRCT) was first described only about 20 years ago. It usually presents as an intraabdominal mass in a young adult, but numerous other presentations have been described. The tumor's morphologic features immediately raise the small round cell tumor differential, including Ewing/PNET, neuroblastoma, rhabdomyosarcoma (RMS), synovial sarcoma, Wilms tumor, and lymphoma. Its occasional presence in an older adult widens the differential to include small cell and other neuroendocrine carcinomas. Its only distinctive feature is growth within strikingly desmoplastic stroma. A unique immunohistochemical profile usually aids in identifying this tumor, however it is fully manifested in only 80% to 90% of cases: neuron-specific enolase positive, EMA-positive, keratin-positive, and desmin-positive. A unique translocation is present in nearly all IADSRCTs: t(11;22)(p13;q12) which results in the fusion of the *EWS* gene to the Wilms tumor gene (*WT1*) on 11p13.

- Clear cell sarcoma of tendons and aponeuroses (malignant melanoma of soft parts) is another *EWS*-associated tumor. Clear cell sarcoma is an unusual tumor that presents in the soft tissue of the extremity in young adults or adolescents. Its comparison to malignant melanoma derives from several shared morphologic, immunohistochemical,

and ultrastructural features. Identification of a molecular rearrangement unique to clear cell sarcoma permits definitive distinction. About 90% of cases demonstrate the t(12;22)(q13;q12) translocation which produces the *EWS/ATF1* fusion gene. Conventional cytogenetics, FISH, or PCR can readily detect the translocation. *ATF1* (activating transcription factor 1) is located at 12q13. A second abnormality, +8, has been described in a significant minority of cases.

Neuroblastoma

- Neuroblastoma tends to affect children younger than 5 years. It presents as an abdominal mass or, less commonly, a posterior mediastinal mass, because it is most often derived from either the adrenal medulla or a portion of the sympathetic chain. Amplification of the *MYCN* (n-Myc) proto-oncogene is found in 30% of neuroblastomas and is a marker of aggressive behavior. *MYCN* is normally found at 2p23-24, and each cell normally has 2 gene copies; amplification refers to an increased number of gene copies per cell. *MYCN* amplification appears to be central to tumor progression and may occur in a variety of ways, including: (1) gene duplication in situ, with expansion of 2p23-34, (2) gene duplication with the formation of extra double minute chromosomes, and (3) gene duplication and insertion into random chromosomes, leading to segmental chromosome gain that may be visible as homogeneously staining regions.

- A greater than 10-fold amplification (>10 copies per cell) is correlated with poor prognosis. The overall proportion of tumors with this degree of *MYCN* amplification is 30%, but 40% in high-stage tumors and only 10% in low-stage tumors. Several modalities are available for detecting *MYCN* duplication, including FISH, chromogenic in situ hybridization, Southern blotting, and quantitative RT-PCR.

- In addition to MYCN amplification, neuroblastomas may display aneuploidy and/or a complex set of structural chromosomal anomalies. Abnormalities of 17q23 are present in more than 50% of cases, deletion of 1p36 in 30% to 40%, and deletion of 11q23 in 40% to 50%. The 1p deletion is associated with poor prognosis. The DNA content (ploidy) of the tumor has been shown to correlate with outcome, particularly in infants. Those with hyperdiploid tumors (DNA index greater than 1.0) have a more favorable outcome (similar to what is seen in acute lymphoblastic lymphoma).

Soft Tissue Tumors>Neuroblastoma

T14.3
Molecular Findings in Soft Tissue Tumors

Tumor	Cytogenetic Finding	Molecular Finding
Ewing/PNET	t(11;22)(q24;q12)	FLI1/EWS
	t(21;22)(q22;q12)	ERG/EWS
	t(7;22)(p22;q12)	ETV1/EWS
	t(17;22)(q12;q12)	E1AF/EWS
	t(2;22)(q33;q12)	FEV/EWS
Neuroblastoma	del(1p), +17	n-MYC
Alveolar rhabdomyosarcoma	t(2;13)(q37;q14)	PAX3/FKHR
	t(1;13)(p36;q14)	PAX7/FKHR
Desmoplastic small round cell tumor	t(11;22)(p13;q12)	EWS/WT1
Alveolar soft part sarcoma	t(X;17) (p11;q25)	ASPL/TFE3
Myxoid liposarcoma	t(12;16)(q13;p11)	TLS/CHOP
Dermatofibrosarcoma protuberans, Giant cell fibroblastoma	t(17;22)(q22;q13) Ring 17	COL1A1/PDGF
Infantile fibrosarcoma, Congenital mesoblastic nephroma	t(12;15)(p12;q25)	ETV6/NTRK3
Low-grade fibromyxoid sarcoma	t(7;16)(q33;p11)	FUS/CREB3L2
Myxoid chondrosarcoma (extraskeletal)	t(9;22)(q22;q12)	TEC/EWS
Liposarcoma, well-differentiated	Ring 12	
Liposarcoma, myxoid, and round cell	t(12;16)(q13;p11)	FUS/CHOP
Clear cell sarcoma	t(12;22)(q13;q12)	ATF1/EWS
Synovial sarcoma	t(X;18)(p11.2;q11.2)	SSX1/SYT
	t(X;18)(p11;q11)	SSX2/SYT
	t(5;18)(q11;q11)	
Inflammatory myofibroblastic tumor	t(1;2)(q25;p23)	TPM3/ALK
	t(2;19)(p23;p13)	TPM4/ALK
Angiomatoid fibrous histiocytoma	t(12;16)(q13;p11)	FUS/ATF1

Rhabdomyosarcoma (RMS)

- RMS occurs as 1 of several subtypes, only 1 of which has a recurring chromosomal anomaly: the *alveolar RMS*.

- The most common finding is the t(2;13)(q35;q14) translocation that results in the apposition of the *PAX3* gene (2q35) and the *FKHR* gene (13q14) to form a *PAX3-FKHR* fusion gene.

- A significant minority of cases have been found instead to have a t(1;13)(p36;q14) translocation involving the *PAX7* gene. Tumors with the *PAX7-FKHR* fusion gene appear to have a much better prognosis than those with *PAX3-FKHR*.

- About a third of alveolar RMS has neither of these anomalies. Many such cases have been described as having mixed alveolar-embryonal histology.

Synovial Sarcoma (SS)

- In classic cases, SS presents as an extremity tumor in an adolescent or young adult. The tumor arises in proximity to a joint, in a paraarticular but almost never intraarticular location. Tumors may be monophasic (spindled) or biphasic (spindled and epithelial). In fact, while thought of as the prototypical biphasic tumor, most are monophasic. This fact sometimes makes the diagnosis difficult, particularly when the tumor arises in unusual locations. The spindle cell component is highly cellular, composed of oblong cells with very little cytoplasm; essentially resembling a highly cellular fibrosarcoma. Key to this distinction is a lack of a well-formed herringbone pattern and the often present hemangiopericytoma-like pattern. Expression of epithelial immunohistochemical markers can help support this suspicion, but these may be weak or absent in the spindle component.

- SS is consistently associated with the t(X;18)(p11;q11) translocation, resulting in the fusion of the *SYT* gene (18q11) with either the *SSX1* or *SSX2* gene (Xp11). There is evidence that the *SSX1* fusion is associated with biphasic histology and *SSX2* with monophasic histology.

Gastrointestinal Stromal Tumor (GIST)

- GISTs, the most common soft tissue tumor of the GI tract, usually arise in the bowel wall in an older adult. The most common site is the stomach. Presentations unassociated with the bowel are common, and presentations outside the abdomen have been reported.

- Endoscopically, GISTs present as dome-shaped masses with central ulceration or umbilication. Histologically, they occupy the submucosa. Any ulceration is usually caused by thinning and rarefaction of the overlying mucosa (though GISTs occasionally directly invade the mucosa). The tumor is composed of a proliferation of either spindled or epithelioid cells in a pattern that may be reminiscent of a smooth muscle tumor, nerve sheath tumor, or, occasionally, carcinoma.

- In the past, GISTs were diagnosed as leiomyomas, leiomyosarcomas, nerve sheath tumors, or autonomic nerve tumors. The breakthrough that allowed unification under the GIST heading was the recognition that most of these tumors represented neoplastic transformation of a single cell type, the interstitial cell of Cajal, which is a mesenchymal cell capable of both neural and myoid differentiation. Cajal cell transformation, furthermore, was found to involve mutation of a tyrosine kinase, most often the *KIT* gene but sometimes the *PDGFR* gene.

- The clinical behavior of a GIST is notoriously difficult to predict, with over 1 in 3 behaving malignantly. Metastases to the liver are common, as are local recurrences. Indicators of aggressive potential include size, mitotic rate, coagulative-type necrosis, mucosal infiltration, and nuclear atypia. The most powerful of these are size and mitotic rate. Interestingly, deletional mutations (as opposed to substitutional) in exon 11 of the *KIT* gene have been associated with aggression.

- With regard to IHC, the most important marker is CD117 (C-KIT). Controversy exists over whether CD117 expression is required for the diagnosis of GIST. Regardless of this debate, the CD117 status may be important in guiding therapy. Depending on definitions of both disease and positivity, CD117 is positive in 90% to 100% of cases. Before CD117, the marker used to support a diagnosis of GIST was CD34, which is positive in 85% to 95% of cases. While it was previously thought that neural differentiation affected GIST prognosis, this belief is no longer widely held. Thus, additional markers (of smooth muscle and neural differentiation) are generally not indicated. Nonetheless, actin will be expressed in around 25% of cases, desmin in 10%, S-100 in 5%.

14: Solid Tumors

Soft Tissue Tumors>Gastrointestinal Stromal Tumor; Kaposi Sarcoma and Human Herpes Virus Type 8; Low-Grade Fibromyxoid Sarcoma and Hyalinizing Spindle Tumor with Giant Rosettes; Liposarcoma

- In nearly all cases, a tyrosine kinase mutation can be demonstrated. Most mutations are in *KIT* (95%), and about 5% are in *PDGFR*. A particular tumor has 1 or the other mutation, and rarely or never both. *KIT*-related tumors tend to have spindled morphology, and *PDGFR*-related tumors have epithelioid morphology. The *KIT* and *PDGFR* genes encode highly homologous tyrosine kinase proteins, and both genes are located on 4q12.

    □ *KIT* mutations are most common in exon 11, followed in order by 9, 13, and 17. Most exon 11 anomalies are point mutations that do not affect the reading frame (ie, not truncation or nonsense deletions). GISTs with most kinds of exon 11 mutations seem to have a better prognosis than those with exon 11 deletions. Note that *KIT* mutations are not unique to GIST and are common in mastocytosis.

    □ *PDGFR* mutations are most common in exon 18, followed by 12 and 14. Most *PDGFR*-associated cases have been gastric, and most have epithelioid morphology.

- GISTs are unresponsive to standard chemotherapy. There has been considerable success, however, with tyrosine kinase inhibitors, especially imatinib mesylate (STI571, Gleevec, Novartis Pharmaceuticals, East Hanover, NJ). Imatinib mesylate is an orally administered agent with the capacity to inhibit a variety of tyrosine kinases, including BCR-ABL, KIT, and *PDGFR*. The mutation site impacts sensitivity to imatinib inhibition; for example, mutations in exon 18 of *PDGFR* are insensitive to imatinib, exon 17 and 9 KIT mutations are relatively insensitive, and exon 11 *KIT* mutations are highly sensitive. As in the treatment of chronic myelogenous leukemia (see chapter 15), resistance emerges in some cases. Resistance is usually associated with the acquisition of additional KIT or PDGFR mutations.

- GIST may be seen in association with the Carney triad (see chapter 13). Less commonly, it is associated with neurofibromatosis type 1 (see chapter 13), and rarely it is familial. Interestingly, NF1-associated GISTs generally lack *KIT* and *PDGFR* mutations, and they are often small and multiple, with a predilection for the small bowel. Inherited germline *KIT* mutations form the basis for the familial GIST syndrome.

Kaposi Sarcoma (KS) and Human Herpes Virus Type 8 (HHV8)

- From the time of its emergence, endemic-type KS had all the hallmarks of an infectious disease: geographic circumscription, association with immunodeficiency, and a tendency to affect those who acquired human immunodeficiency virus (HIV) through sexual transmission, suggesting cotransmission. There are several clinical variants of KS. Classic KS affects elderly Mediterranean men, presenting as 1 or several nodules mainly on the lower extremities. Over a protracted time (>10 years), these spread proximally but rarely involve viscera and rarely cause death. Endemic KS is most often seen in immunocompromised hosts and came to prominence during the acquired immunodeficiency syndrome (AIDS) epidemic. This form of KS affects the skin but with no predictable topography, and it is very likely to involve viscera and progress rapidly. In parts of sub-Saharan Africa, KS is presently the most common tumor of soft tissue.

- Regardless of the clinical type, the vast majority of cases are associated with HHV8 (also called Kaposi sarcoma–related herpes virus or KSHV), which is also the etiologic agent of primary body cavity lymphoma (primary effusion lymphoma [PEL, see chapter 15] and AIDS-associated plasma cell type or multicentric Castleman disease). The virus appears to have incorporated human oncogenes into its genome over time.

Low-Grade Fibromyxoid Sarcoma (LGFMS) and Hyalinizing Spindle Tumor with Giant Rosettes (HSTGR)

- These 2 soft tissue tumors of low malignant potential, both recently described, appear to be morphologic expressions of a single entity.

- A single structural rearrangement—the t(7;16)(q34;p11) translocation—is present in all morphologic presentations of this tumor.

Liposarcoma

- This group of tumors collectively represents the most common type of sarcoma in adults. There are several recognized types: well-differentiated (lipomalike, sclerosing, and pleomorphic) liposarcoma (atypical lipoma), myxoid liposarcoma, round cell liposarcoma, and dedifferentiated/pleomorphic liposarcoma.

- Well-differentiated liposarcomas are often difficult to distinguish from lipoma variants, and their location (superficial versus deep) is frequently the decisive feature. In fact, the term *atypical lipoma* has been advocated for such tumors when they arise in superficial locations (eg, subcutis). Histologically identical tumors, when arising in deep locations (eg, retroperitoneum), should be regarded as malignant and called *well-differentiated liposarcoma*. Well-differentiated liposarcomas often show karyotypic abnormalities, including ring chromosomes and giant marker chromosomes that contain amplified segments derived from 12q13-q15.

- Dedifferentiated liposarcoma is a malignant fibrous histiocytoma (MFH)–like tumor that shows evidence of having derived from a well-differentiated liposarcoma. As would be expected, these have karyotypic anomalies resembling those of well-differentiated liposarcoma with a complex set of additional anomalies.

- Both myxoid and round cell liposarcomas display t(12;16)(q13;p11) and/or t(12;22)(q13;q12).

Extraskeletal Myxoid Chondrosarcoma

- Myxoid chondrosarcoma of soft issue is associated in most cases with the t(9;22)(q22;q12) translocation that results in a *EWS-TEC* fusion gene.

- Less common findings include t(9;17)(q22;q11) and t(9;15)(q22;q21).

- What is striking about nearly all reported structural rearrangements is the involvement of the 9q22 locus, leading to *TEC*-containing fusion genes. This finding appears to be quite sensitive and specific for the diagnosis of extraskeletal myxoid chondrosarcoma.

- *TEN*, also called *NOR1* and *CHN*, encodes a steroid receptor protein.

Breast Cancer

Her2 (Neu, ERB-B2)

- Her2 protein is a transmembrane glycoprotein in the epidermal growth factor receptor (EGFR) family. While it is expressed in various normal epithelia, including breast ductal epithelium, it is found to be overexpressed in about 20% of invasive breast cancers. Gene amplification is the mechanism by which Her2 becomes overexpressed in these tumors, and

chromosome 17 copy number by itself has little impact on Her2 overexpression.

- Her2 positivity (by which is implied Her2 overexpression) has been associated with a number of clinical attributes, including: (1) poor outcome, based on either recurrence rates or mortality, independent of other prognostic markers, (2) high nuclear grade (3) good response to adriamycin-based adjuvant chemotherapy, (4) a poor response to hormonal therapy, independent of estrogen receptor/progesterone receptor (ER/PR) status, and (5) a good response to Her2-targeted therapy, such as Trastuzumab (Herceptin), an anti-Her2 monoclonal antibody.

- The benefit of Her2-targeted therapy appears to apply only to those with 3+ staining by IHC or a positive FISH result. Tumors with 0 or 1+ staining by IHC derive no benefit. Among those with 2+ staining by IHC, about 25% show amplification by FISH.

- With regard to the correlation of histologic features with Her2 status, a few generalizations can be made. As noted already, Her2-positive tumors tend to have a higher nuclear grade; grade 1 tumors are rarely Her2-positive, and the vast majority of Her2-positive tumors have a grade of 3. Furthermore, Her2 overexpression is seen almost exclusively in invasive ductal carcinoma of the usual type. Her2 is rarely overexpressed in ductal carcinoma variants such as mucinous (colloid) and tubular carcinoma, and within the spectrum of lobular carcinoma is seen mainly in pleomorphic variants, if at all. This distribution is in contrast to that of hormone (ER/PR) receptor expression. There is in fact an inverse correlation between Her2 expression and ER/PR expression; however, there is a subset of tumors that express all 3 markers (ER-positive, PR-positive, Her2-positive), and these generally have grade 2 nuclei. Lastly, in breast tumors expressing none of these markers (negative for ER, PR, and Her2), the so-called basal type of tumor is overly represented.

- Much hinges on the result of Her2 testing. Therapeutic benefits can be great (but not all patients who are unequivocally Her2-positive respond); however, a course of therapy is extremely expensive, and there is a risk of serious cardiotoxicity. As with all tests, the pathologist must ensure the validity of the result through meticulous control of the conditions under which the test is performed and interpreted. At the very least, one should participate in interlaboratory proficiency testing and conform to guidelines published jointly by the American Society of Clinical Oncologists (ASCO) and the College of American Pathologists (CAP).

- Her2 testing modalities

  □ Many laboratories use IHC as the initial test of Her2 amplification. In assessing HER-2 expression, only circumferential membranous staining is considered. Expression is usually reported as 0 to 3+, depending on the proportion of cells displaying strong circumferential membranous staining. A 3+ result is defined as strong circumferential staining in more than 30% of tumor cells. Scores of 0 and 1+ are considered negative. 3+ is considered positive. An equivocal result (2+) is defined as complete circumferential membrane staining in more than 10% of cells that is either nonuniform or weak in intensity. Occasionally, a 2+ result can be the result of strong membranous staining in more than 10% but less than 30% of tumor cells.

  □ FISH may be used as either the primary means of Her2 assessment, or as a reflex test in 2+ IHC cases. The test is performed by applying an allele-specific Her2 probe to a section of tumor and may be performed with or without an internal control, a centromeric chromosome 17 (CEP17) probe. When an internal control is used, the number of signals from the Her2 oncogene probe (eg, with an orange label) is compared with the number of signals from the CEP17 probe (eg, with a green label), and a ratio is calculated. Visualization of 2 green and 2 orange signals is expected in a nonamplified cell (a ratio of 1:1). A positive test is defined as an average Her2/CEP17 ratio of 2.2 or more. A negative test is defined as an average Her2/CEP17 ratio of less than 1.8. When no internal control is used, the number of Her2 probe signals per nucleus are simply counted. A positive result is when an average of more than 6 Her2 signals per nucleus is counted. A negative result is fewer than 4 copies of Her2 gene per nucleus.

  □ Equivocal and discordant results may be obtained. An IHC score of 2+ by IHC is considered equivocal, and it is recommended that these tumors be studied by FISH. By FISH, a Her2/CEP17 ratio of 1.8 to 2.2 (or gene copy number of 4.0 to 6.0) is considered equivocal, and it is recommended in these cases that either additional cells are counted or the entire FISH assay is repeated. If an

unequivocal result cannot be achieved after repeat FISH, then IHC is recommended. At this time, it appears that discordant results (eg, 3+ IHC with a negative FISH or 0-1+ IHC with a positive FISH) should be treated according to the FISH assay.

- While having not yet found a place in routine practice, both real-time quantitative PCR (performed on paraffin-embedded tissue) and enzyme-linked immunosorbent assay (ELISA; performed on serum) have recently demonstrated high reproducibility and good correlation with the traditional assays. The ELISA assay for circulating Her2 protein may obviate the need for biopsy of metastatic foci.

EGFR (Her1, ERB-B1)

- The *EGFR* gene is likely to be amplified in breast cancer, similar in most respects to its cousin, Her2. Like Her2, both IHC and FISH may be used to detect EGFR amplification, and interpretation is similar as well.

- The impact on prognosis of *EGFR* overexpression is controversial, but it appears that EGFR-positive tumors may respond to anti-EGFR agents (e.g. Iressa).

TP53 Tumor Suppressor Gene

- The *TP53* gene (17p) encodes the transcription factor p53. It is the normal function of p53 to bind to several specific DNA sequences and enhance their transcription. The genes it normally enhances—such as those that promote apoptosis and others that inhibit entry into the cell cycle—work in concert to control cell division. Clinically significant *TP53* mutations usually affect the DNA-binding domain and result is loss of specificity of p53 protein; thus, this effective promoter of transcription becomes less inclined to promote its usual targets and becomes free to activate other genes.

- Mutated *TP53* encodes proteins that are resistant to degradation (so-called TP53 stabilized mutant protein); thus *TP53* mutations, though associated with decreased p53 functional activity, are associated with increased p53 IHC staining. There is, however, imperfect correlation between IHC and *TP53* mutation status.

- *TP53* mutations correlate with tumor aggressiveness, higher tumor grade, and lower rates of ER/PR expression.

- There is some evidence that *TP53* mutation may reduce the efficacy of chemotherapeutic agents whose mechanism of action involves the induction of apoptosis; eg, adriamycin, 5-fluorouracil.

Steroid Receptor Status

- The steroid receptors ER and PR, like all steroid receptors, reside in the nucleus and, when bound to steroid hormone, activate transcription of specific genes.

- There is an alpha form and a beta form for both ER and PR. In the case of ER, these are encoded by separate largely, but not entirely, homologous genes. In contrast, PRα and PRβ are encoded by the same gene, one with more 3′ (amino-terminal) material than the other. In routine immunohistochemical assays for ER, only ERα is measured; whereas the PR assay measures both PRα and PRβ.

- A clinical response to hormonal therapy (tamoxifen, aromatase inhibitors, or luteinizing hormone–releasing hormone agonists) is largely, but not entirely, dependent on the expression of steroid hormone receptors. In fact, about 70% of tumors expressing both ER and PR will respond to hormonal therapy, and only about 5% of tumors negative for ER and PR will respond. ER-positive, PR-negative tumors respond at roughly the same rate as those positive for both; however, ER-negative, PR-positive tumors respond in only about 15% of cases.

Cervical Cancer

Human Papillomavirus (HPV)

- The relationship of HPV to cervical cancer is now well established. However, HPV itself is not a simple matter, because there are over 100 HPV types and a complex interplay of HPV DNA with human DNA.

- The risk of cervical cancer is related to the type of infecting HPV. The HPV types that are considered carcinogenic are referred to as high-risk HPV (HRHPV) and include HPV 16, 18, 31, 33, 35, 39, 45, 51, 52, 56, 58, 59, 68, 73, and 82. Others, such as 6 and 11, are extremely common causes of human infection but do not pose a great cancer risk. The likelihood of malignant transformation appears to relate to 2 variables: (1) the ease with which the viral genome becomes integrated into the host genome, and (2)

the particular gene sequence (alleles) of the viral E6 and E7 genes. That is, HPV infections that result in benign processes are usually associated with an episomal viral DNA, whereas HPV infections that result in malignancy are usually associated with integration of the viral DNA into the host genome. Such integration results in unchecked transcription of 2 viral genes in particular—E6 and E7—that trigger malignant transformation. The E6 and E7 gene products act through several mechanisms, important among them being the inhibition of the retinoblastoma (Rb) and p53 tumor suppressor proteins. Some viral E6/E7 alleles encode potent inhibitors, and some encode weak inhibitors.

- While E6 and E7 appear to be important, and probably necessary for the development of cervical carcinoma, it seems that other conditions must also be met. This contention is based on the observation that many more women are infected with HPV, including high-risk HPV, than develop cervical cancer. The additional mechanisms may include HPV-independent somatic DNA events (such as *FHIT* mutation), host immune status, and/or germline DNA polymorphisms.

- The approach most widely advocated for HPV screening is cervical cytology. When a cytologic diagnosis of either low- or high-grade squamous intraepithelial lesion (LSIL or HSIL) is rendered, colposcopy is indicated. When a cytologic diagnosis of atypical squamous cells (ASC) is rendered, molecular testing for the presence of high-risk HPV (HRHPV) is indicated, followed by colposcopy and biopsy if this is positive. In all 3 instances, the purpose of colposcopy is to exclude a high grade lesion. Several assays are currently available for the molecular detection of HPV in cervical samples, most of which are performed on the same liquid-based collection system used to prepare the slide for cytologic screening.

- The most common assay is a solution-phase hybridization using labeled RNA probes. Successful hybridization of the probes (with any viral DNA present in the sample) is detected by enzymatic reaction. This assay may be used to detect HRHPV specifically, or it may be used to detect low-risk HPV. Such assays have much higher sensitivity than cytology, but they are positive in a large number of women with no lesion (low specificity); hence the recommendation for testing only in the presence of an atypical cytology.

■ An available alternative, not widely applied at this time, is the use of markers directly on cytologic or histologic slides. This allows correlation of the signal with morphologic findings, possibly offering some advantages. Potential markers include FISH probes for HRHPV and a number of surrogate HRHPV markers, such as p16INK4a and Ki-67. P16INK4a is a tumor suppressor protein that exerts itself through interaction with Rb and is lost in various tumors (through mutation, hypermethylation, or deletion). P16INK4a transcription is suppressed, through a feedback loop, by Rb, which, due to the action of E6/E7, is markedly reduced in cells infected with HRHPV. Thus p16INK4a is markedly elevated in these cells (because of loss of negative feedback). Overexpression of p16INK4a can be demonstrated by IHC in nearly all malignant and dysplastic cells infected with HRHPV. Low-risk HPV-infected and benign lesions do not show overexpression. Ki-67 (MIB-1) is expressed in cells that are progressing through the cell cycle. Thus, like proliferating cell nuclear antigen (PCNA), Ki-67 is a proliferation marker. Neither marker is linked as closely to HRHPV as p16INK4a, but both markers are useful to distinguish high-grade lesions from cytologic and histologic mimics.

Colorectal Cancer

Pathogenesis

■ Colorectal carcinomas arise in adenomatous polyps and rarely (if ever) from normal mucosa. This assertion is supported by several lines of evidence, among the most powerful of which is the finding that timely removal of polyps, ie, interruption of the adenoma-carcinoma sequence, significantly reduces the incidence of adenocarcinoma.

■ In normal colonic mucosa, the base of the crypt is the site of cell division, and the luminal surface is the site of apoptosis. A balance between the rates of these processes prevents overcrowding, and a loss of balance leads to a polyp—hyperplastic or adenomatous. Increased entry into the cell cycle, a reduced rate of apoptosis, or both cause a shift in favor of proliferation, the earliest morphologic reflection of which are the so-called aberrant crypt foci. These lesions arise in flat mucosa and precede polyps. As

molecular changes accumulate, low-grade dysplasia (adenoma) may give way to high-grade dysplasia and carcinoma.

■ There appear to be 2 major pathways for the development of colorectal carcinoma **T14.4**, each associated with a morphologically distinctive type of premalignant polyp, and each with a clinicopathologically distinctive type of invasive carcinoma.

■ The first, referred to here as the APC pathway, leads to around 85% of colorectal carcinoma cases. It is initiated by truncating mutations in the adenomatous polyposis coli (*APC*) gene. In its early stages, this pathway leads to the formation of tubular adenomas, and, less commonly, tubulovillous or villous adenomas. Malignancies forming through this pathway take the form of conventional gland-forming colorectal adenocarcinoma.

■ The second, referred to here as the MMR pathway, leads to about 15% of colorectal carcinoma cases. It is initiated by aberrations in 1 of the mismatch repair (*MMR*) genes. Early lesions along the MMR pathway take the form of serrated adenomas, and malignancies resulting from this pathway have a distinct high-grade, non–gland-forming morphology.

■ Other pathways have been less well elucidated, including the colitis-carcinoma sequence and the flat dysplasia-carcinoma sequence.

T14.4
Colorectal Carcinoma Pathogenesis

Feature	APC Pathway	MMR Pathway
Usual initiating event, inherited cases	*APC* gene mutation	*MSH2* or *MLH1* gene mutation
Usual initiating event, sporadic cases	*APC* gene mutation (uncommonly *B-catenin* mutation)	*MLH1* CpG-island hypermethylation
Progression	*KRAS* mutation Wnt signaling pathway disruption Chromosomal instability	Microsatellite instability *BRAF* mutation or *KRAS* mutation
Polyp type, sporadic cases	Tubular adenoma	Sessile serrated adenoma
Polyp type, inherited cases	Tubular adenoma	Tubular adenoma
Ploidy	Aneuploid	Diploid

Molecular Features of the APC Pathway

- The APC pathway has also been called the tumor suppressor or chromosomal instability pathway (note that chromosomal instability should be distinguished from microsatellite instability [MSI]; tumors in the APC pathway are microsatellite stable [MSS]). Accounting for around 85% of cases, the APC pathway involves a series of molecular events initiated by aberrations in the adenomatous polyposis coli (*APC*) gene (5q). Acquired (somatic) mutations account for about 98% to 99% of such cases, and inherited (germline) mutations 1% to 2% (inherited *APC* mutations are the cause of familial adenomatous polyposis [FAP] and related syndromes [see chapter 13]).

- The earliest molecular event in this pathway is a somatic or germline mutation in 1 *APC* gene. The next event, requisite for the formation of a morphologically distinct adenoma, is mutation of (or loss of heterozygosity of) the second *APC* gene. With regard to the initial *APC* mutation, most of these occur in a region of the gene known as major cluster region (MCR), found between codons 1061 and 1309, and result in protein truncation. The MCR precedes the domains involved in interactions with (and downregulation of) β-catenin and axin.

- There are several intracellular consequences, mediated through a variety of mechanisms, of a truncated APC protein. First, control over entry into the cell cycle is lost. Second, induction of apoptosis is impaired. Third, the process of mitosis is disorderly, resulting in a great tendency for chromosomal instability and aneuploidy.

- 1 important mechanism relates to the central role of APC in a signaling cascade known as the wingless-type (Wnt) signaling pathway. While extremely complex, a highly simplified version may be summarized as follows:

  - In a cell that has not been stimulated by extracellular Wnt protein, intracellular β-catenin levels are kept low. Low levels are maintained by (1) binding available β-catenin in a complex that forms on a backbone of the protein Axin, along with numerous other proteins including APC, and (2) binding of β-catenin to ubiquitin and thus marking it for destruction. Both these mechanisms—the binding to axin and the binding to ubiquitin—are mediated by APC protein.

  - When the transmembrane receptor (called Frizzled protein) binds its ligand (Wnt protein), a series of events ensues that lead ultimately to increased free intracellular β-catenin. Essentially, APC undergoes a conformational change due to dephosphorylation, the axin complex breaks down, and less β-catenin is bound to ubiquitin.

  - Increased β-catenin promotes the transcription of a number of genes. In the nucleus, it complexes with 2 transcription factors: T-cell factor (TCF) and lymphoid-enhancing factor (LEF). This complex enhances the transcription of a set of genes normally under the influence of active repression—genes known for their tendency to promote tumorigenesis—including *cMyc*, *BCL1* (cyclin D1), *MDR1* (multi-drug resistance 1), *PPAR-d* (peroxisome proliferator-activated receptor d), and *COX-2*.

  - Recall that truncating mutations in APC usually result in loss of the β-catenin binding site. The result is an inability of the cell to replicate the unstimulated low β-catenin state. The result is essentially a constitutively activated Wnt signaling pathway and a high rate of transcription of the normally repressed genes listed earlier.

- Further progression toward malignancy seems to require additional mutations. In particular, a *KRAS* gene mutation is affected in the vast majority of tumors derived from APC pathway and may represent the step immediately following mutation of the second *APC* gene. Additional anomalies common to tumors deriving from this pathway include mutations of *TP53*, *DCC* (deleted in colon cancer, 18q), *SMAD4*, *SMAD2*, and *TGFβRII*.

- A small minority of adenomas and colon cancers has a normal *APC* genotype and in fact has mutations in *β-catenin* which render the *β-catenin* product resistant to the action of normal APC protein.

Molecular Features of the MMR Pathway

- The MMR pathway, which has also been called the microsatellite instability (MSI) or mutator pathway, is involved in about 15% of cases. It is initiated by aberrations in 1 of the mismatch repair (MMR) genes. Acquired (somatic) aberrations account for about 95% of cases, and inherited (germline) mutations about 5%. Inherited MMR gene mutations are the cause of hereditary nonpolyposis colorectal carcinoma (HNPCC) and related syndromes (see chapter 13).

- A mismatch in this context refers to an anomalous base-pairing (ie, something other than the normal A-T and G-C pairings). Such errors occur at a low rate in DNA replication, and they are normally corrected by the action MMR proteins. The nomenclature of MMR proteins derives from early studies involving the analogous repair process in bacteria, known as the mutator pathway. In the mutator mechanism, 2 proteins called MutS and MutL mediate the necessary repair functions. Human proteins with homology to the bacterial proteins, when discovered, were called either MutS homologs (MSH) or MutL homologs (MLH). Presently, 9 human homologs are recognized: the MSH proteins including MSH2, MSH3, MSH4, MSH5, and MSH6, and the MLH proteins including MLH1, MLH3, PMS1, and PMS2.

- The mechanism of *MMR* gene inactivation differs in familial and sporadic MMR tumors. While most cases of HNPCC are caused by germline *MMR* gene mutations, such mutations seldom are found in sporadic MMR tumors. In fact, the actual coding sequences in the *MMR* genes are normal in the vast majority of sporadic MMR tumors. Despite this, the level of at least 1 of the MMR proteins is markedly diminished in such tumors. The cause of this apparent discrepancy, and the molecular defect in most sporadic MMR tumors, is hypermethylation of the promoter region of an *MMR* gene, leading to reduced transcription. The *MLH1* gene promoter contains CpG islands found to be heavily methylated in most sporadic MMR colon cancers. Of course, to cause tumorigenesis, promoter hypermethylation must affect both copies of the gene. The cause of this hypermethylation is presently unknown.

- The consequence of defective MMR is a manyfold increase in the rate of spontaneous mutations, particularly in segments of DNA-containing microsatellites. Most microsatellites, including those tested to assess for MSI, lie within noncoding DNA. However, a subset of genes contain microsatellites in coding regions, and as would be expected, these genes are the first to be affected in the MMR pathway. Such genes include *BRAF, KRAS, TGFβRII* (type II TGF-β receptor II), *p16INK4a*, and *BAX*. While anomalies in the MMR genes initiate this pathway, mutations in these subsequent genes permit progression to malignancy.

Clinicopathologic Features of APC Pathway Tumors

- APC pathway tumors tend to arise in the left colon and rectum. Nearly 60% of lesions present in the rectosigmoid, and only about 10% arise in the cecum and ascending colon.

- Due in part to the narrowness of the lumen in this segment of the colon, the tumors tend to grow circumferentially and present as annular "napkin-ring" lesions that may cause obstruction. Endophytic (invasive) growth is usually out of proportion to exophytic growth.

- Histologically, the tumors usually maintain the ability to form glands, and the neoplastic cells are often tall and columnar. The advancing edge of the tumor is usually infiltrative (rather than pushing), and peri-tumoral lymphocytes are not a prominent feature. In the glands, there is often central necrosis admixed with the karyorrhectic débris of degenerating neutrophils (so-called dirty necrosis).

- A subset of APC tumors have mucinous differentiation (colloid carcinoma), an appearance more often associated with MMR tumors. Mucinous APC tumors, however, behave more like conventional APC tumors, and they do not have the favorable prognosis of an MMR tumor.

- APC-associated adenomas, like the APC carcinomas into which they develop, are usually left-sided lesions. Whether tubular, villous, or tubulovillous, they are lined by mildly dysplastic columnar epithelium with a relative paucity of goblet cells. The architecture is disordered, with branching and cystic dilation not normally seen in benign colonic mucosa. Adjacent glands/crypts are separated from one another by lamina propria.

Clinicopathologic Features of MMR Pathway Tumors

- MSI tumors that form in association with HNPCCs present at a mean age of about 45 years, whereas sporadic MSI tumors present at a mean age of about 75 years.

- MSI tumors tend to be located in the right colon (cecum and ascending), and often present as large sessile lesions but rarely causing obstruction. There tends to be more exophytic growth than endophytic (invasive) growth, and despite their large size they usually present at a low stage relative to APC tumors.

- Histologically, they often present as mucinous (colloid) carcinomas. The degree of differentiation varies, from well-differentiated gland-forming tumors to poorly differentiated trabecular tumors, and some have a significant signet ring cell component. Importantly, the gland-forming MMR tumors lack central "dirty" necrosis.

- The tumors have prominent tumor-infiltrating lymphocytes (TIL) and/or a peri-tumoral "Crohn-like" nodular lymphoid reaction.

- A "pushing" rather than infiltrating tumor margin is characteristic. Because of this circumscribed appearance, a usually high nuclear grade, and infiltrating lymphocytes, the tumors have been described as medullary-like (referring to medullary breast carcinoma).

- Individual histologic features, as described earlier, predict MSI with moderate specificity and sensitivity. The most accurate morphologic predictor of MSI in several studies has been tumor-infiltrating lymphocytes (TILs), with definitions varying from straightforward (>2 per high-power field) to awkward (40 CD3-positive lymphocytes per 0.94 mm^2).

- MSI tumors run a relatively favorable clinical course, with a lower incidence of metastasis, and longer overall survival compared with APC tumors.

- Furthermore, MSI tumors show relative resistance to, and appear to not benefit from, adjuvant chemotherapy with 5-fluorouracil. They may be similarly resistant to alkylating agents, cisplatin, and doxorubicin. Thus, MSI testing may be indicated to determine whether chemotherapy is to be administered.

- The sessile serrated adenoma must be distinguished from tubular adenoma (usually an easy distinction), uncommon "traditional serrated adenoma," and the very common hyperplastic polyp (not so easy). The serrated adenoma is a bit of a mystery to many experienced pathologists, who for many years have classified these lesions as hyperplastic polyps. In fact, one can infer from the literature that about 20% of "hyperplastic polyps" diagnosed over 10 years ago are in fact serrated adenomas. Furthermore, during the elucidation of sessile serrated adenoma, there was an apparent explosion in serrated adenoma types, including the traditional serrated adenoma and others, adding to the confusion.

- An excellent illustration of sessile serrated adenoma morphology is a lesion we have been content to call

an adenoma for quite some time, the appendiceal adenoma. Like the appendiceal adenoma (and like the hyperplastic polyp) the serrated adenoma has a serrated superficial outline and lacks the arresting nuclear stratification and dark basophilia of a tubular adenoma. However, unlike hyperplastic polyps, these lesions have several features that make them distinct:

- Crypt basilar dilation and horizontally oriented crypts, which are not seen in hyperplastic polyps. The crypt bases in hyperplastic polyps are tapering when longitudinally sectioned, circular with small lumens when cross-sectioned.

- Serrated architecture that becomes apparent in the basilar and mid-crypt regions, whereas this change is seen only in mid to superficial crypt regions in hyperplastic polyps.

- Dysmaturation (persistence of immature regenerative zone–like cytologic features high into the mid and superficial aspects of the crypt), in contrast to confinement of these cytologic changes to the lower third of crypts in hyperplastic polyps. Often this change is apparent as a high proliferation zone confined to 1 side of a crypt or simply higher on 1 side of a crypt than the other. Dysmaturation is also reflected in the location of mitoses high in the crypts or even at the luminal surface.

- The distinction from traditional serrated adenoma appreciated a low magnification: the traditional serrated adenoma shows uniform serration, villiform architecture, and uniform cytology (tall, eosinophilic cells with centrally placed nuclei); in contrast, the sessile serrated adenoma shows haphazard serration, sessile architecture, and a mixture of cell types. If examined closely, additional differences include a low mitotic rate in the traditional serrated adenoma.

Molecular Testing for APC Defects

- Molecular testing is not usually indicated unless FAP is suspected (see chapter 13).

- Nearly all tumorigenic mutations in *APC* result in *premature truncation* of the APC protein. A large variety of mutations have been described, such that directed mutation scanning is impractical. A protein truncation assay is available for detecting significant mutation effects, however. This is based on the vitro transcription and translation of the APC gene. The recovered protein product is then subjected to electrophoresis to determine its size.

14: Solid Tumors

Colorectal Cancer>Molecular Testing for MMR Defects; Fecal DNA for Colon Cancer Screening |
Tyrosine Kinases>Physiologic Features of Tyrosine Kinases

Molecular Testing for MMR Defects

- 3 types of testing may be used to assess for *MMR* gene defects: MSI testing, IHC for *MMR* gene products, and genotyping.

  - MSI testing requires comparison of neoplastic and nonneoplastic tissue. A microsatellite is a DNA sequence, normally present in the genome, which consists of nucleotide repeats; eg, a stretch of several CA dinucleotides. The number of repeats is normally stable; that is, from 1 cell to the next the number is the same. MSI refers to a gain or loss in the number of repeats in tumor DNA compared with the number of repeats in the DNA of nontumor tissue. MSI testing is performed by extracting DNA from paraffin-embedded nonneoplastic and neoplastic tissue (either a carcinoma or an adenoma). PCR using a set of primers is used to amplify 5 specific microsatellite regions—BAT25, BAT26 (both of which are regions of mononucleotide repeats), D2S123, D5S346, and D17S250 (regions of dinucleotide repeats). These regions from the tumor are compared with those from adjacent nonneoplastic tissue to assess for differences in length, indicative of MSI. Tumors are classified as MSI-High (MSI-H) when differences are present in 2 or more (≥40%) of the markers, MSI-Low (MSI-L) when present in 1 marker (≥20%), and microsatellite stable (MSS) when all markers are unchanged.

  - IHC testing is performed on neoplastic and nonneoplastic tissue for expression of the proteins encoded by MMR genes. At least MLH1 and MSH2 should be included in such a panel. While the analysis may be performed on either a carcinoma or an adenoma, sensitivity in adenomas is only about 60%. Dim or absent staining is indicative of gene mutation/inactivation. IHC appears to have good sensitivity (>90%) and specificity (nearly 100%) for MSI.

- If a tumor is found to have MSI (either MSI-L or MSI-H) or underexpression of an *MMR* gene by IHC, this raises the question of HNPCC. The only way to fully exclude HNPCC is testing for germline mutations (although a family history may provide an answer).

- Regardless of whether the patient has HNPCC, the presence of MSI implies the aforementioned clinicopathologic features described.

- Testing for MSI in benign polyps may seem like a good idea, but it has certain limitations, depending on whether the polyp forms as part of HNPCC. In sporadic MMR-associated adenomas and hyperplastic polyps, a finding of MSI-H or MSI-L is rare (unless there is either high-grade dysplasia or carcinoma arising within them). In contrast, in HNPCC MMR-associated adenomas, a majority have MSI-H even in the absence of high-grade dysplasia/carcinoma. MSI-L is found in about 10% of HNPCC-associated hyperplastic polyps, and MSI-H is rare in these lesions.

Fecal DNA for Colon Cancer Screening

- It has been demonstrated that mutations in oncogenes such as *KRAS* can be detected in the stool of patients with colorectal cancer. Because *APC* mutations are more generally present in colorectal neoplasia, however, this represents a more attractive target. As alluded to earlier, protein truncation assays are much more practical than genotyping assays for *APC* anomalies, since detecting the huge variety of APC mutations would require complete gene sequencing in most cases.

- Other studies have evaluated multitarget probes for oncogene DNA mutations. Yet another line of study involves evaluation of the quantity of intact DNA in feces; that is, the capacity of DNA isolated from stool to yield intact gene copies by PCR. In this case, the genes undergoing amplification may be a globin chain gene entirely unassociated with carcinogenesis. Apparently, colorectal neoplasms are associated with a significantly higher quantity of intact fecal DNA in these studies.

- When directly compared, stool DNA assays have performed significantly better than fecal occult blood. However, sensitivity and specificity were not high, and the studies have been small.

Tyrosine Kinases

Physiologic Features of Tyrosine Kinases

- Tyrosine kinases are enzymes that catalyze the phosphorylation of proteins, usually by transferring a phosphate group from adenosine triphosphate (ATP) (or guanosine triphosphate [GTP]) to a tyrosine residue. An enzyme that reverses phosphorylation is called a phosphatase. In cell biology, phosphorylation is 1 of the key mechanisms used to activate enzymes and is important in perpetuating signaling and/or metabolic cascades.

- There are 2 main types of tyrosine kinases: receptor protein kinases and cytosolic (cellular) protein kinases.

- Receptor protein kinases have 3 major domains: an extracellular (receptor or ligand-binding) domain, a transmembrane (anchoring) domain, and intracellular (catalytic) domain. Binding to ligand (often a hormone) leads to dimerization of receptor protein kinases, and dimerization causes activation. Activation leads to phosphorylation of tyrosine residues located on free intracellular proteins. There are several classes of receptor protein kinase, including the EGFR (epidermal growth factor receptor) family, insulin receptor family, platelet-derived growth factor (PDGF) family, *RET* family, and ERBB family. Alternate names for these families are RTK (receptor tyrosine kinase) class I, class II, etc.

- Cytosolic (or cellular) protein kinases are composed of a tyrosine kinase domain with or without additional domains. They are often themselves activated by oligomerization (dimerization, etc), which leads to mutual phosphorylation, producing active tyrosine kinases that go on to phosphorylate other proteins. Cytosolic protein kinases are grouped into 8 families: SRC, JAK, ABL, FAK, FPS, CSK, SYK and BTK.

Tyrosine Kinases in Cancer

- If a tyrosine kinase becomes dysregulated, especially if constitutively activated, it can drive the proliferation of a cell. Many examples of this phenomenon are discussed in the preceding text. The main bases for dysregulation are translocation, mutation, and amplification.

- Fusion of a tyrosine kinase gene with another gene, by chromosomal translocation, is the mechanism for activation of the ABL tyrosine kinase. The fused gene, *BCR*, contains a tetramerization domain which promotes oligomerization of the fusion gene product, leading to spontaneous tyrosine kinase activation.

- Gene mutations, particularly if they succeed in knocking out inhibitory regulatory domains, can cause constitutive tyrosine kinase activation. This mechanism is exemplified by EGFR activation in non–small cell lung cancer.

- Tyrosine kinase overexpression is the mechanism by which Her2 (ErbB2) drives breast tumors.

- EGFR family
  - The EGFR family has 4 members: ErbB-1 (EGFR), ErbB-2 (HER-2), ErbB-3, and ErbB-4.

  - EGFR (ErbB-1) is overexpressed in a wide variety of human malignancies, including over 50% of non–small cell lung cancers, squamous cell carcinomas of the head and neck, intestinal adenocarcinomas, pancreatic adenocarcinomas, breast carcinomas, ovarian carcinomas, and gliomas.

  - Several EGFR inhibitors have been developed. These may be EGFR-specific or cross-react with other EGFR family tyrosine kinases. These are not monoclonal antibodies but rather small molecules capable of crossing the cell membrane, and act by binding to the ATP-binding site on the intracellular (catalytic) domain.

  - EGFR inhibitors (gefitinib, erlotinib) have demonstrated moderate efficacy in the treatment of non–small cell lung cancer. Response appears to be significantly associated with EGFR expression by IHC, EGFR gene copy number, or EGFR gene mutation status. Responsiveness also correlates with a set of clinical parameters, with response being highest in *women, nonsmokers, those with adenocarcinoma histologic type, and those of Asian heritage.*

  - EGFR gene mutations usually are either (1) small deletions located in a restricted portion of the gene, affecting amino acids 747-750, or (2) point mutations, usually affecting codon 858 (L858R). The finding of either type of mutation implies a sensitivity to EGFR inhibitors.

References

Aldape K, Burger PC, Perry A. Clinicopathologic aspects of 1p/19q loss and the diagnosis of oligodendroglioma. *Arch Pathol Lab Med* 2007; 131: 242-251.

Altiok S. Molecular markers in cervical cytology. *Clin Lab Med* 2003; 23: 709-728.

Andersson J, Sihto H, Meis-Kindblom JM, et al. NF1-associated gastrointestinal stromal tumors have unique clinical, phenotypic, and genotypic characteristics. *Am J Surg Pathol* 2005; 29: 1170-1176.

Antonescu CR, Tschernyavsky SJ, Woodruff JM, et al. Molecular diagnosis of clear cell sarcoma: detection of EWS-ATF1 and MITF-M transcripts and histopathological and ultrastructural analysis of 12 cases. *J Mol Diag* 2002; 4: 44-52.

Argani P, Antonescu CR, Couturier J, et al. PRCC-TFE3 renal carcinomas morphologic, immunohistochemical, ultrastructural, and molecular analysis of an entity associated with the t(X;1)(p11.2;q21). *Am J Surg Pathol* 2002; 26: 1553-1566.

Argani P, Lae M, Hutchinson B, Reuter VE, et al. Renal carcinomas with the t(6;11)(p21;q12): clinicopathologic features and demonstration of the specific alpha-tfeb gene fusion by immunohistochemistry, RT-PCR, and DNA PCR. *Am J Surg Pathol* 2005; 29: 230-240.

Balakumaran BS, Febbo PG. New insights into prostate cancer biology. *Hematol Oncol Clin North Am* 2006; 20: 773-796.

Biegel JA, Conard K, Brooks JJ. Translocation (11;22)(p13;q12): primary change in intraabdominal desmoplastic small round cell tumor. *Genes Chromosomes Cancer* 1993; 7: 119-121.

Bijwaard KE, Fetsch JF, Przygodzki R, et al. Detection of SYT-SSX fusion transcripts in archival synovial sarcomas by real-time reverse transcriptase-polymerase chain reaction. *J Mol Diag* 2002; 4: 59-64.

Boynton KA, Summerhayes IC, Ahlquist DA, et al. DNA integrity as a potential marker for stool-based detection of colorectal cancer. *Clin Chem* 2003; 49: 1058-1065.

Bruder E, Passera O, Harms D, et al. Morphologic and molecular characterization of renal cell carcinoma in children and young adults. *Am J Surg Pathol* 2004; 28: 1117-1132.

Brunelli M, Eble JN, Zhang S, et al. Eosinophilic and classic chromophobe renal cell carcinomas have similar frequent losses of multiple chromosomes from among chromosomes 1, 2, 6, 10, and 17, and this pattern of genetic abnormality is not present in renal oncocytoma. *Mod Pathol* 2005; 18: 161-169.

Burgart LJ. Testing for defective dna mismatch repair in colorectal carcinoma: a practical guide. *Arch Pathol Lab Med* 2005; 129: 1385-1389.

Burstein HJ. The distinctive nature of HER2-positive breast cancers. *N Engl J Med* 2005; 353(16): 1652-1654.

Carter BS, Beaty TH, Steinberg GD, et al. Mendelian inheritance of familial prostate cancer. *Proc Natl Acad Sci USA* 1992; 89: 3367-3371.

Chapusot C, Martin L, Puig PL, et al. What is the best way to assess microsatellite instability status in colorectal cancer? study on a population base of 462 colorectal cancers. *Am J Surg Pathol* 2004; 28: 1553-1559.

Chung EB, Enzinger FM. Malignant melanoma of soft parts: a reassessment of clear cell sarcoma. *Am J Surg Pathol* 1983; 7: 405-413.

Cossu-Rocca P, Eble JN, Delahunt B, et al. Renal mucinous tubular and spindle carcinoma lacks the gains of chromosomes 7 and 17 and losses of chromosome Y that are prevalent in papillary renal cell carcinoma. *Mod Pathol* 2006; 19: 488-493.

DeAngelis LM. Brain tumors. *N Engl J Med* 2001; 344: 114-123.

Deutsch E, Maggiorella L, Eschwege P, et al. Environmental, genetic, and molecular features of prostate cancer. *Lancet Oncol* 2004; 5: 303-313.

DiGiuseppe JA, Sauvageot J, Epstein JI. Increasing incidence of minimal residual cancer in radical prostatectomy specimens. *Am J Surg Pathol* 1997; 21: 174-178.

References

Dim DC, Cooley LD, Miranda RN. Clear cell sarcoma of tendons and aponeuroses. *Arch Pathol Lab Med* 2007; 131: 152-156.

Dolan M, Snover D. Comparison of immunohistochemical and fluorescence in situ hybridization assessment of HER-2 status in routine practice. *Am J Clin Pathol* 2005; 123: 766-770.

Dong SM, Lee EJ, Jeon ES, et al. Progressive methylation during the serrated neoplasia pathway of the colorectum. *Mod Pathol* 2005; 18: 170-178.

Downs-Kelly E, Yoder BJ, Stoler M, et al. The influence of polysomy 17 on HER2 gene and protein expression in adenocarcinoma of the breast: a fluorescent in situ hybridization, immunohistochemical, and isotopic mRNA in situ hybridization study. *Am J Surg Pathol* 2005; 29: 1221-1227.

Duffy MJ. Predictive markers in breast and other cancers: a review. *Clin Chem* 2005; 51: 494-503.

Eble JN, Sauter G, Epstein JI, Sesterhenn IA, eds. Tumours of the Urinary System and Male Genital Organs. Lyon, France: *World Health Organization IARC Press*, 2004.

Kazama Y, Watanabe T, Kanazawa T, et al. Mucinous colorectal cancers with chromosomal instability: a biologically distinct and aggressive subtype. *Diagn Mol Pathol* 2006; 15: 30-34.

Enzinger F. Clear cell sarcoma of tendons and aponeuroses: an analysis of 21 cases. *Cancer* 1968; 18: 1163-1172.

Evans HL. Low-grade fibromyxoid sarcoma: a report of two metastasizing neoplasms having a deceptively benign appearance. *Am J Clin Pathol* 1987; 88: 615-619.

Evans HL. Low-grade fibromyxoid sarcoma: a report of 12 cases. *Am J Surg Pathol* 1993; 17: 595-600.

Fradet Y, Saad F, Aprikian A, et al. UPM3, a new molecular urine test for the detection of prostate cancer. *Urology* 2004; 64: 311-316.

Goldstein NS, Begin LR, Grody WW, et al. Minimal or no cancer in radical prostatectomy specimens: report of 13 cases of the 'vanishing cancer phenomenon'. *Am J Surg Pathol* 1995; 19: 1002-1009.

Goldstein NS, Bhanot P, Odish E, et al. Hyperplastic-like colon polyps that preceded microsatellite-unstable adenocarcinomas. *Am J Clin Pathol* 2003; 119: 778-796.

Gologan A, Sepulveda AR. Microsatellite instability and DNA mismatch repair deficiency testing in hereditary and sporadic gastrointestinal cancers. *Clin Lab Med* 2005; 25: 179-196.

Gras E, Matias-Guiu X, Catasus L, et al. Application of microsatellite PCR techniques in the identification of mixed up tissue specimens in surgical pathology. *J Clin Pathol* 2000; 53: 238-240.

Greenson JK, Bonner JD, Ben-Yzhak O, et al. Phenotype of microsatellite unstable colorectal carcinomas well-differentiated and focally mucinous tumors and the absence of dirty necrosis correlate with microsatellite instability. *Am J Surg Pathol* 2003; 27: 563-570.

Gryfe R, Kim H, Hsieh ET, et al. Tumor microsatellite instability and clinical outcome in young patients with colorectal cancer. *N Engl J Med* 2000; 342: 69-77.

Gupta M, Djalilvand A, Brat DJ. Clarifying the diffuse gliomas: an update on the morphologic features and markers that discriminate oligodendroglioma from astrocytoma. *Am J Clin Pathol* 2005; 124: 755-768.

Hill DA, O'Sullivan MJ, Zhu X, et al. Practical application of molecular genetic testing as an aid to the surgical pathologic diagnosis of sarcomas: a prospective study. *Am J Surg Pathol* 2002; 26: 965-977.

Hsieh K, Albertsen PC. Populations at high risk for prostate cancer. *Urol Clin North Am* 2003; 30: 669-676.

Imperiale TF, Ransohoff DF, Itzkowitz SH, et al. Fecal DNA versus fecal occult blood for colorectal-cancer screening in an average-risk population. *N Engl J Med* 2004; 351: 2704-2714.

Jimenez RE, Wallis T, Tabasczka P, et al. Determination of Her-2/Neu status in breast carcinoma: comparative analysis of immunohistochemistry and fluorescent in situ hybridization. *Mod Pathol* 2000; 13: 37-45.

Joensuu H, Roberts PJ, Sarlomo-Rikala M, et al. Effect of the tyrosine kinase inhibitor STI571 in a patient with a metastatic gastrointestinal stromal tumor. *N Engl J Med* 2001; 344(14): 1052-1056.

References

Jones JS. DNA-based molecular cytology for bladder cancer surveillance. *Urology* 2006; 67(suppl 3A): 35-47.

Jones TD, Eble JN, Cheng L. Application of molecular diagnostic techniques to renal epithelial neoplasms. *Clin Lab Med* 2005; 25: 279-303.

Kelley TW, Tubbs RR, Prayson RA. Molecular diagnostic techniques for the clinical evaluation of gliomas. *Diagn Mol Pathol* 2005; 14: 1-8.

Kennedy MM, Cooper K, Howells DD, et al. Identification of HHV8 in early Kaposi's sarcoma: implications for Kaposi's sarcoma pathogenesis. *J Clin Pathol: Mol Pathol* 1998; 51: 14-20.

Klaassen CH, Jeunink MA, Prinsen CF, et al. Quantification of human DNA in feces as a diagnostic test for the presence of colorectal cancer. *Clinical Chemistry* 2003; 497: 1185-1187.

Kobayashi S, Boggon TJ, Dayaram T, et al. EGFR mutation and resistance of non-small-cell lung cancer to gefitinib. *N Engl J Med* 2005; 352: 786-792.

Konigshoff M, Wilhelm J, Bohle RM, et al. HER-2/neu gene copy number quantified by real-time PCR: comparison of gene amplification, heterozygosity, and immunohistochemical status in breast cancer tissue. *Clin Chem* 2003; 49: 219-229.

Krause DS, Van Etten RA. Tyrosine kinases as targets for cancer therapy. *N Engl J Med* 2005; 353: 172-187.

Lae ME, Roche PC, Jin L, et al. Desmoplastic small round cell tumor: a clinicopathologic, immunohistochemical, and molecular study of 32 tumors. *Am J Surg Pathol* 2002; 26: 823-835.

La P, Tan LK, Chen B. Correlation of HER-2 status with estrogen and progesterone receptors and histologic features in 3,655 invasive breast carcinomas. *Am J Clin Pathol* 2005; 123: 541-546.

Lane KL, Shannon RJ, Weiss SW. Hyalinizing spindle cell tumour with giant rosettes: a distinctive tumor closely resembling low-grade fibromyxoid sarcoma. *Am J Surg Pathol* 1997; 21: 1481-1488.

Lefevre M, Couturier J, Sibony M, et al. Adult papillary renal tumor with oncocytic cells: clinicopathologic, immunohistochemical, and cytogenetic features of 10 cases. *Am J Surg Pathol* 2005; 29: 1576-1581.

Li SC, Burgart L. Histopathology of serrated adenoma, its variants, and differentiation from conventional adenomatous and hyperplastic polyps. *Arch Pathol Lab Med* 2007; 131: 440-445.

Longacre TA, Fenoglio-Preiser CM. Mixed hyperplastic adenomatous polyps/serrated adenomas: a distinct form of colorectal neoplasia. *Am J Surg Pathol* 1990; 14: 524-537.

Marks LS, Fradet Y, Deras IL, et al. PCA3 molecular urine assay for prostate cancer in men undergoing repeat biopsy. *Urology* 2007; 69: 532-535.

Medeiros F, Corless CL, Duensing A, et al. KIT-negative gastrointestinal stromal tumors: proof of concept and therapeutic implications. *Am J Surg Pathol* 2004; 28: 889-894.

Miettinen M, Lasota J. Gastrointestinal stromal tumors: review on morphology, molecular pathology, prognosis, and differential diagnosis. *Arch Pathol Lab Med* 2006; 130: 1466-1478.

Miettinen M, Sobin LH, Lasota J. Gastrointestinal stromal tumors of the stomach: a clinicopathologic, immunohistochemical, and molecular genetic study of 1765 cases with long-term follow-up. *Am J Surg Pathol* 2005; 29: 52-68.

Moskaluk CA. Vanishing prostate cancer syndrome: symptom of a larger clinical issue. *Am J Surg Pathol* 2005; 29: 561-563.

Munoz N, Bosch X, de Sanjose S, et al. Epidemiologic classification of human papillomavirus types associated with cervical cancer. *N Engl J Med* 2003; 348: 518-527.

Nelson WG, DeMarzo AM, DeWeese TL. The molecular pathogenesis of prostate cancer: focus on the earliest steps. *Eur Urol* 2001; 39: 8-11.

Nigro JM, Takahashi MA, Ginzinger DG, et al. Detection of 1p and 19q loss in oligodendroglioma by quantitative microsatellite analysis, a real-time quantitative polymerase chain reaction assay. *Am J Pathol* 2001; 158: 1253-1262.

References

Oakley GJ, Tubbs RR, Crowe J, et al. HER-2 amplification in tubular carcinoma of the breast. *Am J Clin Pathol* 2006; 126: 1-4.

O'Brien MJ, Yang S, Clebanoff JL, et al. Hyperplastic (serrated) polyps of the colorectum: relationship of CpG island methylator phenotype and K-ras mutation to location and histologic subtype. *Am J Surg Pathol* 2004; 28: 423-434.

O'Brien MJ, Yang S, Mack C, et al. Comparison of microsatellite instability, CpG island methylation phenotype, BRAF and KRAS status in serrated polyps and traditional adenomas indicates separate pathways to distinct colorectal carcinoma end points. *Am J Surg Pathol* 2006; 30: 1491-1501.

Ogino S, Brahmandam M, Cantor M, et al. Distinct molecular features of colorectal carcinoma with signet ring cell component and colorectal carcinoma with mucinous component. *Mod Pathol* 2006; 19: 59-68.

Paner GP, Lindgren V, Jacobson K, et al. High incidence of chromosome 1 abnormalities in a series of 27 renal oncocytomas: cytogenetic and fluorescence in situ hybridization studies. *Arch Pathol Lab Med* 2007; 131: 81-85.

Parham DM, Ellison DA. Rhabdomyosarcomas in adults and children: an update. *Arch Pathol Lab Med* 2006; 130: 1454-1465.

Patel RM, Downs-Kelly E, Weiss SW, et al. Dual-color, break-apart fluorescence in situ hybridization for EWS gene rearrangement distinguishes clear cell sarcoma of soft tissue from malignant melanoma. *Mod Pathol* 2005; 18: 1585-1590.

Pritchard KI, Shepherd LE, O'Malley FP, et al. HER2 and responsiveness of breast cancer to adjuvant chemotherapy. *N Engl J Med* 2006; 354: 2103-2111.

Reid R, de Silva M, Paterson L, et al. Low-grade fibromyxoid sarcoma and hyalinizing spindle cell tumor with giant rosettes share a common t(7;16)(q34;p11) translocation. *Am J Surg Pathol* 2003; 27: 1229-1236.

Ribic CM, Sargent DJ, Moore MJ, et al. Tumor microsatellite-instability status as a predictor of benefit from fluorouracil-based adjuvant chemotherapy for colon cancer. *N Engl J Med* 2003; 349: 247-257.

Ridolfi RL, Jamehdor MR, Arber JM. HER-2/neu testing in breast carcinoma: a combined immunohistochemical and fluorescence in situ hybridization approach. *Mod Pathol* 2000; 13: 866-873.

Ruijter E, Van De Kaa C, Miller G, et al. Molecular genetics and epidemiology of prostate carcinoma. *Endocrine Rev* 1999; 20: 22-45.

Santos GC, Zielenska M, Prasad M, et al. Chromosome 6p amplification and cancer progression. *J Clin Pathol* 2007; 60: 1-7.

Schaid DJ, McDonnell SK, Blute ML, et al. Evidence for autosomal dominant inheritance of prostate cancer. *Am J Hum Genet* 1998; 62: 1425-1438.

Schmidt H, Bartel F, Kappler M, et al. Gains of 13q are correlated with a poor prognosis in liposarcoma. *Mod Pathol* 2005; 18: 638-644.

Schuetz AN, Yin-Goen Q, Amin MB, et al. Molecular classification of renal tumors by gene expression profiling. *J Mol Diagn* 2005; 7: 206-218.

Simard J, Dumont M, Soucy P, et al. Perspective: prostate cancer susceptibility genes. *Endocrinology* 2002; 143: 2029-2040.

Sjögren H, Meis-Kindblom JM, Orndal C, et al. Studies on the molecular pathogenesis of extraskeletal myxoid chondrosarcoma: cytogenetic, molecular genetic, and cDNA microarray analyses. *Am J Pathol* 2003; 162: 781-792.

Snover DC, Jass JR, Fenoglio-Preiser C, et al. Serrated polyps of the large intestine: a morphologic and molecular review of an evolving concept. *Am J Clin Pathol* 2005; 124: 380-391.

Tabernero MD, Espinosa AB, Maíllo A, et al. Characterization of chromosome 14 abnormalities by interphase in situ hybridization and comparative genomic hybridization in 124 meningiomas: correlation with clinical, histopathologic, and prognostic features. *Am J Clin Pathol* 2005; 123: 744-751.

Takazawa Y, Sakurai S, Sakuma Y, et al. Gastrointestinal stromal tumors of neurofibromatosis type I (von Recklinghausen's disease). *Am J Surg Pathol* 2005; 29: 755-763.

References

Thorner PS, Ho M, Chilton-MacNeill S, et al. Use of chromogenic in situ hybridization to identify MYCN gene copy number in neuroblastoma using routine tissue sections. *Am J Surg Pathol* 2006; 30: 635-642.

Torlakovic E, Skovlund E, Snover DC, et al. Morphologic reappraisal of serrated colorectal polyps. *Am J Surg Pathol* 2003; 27: 65-81.

Traverso G, Shuber A, Levin B, et al. Detection of APC mutations in fecal DNA from patients with colorectal tumors. *N Engl J Med* 2002; 346: 311-320.

Trpkov K, Gao Y, Hay R, et al. No residual cancer on radical prostatectomy after positive 10-core biopsy: incidence, biopsy findings, and dna specimen identity analysis. *Arch Pathol Lab Med* 2006; 130: 811-816.

Tse C, Brault D, Gligorov J, et al. evaluation of the quantitative analytical methods real-time PCR for HER-2 gene quantification and ELISA of serum HER-2 protein and comparison with fluorescence in situ hybridization and immunohistochemistry for determining HER-2 status in breast cancer patients. *Clin Chem* 2005; 51: 1093-1101.

Vlahovic G, Crawford J. Activation of tyrosine kinases in cancer. *The Oncologist* 2003; 8: 531-538.

Von Mehren M, Watson JC. Gastrointestinal stromal tumors. *Hematol Oncol Clin North Am* 2005; 19: 547-564.

Winawer SJ, Zauber AG, Ho MN, et al. Prevention of colorectal cancer by colonoscopic polypectomy. The National Polyp Study Workgroup. *N Engl J Med* 1993; 329: 1977-1981.

Woenckhaus M, Grepmeier U, Wild PJ, et al. Multitarget FISH and LOH analyses at chromosome 3p in non–small cell lung cancer and adjacent bronchial epithelium. *Am J Clin Pathol* 2005; 123: 752-761.

Wolff AC, Hammond ME, Schwartz JN, et al. American Society of Clinical Oncology/College of American Pathologists guideline recommendations for human epidermal growth factor receptor 2 testing in breast cancer. *Arch Pathol Lab Med* 2007; 131: 18-43.

Worsham MJ, Wolman SR, Zarbo RJ. Molecular approaches to identification of tissue contamination in surgical pathology sections. *J Mol Diagn* 2001; 3: 11-15.

Wright TC Jr, Cox JT, Massad LS, et al. 2001 Consensus guidelines for the management of women with cervical cytological abnormalities. *JAMA* 2002; 287: 2120-2129.

Wright CL, Stewart ID. Histopathology and mismatch repair status of 458 consecutive colorectal carcinomas. *Am J Surg Pathol* 2003; 27: 1393-1406.

Yamamoto H, Oda Y, Kawaguchi K, et al. C-kit and PDGFRA mutations in extragastrointestinal stromal tumor (gastrointestinal stromal tumor of the soft tissue). *Am J Surg Pathol* 2004; 28: 479-488.

Yang S, Farraye FA, Mack C, et al. BRAF and KRAS mutations in hyperplastic polyps and serrated adenomas of the colorectum relationship to histology and CpG island methylation status. *Am J Surg Pathol* 2004; 28: 1452-1459.

Yatabe Y, Kosaka T, Takahashi T, et al. EGFR mutation is specific for terminal respiratory unit type adenocarcinoma. *Am J Surg Pathol* 2005; 29: 633-639.

Chapter 15

Neoplastic Hematology

B-Cell Neoplasms

Gene Rearrangement

- B and T cells undergo somatic gene rearrangements to produce the genes that will ultimately encode their respective immunoglobulin (Ig) and T-cell receptor (TCR) proteins. The primitive B cell has genes in germline configuration; that is, the coding sequences (V, D, J, and C) for the immunoglobulin heavy (IgH) chain are separated by considerable distances on chromosome 14. In fact, there are several sequences in each coding class—over 100 different variable (V) sequences, and several diversity (D), joining (J), and constant (C) sequences. Analogously, the germline kappa (κ) light chain gene segments, on chromosome 2, consist of separately located V, J, and C segments (no D), and the germline lambda (λ) light chain gene segments, on chromosome 22, are V, J, and C. All these segments become linked closely enough together to produce a functional protein through a process of somatic gene rearrangement.

- In early B-cell maturation, the IgH gene rearranges; that is, in a random fashion a variable quantity of genetic material is deleted between random V, D, J, and C sequences such that they become joined. This results in a functional IgH gene, and because this happens independently in all the maturing B cells, it results in a polyclonal population of maturing B cells with a wide array of IgH gene sequences. Successful IgH rearrangement is followed by rearrangement of the kappa (κ) light chain genes. If the kappa rearrangement is nonproductive, which happens in about one third of instances, then lambda (λ) rearranges. Finally, with all the rearranging complete, the cell begins to make immunoglobulin in its cytoplasm (cytoplasmic immunoglobulin (cIg) positive). Later, it will incorporate this immunoglobulin into its cell membrane (surface immunoglobulin [sIg] positive) and will be defined as a mature B cell. 3 consequences of the nature of this process should be appreciated: (1) there develops a wide range of B cells with a wide range of antibody specificities, (2) the normal kappa:lambda ratio turns out with remarkable consistency to be about 2:1, and (3) every mature B cell has a rearranged IgH and kappa gene, and about a third of B cells also have a rearranged lambda gene.

- Thus, a clonal IgH or kappa rearrangement is supportive of a diagnosis of neoplasia. The finding of only germline genes or no clonal rearrangements is indicative of (1) a benign lymphoid proliferation (2) a lymphoid neoplasm composed of very early lymphoid cells, eg, some cases of precursor-B-ALL or ALCL, or (3) nonlymphoid neoplasm.

- Some caveats are worth noting. First, for unclear reasons, a number of B-cell neoplasms will display, in addition to rearrangement of Ig genes, rearrangement of TCR genes (lineage infidelity). A number of T-cell neoplasms will do the same (T15.1). Second, clonal populations can be detected where no neoplasm exists, particularly in immunocompromised individuals. In general, a clone representing more than 1% to 5% of cells is required for a confident diagnosis of malignancy. This threshold happens to be the lower limit of detection for Southern blot hybridization.

- The techniques in wide use for detection of clonal IgH gene rearrangements include Southern blot analysis (SBA) and polymerase chain reaction (PCR). In PCR for IgH, DNA is amplified using a number

T15.1
Rate of Detection of Clonal Receptor Gene Rearrangements in Lymphoid Neoplasms

Neoplasm	Clonal IgH rearrangement (%)	Clonal TCR rearrangement (%)
Mature B-NHL	>99	5-7
Mature T-NHL	4-6	>90
B-ALL	>99	20-40
T-ALL	10-15	85-95

B-ALL = B-cell acute lymphoblastic leukemia; B-NHL = B-cell non-Hodgkin lymphoma; IgH = immunoglobulin heavy chain; T-ALL = T-cell acute lymphoblastic leukemia; TCR = T-cell receptor; T-NHL = T-cell non-Hodgkin lymphoma.

of consensus primers that are designed to amplify several members of the V gene class and several of the J gene class. The amplicon is then subjected to electrophoresis, and if there is a major population of lymphocytes having the same IgH gene rearrangement, it will appear as a distinct band. A mixture of polyclonal B cells will produce a ladderlike distribution of bands. In SBA for IgH, restriction endonucleases are used to cut DNA into restriction fragments. The restriction fragments are then subjected to electrophoresis. If there is a major population with the same IgH gene rearrangement, it will appear as a distinct nongermline band, whereas a mixture of polyclonal B cells will produce only germline bands.

- While SBA is still considered the gold standard, it requires high-quality DNA samples and is labor-intensive. As a result, it is being replaced by PCR which can be automated and performed on formalin-fixed, paraffin-embedded material. PCR is not perfect, however, because the results are dependent on a host of considerations, especially the choice of primers.

Small Lymphocytic Lymphoma/Chronic Lymphocytic Leukemia (SLL/CLL)

- For practical purpose, SLL/CLL is defined by its immunophenotype, when present in association with the appropriate morphologic features. Typical SLL/CLL expresses CD19, CD20 (dim), CD22, CD5, CD23, sIg (dim), CD43, CD79, and CD11c (dim to moderate). It is negative for FMC-7, CD10, bcl-1, and bcl-6.

- It was previously thought, as a result of studies based on conventional cytogenetic techniques, that fewer than half of all cases had chromosomal aberrations and that the most common of these was trisomy 12. The neoplastic cells do not divide readily, and adequate cytogenetic studies require mitogen stimulation; even so, only 30% to 50% of CLL clones show anomalies by conventional cytogenetics alone. It is now known, through the combined application of conventional cytogenetics and fluorescence in situ hybridization (FISH), that only 20% of cases have a normal karyotype, and the most common chromosomal anomaly, present in over half of the cases, is deletion of 13q14 (13q-). About 20% have deletion of 11q (11q-), 15% have trisomy 12 (+12), 10% have deletion of 17p (17p-), and fewer than 10% have deletion of 14q (14q-), or 6q (6q-). About 30% have more than 1 abnormality (complex abnormalities).

- Prediction of disease progression is of major importance. CLL is an extremely common disease and is often indolent, with most cases arising in old age and most affected patients dying of other causes. Thus, treatment is frequently withheld. Some cases, however, are aggressive, and there is much interest in finding markers that can predict this outcome so that the appropriate therapy can be initiated.

- Among the traditional factors associated with a worsened prognosis are advanced stage (assessed in accordance with either the Rai or the Binet staging system), B symptoms (fever, weight loss, and night sweats), atypical cytomorphologic findings, peripheral lymphocyte doubling time of 1 year or less, high initial lymphocyte count (especially >30,000), and a diffuse pattern of marrow infiltration.

- With regard to immunophenotype, a worse prognosis has been associated with bright CD20, bright sIg, CD38 expression, and ZAP-70 expression. These features are strongly associated with atypical morphology and trisomy 12. Furthermore, many of these features have been correlated with an unmutated IgH variable region.

- With regard to chromosome status, as determined by cytogenetics or FISH, some generalities are worth noting:

  □ The best prognosis overall has been associated with a normal karyotype or isolated abnormalities of 13q.

  □ An intermediate prognosis is associated with trisomy 12.

  □ The worst prognosis is associated with 17p- and 11q-.

  □ The t(14:19)(q32;q13) translocation results in juxtaposition of the *BCL-3* gene and the immunoglobulin heavy chain gene, leading to enhanced expression of bcl-3 protein. This genetic change is present in 5% of cases of CLL and is rare in other types of B-cell leukemia/lymphoma (bcl-3 protein overexpression is significantly more common than the t(14;19) rearrangement, being found in about 10% of B-cell lymphomas overall, 20% of B-CLL and T-cell lymphomas, and 40% of Hodgkin lymphomas). The t(14;19) translocation has been associated with atypical morphologic features, trisomy 12, and aggressive disease.

- The mutation status of Ig heavy chain gene variable region (IgVH) appears to be a pivotal prognostic factor. Somatic hypermutation of IgVH is a physiologic feature of postgerminal center B cells ("memory" B cells) and is seen in about half of CLL cases; thus, it appears that there may be 2 types of CLL, 1 arising from pregerminal center B cells (unmutated IgVH), and 1 from postgerminal center cells (hypermutated IgVH). IgVH hypermutation is associated with prolonged survival, and unmutated IgVH is associated with shortened survival. Mutation analysis is not widely available, however, and CD38 and/or ZAP-70 (both tending to be positive in unmutated cases) may serve as surrogate markers. For a designation of CD38-positive, at least 30% of neoplastic cells should express CD38.

Mantle Cell Lymphoma (MCL)

- MCL is an aggressive lymphoma of small lymphocytes. The diagnosis is made, in the appropriate morphologic context, when the characteristic immunophenotype is demonstrated and/or when the diagnostic t(11;14) translocation is documented.

- MCL expresses CD19, CD20 (bright), CD22, FMC-7, CD5, sIg (bright), and CD43. In histologic sections, there is nuclear expression of bcl-1 (cyclin D1, prad 1). MCL is negative for CD23 and CD11c (crucial for distinction from SLL/CLL).

- The t(11;14)(q13;q32) translocation

  □ This rearrangement is associated with translocation of the *IgH* (14q32) gene JH sequence to the *CCND1* (11q13) gene. Consequentially, there is increased transcription of *CCND1* (*BCL1*, *PRAD1*), leading to loss of cell cycle control. The product of the *CCND1* gene, cyclin D1 (prad-1, bcl-1), is a protein that appears to stimulate entrance into the G1-phase of the cell cycle.

  □ The rate at which the t(11;14) translocation or *CCND1* rearrangements is found in MCL depends on the method used. The major translocation cluster (MTC) region of chromosome 11 (not located in the *CCND1/BCL1/PRAD1* gene) is involved in 40% to 50% of cases, but the remaining translocations involve a multitude of different breakpoints that are not amplified by a single standard PCR primer. Thus, the sensitivity of PCR for the translocation is low (<50%). SBA is similarly limited. The use of multiple SBA probes or multiple primers (multiplex PCR) can raise this detection rate to about 70%. FISH assays, however, can detect nearly 100% of rearrangements and are therefore the clear choice for molecular detection of t(11;14)/BCL1–IgH fusions in MCL.

  □ Immunohistochemistry for bcl-1, though presenting some technical challenges, performs better than PCR or SBA as well. Nuclear expression of bcl-1 is relatively specific for MCL (observed also in HCL which is rarely considered in the same context).

- Most MCLs have structural anomalies in addition to t(11;14). The most common second abnormality affects chromosome 13.

- There is a subset of MCLs with a penchant for peripheral blood involvement; these tend to have cytogenetic aberrations involving chromosome 17, 21, and 8 (in addition to the requisite t(11;14)).

Follicular Lymphoma (FL)

- The immunophenotypic features that support a diagnosis of FL include expression of CD19 (dim to bright), CD20 (bright), FMC-7, CD22, CD10, sIg (bright), bcl-2, and bcl-6. FL is usually negative for CD5, CD43, and CD11c. However, many of the morphologic and immunophenotypic features of FL are highly variable; for example, one sees a wide range of cytomorphology and architecture, and the expression of CD23, CD19, CD10, bcl-6, and bcl-2 is unpredictable. Furthermore, none of these features is specific for FL.

- PCR finds a relatively low rate of IgH gene rearrangement in FL. This is because of a high rate of IgH hypermutation in follicle center cells and leads to an overall sensitivity of only 40% to 50% for PCR. Somatic hypermutation does not affect the sensitivity of Southern blot, however, so that nearly 100% of follicular lymphomas show an IgH rearrangement by Southern blot.

- In virtually all cases, the t(14;18)(p32;q21) translocation forms the basis for FL.

  □ This translocation juxtaposes the *BCL2* gene on chromosome 18 with the J region of the immunoglobulin heavy-chain gene (JH) on chromosome 14 with resulting overexpression of the bcl-2 antiapoptotic protein.

  □ Most of the t(14;18) translocations occur in a 150–base pair region of *BCL2* called the major breakpoint region (MBR). PCR, SBA, or FISH can detect this translocation. About 5% to 10% of t(14;18) translocations involve a region of *BCL2* called the minor cluster region (MCR). Finding this translocation by means of PCR requires a different set of primers and by SBA requires a different set of probes.

- ☐ The t(14;18) abnormality is the most common translocation encountered in B-lineage lymphoma. This anomaly is also found in a significant minority of diffuse large B-cell lymphomas (DLBCL) and in a small proportion of non-FL low-grade B-cell lymphomas. In DLBCL, the presence of the t(14;18) rearrangement has been associated with a "germinal center" phenotype. In SLL/CLL, a variable cluster region (VCR) of the *BCL2* gene is occasionally involved and may rearrange to 2 (kappa) or 22 (lambda) in addition to 14 (JH).

- ☐ Note that while *BCL2* gene rearrangement is nearly always associated with overexpression of bcl-2 protein, the converse is not true. Many B-cell neoplasms overexpress bcl-2, and most of these do not have structural *BCL2* gene rearrangements. These other neoplasms appear to have deregulated *BCL2* loci on other bases.

- ☐ Lastly, note that the t(14;18) translocation can be found occasionally in normal adults.

- ■ Many clinicians have incorporated minimal residual disease (MRD) monitoring into the treatment of FL. Real-time (RT) PCR for the *IgH-BCL2* is replacing the more labor-intensive and contamination-prone nested PCR as the method-of-choice for MRD detection. RT-PCR is about 1 log less sensitive than nested PCR, however. Unlike MRD testing in chronic myelogenous leukemia (CML), nonneoplastic *IgH-BCL2*–bearing cells are a potential cause of false-positive MRD testing (in contrast, there is no normal population of *BCL-ABL*–bearing cells).

Marginal Zone Lymphoma (MZL)

- ■ Marginal zone B-cell lymphomas may present as:

- ☐ Nodal marginal zone B-cell lymphoma, presenting histologically as a proliferation of monocytoid B cells in a diffuse, sinusoidal, or interfollicular pattern, usually with follicular permeation. Plasma cells with intranuclear Dutcher bodies can often be found.

- ☐ Extranodal marginal zone B-cell lymphoma of mucosa-associated lymphoid tissue (MALT lymphoma), presenting as a mixture monocytoid B cells, plasma cells (some of which can be found to contain Dutcher bodies), and lymphoepithelial lesions.

- ☐ Splenic marginal zone lymphoma. The leukemic phase of splenic MZL is synonymous with splenic lymphoma with villous lymphocytes.

- ■ The MZL immunophenotype is distinctive only for what it lacks. Commonly expressed are CD19, CD20, FMC-7, and sIg, whereas CD5, CD23, CD10, and CD11c are negative. Plasma cells within infiltrate contain monoclonal cytoplasmic light chains.

- ■ In extranodal marginal zone (MALT) lymphomas, a wide range of molecular findings have been reported (**T15.2**), some appearing site-specific or at least site-prevalent.

- ☐ The t(11;18) translocation is the most common finding in MALT lymphomas overall, and it is associated with rearrangement of the *API2* and *MALT1* genes. *API2-MALT1* translocation tumors have been identified mainly in the stomach and lung.

- ☐ The t(1;14) translocation results in a *BCL10-IgH* gene fusion. *BCL10-IgH* translocation tumors have been found largely in ocular, parotid, and cutaneous sites.

- ☐ The translocations have not been found in nodal or splenic marginal zone lymphomas, and interestingly they have not been found in high-grade gastric MALTs.

- ■ There appears to be an association between *Chlamydia psittaci* infection and ocular (lacrimal) MALT lymphoma, between *Helicobacter pylori* and gastric MALT lymphoma, and between *Borrelia burdorferi* and cutaneous MALT lymphoma.

Hairy Cell Leukemia (HCL)

- ■ HCL is often subtle, whether presenting in the peripheral blood or marrow. Furthermore, very few of its features are entirely unique, including tartrate-resistant acid phosphatase (TRAP) expression and immunophenotypic features. The most specific markers are CD103 and DBA.44. The recently described unique genetic marker, Annexin A1, may prove to be a useful diagnostic marker.

T15.2
Chromosomal Anomalies in Mucosa-Associated Lymphoid Tissue Lymphoma

Finding	Associated Sites	Note
Normal karyotype	All sites	About 40% overall
t(11;18)	Stomach, small bowel, lung	About 15% overall, does not respond to *Helicobacter pylori* eradication
t(14;18)	Eye, skin, salivary, lung	About 10% overall
t(3;14)	Thyroid, eye, skin	About 10% overall
+3	All sites	About 10% overall
+8	All sites	About 10% overall
t(1;14)	Small bowel	About 2% overall, possibly a more aggressive clinical course

- In addition to these, HCL usually expresses CD19, CD20 (bright), CD22, sIg, CD11c (bright), CD25, and cyclin D1 (shared only with MCL). Many are also CD2-positive. Negative markers include CD5, CD43, CD23, and CD10 (about 10% are CD10-positive).

- There are no known signature molecular findings, and cytogenetic studies are often difficult in HCL because of the low cellularity and low proliferative rate.

- Noted cytogenetic abnormalities include duplications of a region in 14q, t(14;18), and abnormalities of a region of chromosome 5. The finding of cyclin-D1/bcl-1 overexpression in many cases of HCL does not appear to be associated with structural rearrangements of the bcl-1 locus (11q13).

- Like some examples of CLL, hairy cells have hypermutated IgVH genes, resembling a postgerminal center (memory) B cell.

Lymphoplasmacytic Lymphoma (LPL)/Waldenström Macroglobulinemia

- LPL has morphologic resemblance to SLL/CLL, but consists in part of a population of cells with plasmacytoid differentiation. Fully developed plasma cells and Dutcher bodies can usually be found and an IgM monoclonal spike is usually detectable.

- LPL is positive for CD19, CD20, CD38, SIg, and cIg. CD5 is sometimes expressed, as is CD43. It is negative for CD10 and CD23.

- A recently described t(9;14)(p13;q32), involving the *PAX-5* gene, appears to be a reproducible finding in LPL. *PAX-5* encodes a B-cell–specific transcription factor that is involved in the control of B-cell differentiation (eg, into plasma cells). While the chromosome 14 breakpoint involved in *BCL1* and *BCL2* rearrangement is usually within the JH sequence, the *PAX-5* rearrangement involves the C region of the IgH gene. SBA, PCR, or FISH may be used to detect *PAX-5* rearrangements.

Diffuse Large B-cell Lymphoma (DLBCL)

- The *BCL-6* gene (3q) is normally expressed in germinal center B lymphocytes (unlike *BCL-2*, which is expressed only in neoplastic germinal center B lymphocytes). In DLBCL, *BCL-6* is rearranged in 30% of cases, with numerous partners. A common *BLC-6* rearrangement is t(3;14)(q27;q32), joining *BCL-6* with the IgH locus. While bcl-6 protein is over-expressed in most FLs, its gene is rearranged in only 10%; in this 10% subset, grade 3 FL are overrepresented.

- BCL-6 is 1 of 6 genes—*BCL6, LMO2, FN1, BCL2, CCND2,* and *SCYA3*—whose expression appears to significantly impact prognosis DLBCL. In 1 study, *BCL6, LMO2,* and *FN1* expression predicted prolonged survival, whereas *BCL2, CCND2,* and *SCYA3* predicted shortened survival.

- Based on the profile of expressed genes, at least 2 major types of DLBCL have been distinguished: the germinal center B-cell (GCBC) type DLBCL, and the activated B-cell (ABC) type. ABC-DLBCL has frequent expression of BCL2, CCND2, and SCYA3 (frequent anomalies of chromosome 3, 18q, and 6q). The GCB-DLBCL has frequent expression of BCL6, LMO2, and FN1 (frequent anomalies of 12q, 9p, and 2p).

- The germinal center B-cell–like (GCB) type is associated with a relatively good outcome after chemotherapy, whereas the activated B-cell-like (ABC) type is associated with a poor clinical outcome.

Burkitt Lymphoma (BL)/Leukemia

- 3 clinicopathologic types of BL are recognized

  □ African (endemic) BL often presents as a jaw mass and is strongly associated with Epstein-Barr virus (EBV).

  □ Western (sporadic) BL often presents in intraabdominal locations, particularly the ileocecal valve, and is not strongly associated with EBV.

  □ Immunodeficiency-associated BL (so-called Burkitt-like lymphoma) most often presents nodally.

- A common immunophenotype is shared among the BL types, with expression of CD19, CD20, CD22, CD10, bcl-6, sIg, and c-myc protein. They are negative for CD5, CD23, TdT, and CD34. PCNA (Ki67) is expressed in more than 99% of cells. BL lacks expression of bcl-2.

- Molecular rearrangements involving the *C-MYC* gene of chromosome 8, t(8;14), t(2;8), or t(8;22), are nearly always identified. Most commonly, the *C-MYC* gene is translocated to the IgH locus as a result of t(8;14); however, in many cases it is rearranged with Igκ (2p12) or Igλ (22q11). The result of these translocations is c-myc protein overexpression. C-myc and its partner protein, called Max, combine to activate a number of genes involved in driving the cell into the cell cycle.

Primary Effusion Lymphoma (PEL)

- PEL present with effusions composed of large atypical lymphocytes, some with immunoblastic or plasmablastic cytology, often with cytoplasmic vacuolization. In some cases, there is secondary development of solid lesions (in lymph node or soft tissue), and in rare cases, PEL presents exclusively as solid infiltrates. PEL is found in immunosuppressed individuals, particularly those infected with HIV.

- The immunophenotype is distinctly unusual: the cells are negative for typical B-cell, T-cell, and myeloid antigens (CD20, CD79, CD19, CD10, CD3, CD5, CD13, CD14, CD33). While the cells are usually CD45-positive, some are not. Often positive are CD30, CD38, CD138, and epithelial membrane antigen (EMA).

- Despite negative B-cell antigens, most PELs exhibit clonal immunoglobulin gene rearrangements, indicative of B-cell differentiation. While many are found to have clonal EBV DNA, PEL is uniformly associated with human herpesvirus 8 (Kaposi sarcoma–associated herpes virus), the virus implicated in Kaposi sarcoma and multicentric Castleman disease. Like Kaposi sarcoma, PEL is disproportionately a disease of homosexual males with HIV. Human herpesvirus 8 can be displayed in all cases by either immunohistochemistry or molecular studies.

Posttransplant Lymphoproliferative Disorder (PTLD)

- PTLD is a morphologically heterogeneous group of lymphoproliferative disorders that arises in association with EBV infection in immunosuppressed transplant recipients. Most cases of PTLD occur in the first year after transplantation (when immunosuppression is the most profound). PTLD is thought to result from a deficient EBV-specific immune response somewhat analogous to Duncan disease (see chapter 9).

- About 10% of PTLDs appear to be independent of EBV. These cases seem to be a distinct entity that presents later and is highly aggressive.

- Following transplantation, the risk factors for EBV-associated PTLD include profound immunosuppression, pretransplant EBV negativity, and the identity of the transplanted organ (risk is highest for, in decreasing order, small bowel, lung, heart, liver, and kidney).

- PTLD may present in a variety of ways ranging from an illness resembling infectious mononucleosis to fulminant lymphoproliferation. The histopathology also presents a spectrum, ranging from reactive polyclonal proliferations to high-grade non-Hodgkin lymphomas. Presently, the World Health Organization (WHO) recognizes 3 categories: (1) early lesions, (2) polymorphic PTLD, and (3) monomorphic (lymphomatous) PTLD. The monomorphic PTLD most often takes the form of a DLBCL. *BCL-6* gene mutations have been identified in about half of cases.

261

15: Neoplastic Hematology

B-cell Lymphoma>Posttransplant Lymphoproliferative Disorder; Nodular Lymphocyte Predominant Hodgkin Lymphoma I
Acute Lymphoblastic Leukemia and Lymphoma>Classification; Molecular Findings

- Posttransplant monitoring of the EBV-DNA viral load by PCR may be very important. Several studies suggest that an elevated EBV-DNA viral load is predictive of PTLD.

Nodular Lymphocyte Predominant Hodgkin Lymphoma (NLPHL)

- NLPHL presents as lymph node effacement by a nodular or vaguely nodular proliferation of small lymphocytes and histiocytes. Classic Reed-Sternberg cells are very rare, and there is instead the characteristic L&H cell, a cell having abundant cytoplasm and a large vesicular convoluted (popcorn) nucleus. Progressive transformation of germinal centers is thought to be a precursor lesion for NLPHL.

- Immunophenotypically, the L&H cells are positive for CD45, CD20, bcl-6, and EMA. They are negative for CD30 and CD15. Background lymphocytes are predominantly CD20-positive B-cells, but a wreath of CD3-positive, 57-positive T cells surrounds the L&H cells.

- NLPHL is essentially a B-cell lymphoma which consistently demonstrates a clonally rearranged immunoglobulin (Ig) gene. The abnormal juxtaposition of *IgH* and *BCL6* is a reproducible finding in this lymphoma, a result of a t(3;14) (q27;q32) translocation. Interestingly, BCL6 is involved in many cases of follicular lymphoma.

Acute Lymphoblastic Leukemia (ALL) and Lymphoma

Classification

- B-lineage ALL (precursor B-ALL) represent about 80% of acute lymphoblastic *leukemia*, but only about 20% of lymphoblastic *lymphoma*. Precursor B-ALL is typically defined as a proliferation of blasts that express CD34, CD99, CD19, HLA-DR, and TdT (nuclear). CD20 is variable but usually negative, and sIg is negative (in contrast to Burkitt leukemia/lymphoma). CD19 is the earliest B-lineage–specific antigen; thus, lack of CD19 essentially excludes B lineage ALL. 30% to 50% express at least 1 myeloid antigen, usually CD13 or CD33, usually dimly. ALL with t(1;19) has a characteristic blast immunophenotype, with positive CD19, CD9, and CD10, but negative CD34 and CD20.

- T-lineage ALL (precursor T-ALL) represents about 20% of acute lymphoblastic *leukemia*, and about 80% of lymphoblastic *lymphomas*. Precursor T-ALL expresses CD34, CD99, CD7, CD2, CD5, CD3 (cytoplasmic), and TdT (nuclear). It is negative for HLA-DR. CD4 and CD8 are often both positive or both negative.

Molecular Findings

- More than 70% of ALLs have chromosomal abnormalities **T15.3**, numerical or structural.

- Among these, so-called high hyperdiploidy (>51 chromosomes) is associated with a favorable prognosis.

- Also favorable is t(12;21), the *TEL-AML1* also known as *ETV6-AML1* rearrangement.

- Hypodiploidy (<46 chromosomes) is associated with a relatively poor prognosis, and the prognosis worsens the fewer the chromosomes. Cases with 45 chromosomes comprise the largest share in this group. Cases having 33 to 44 chromosomes are rare but have a poorer overall outcome than those with 45, and cases with so-called near-haploidy (23-29 chromosomes) are rarer and gloomier still, with a median survival of less than 1 year.

- The t(9;22)(q34;q11), the *BCR/ABL* translocation, is present in 5% of childhood ALL and 20% of adult ALL, and is distinctly unfavorable. At the cytogenetic level, the t(9;22) of ALL appears identical to that of CML. However, at the molecular level, the translocations differ. The major breakpoint (M-bcr) rearrangement results in a chimeric protein of 210kD and is common in CML. The minor breakpoint (m-bcr) rearrangement results in a chimeric protein of 190 kD and is common in ALL. PCR and FISH are capable of distinguishing these rearrangements.

- Other findings that connote a poor prognosis are t(1;19), 11q23 (*MLL*) rearrangements, and abnormalities in the short arm of chromosome 9 (*P16INK4A*).

- The t(4;11)(q21;q23) translocation is present in about 5% of cases and is associated with expression of CD15 and lack of CD10.

- Minimal residual disease (MRD) monitoring in precursor B-ALL is often based on patient-specific Ig heavy chain gene rearrangements. This locus is sequenced by PCR at the time of diagnosis. Sequence-specific oligonucleotide primers are then designed for future use.

15: Neoplastic Hematology

Acute Lymphoblastic Leukemia (ALL) and Lymphoma>Molecular Findings; Coexistent Chronic Eosinophilic Leukemia and T-Lymphoblastic Lymphoma I Plasma Cell Neoplasms>Molecular Findings and Prognosis in Multiple Myeloma

T15.3
Structural and Numerical Chromosomal Anomalies in Acute Lymphoblastic Leukemia

Finding	Genes	Notes
Hyperdiploidy (>50 chromosomes)	—	Good prognosis
t(12;21)(p13;q22)	TEL/AML1	Good prognosis
t(1;19)(q23;p13)	PBX1/E2A	Variable impact on prognosis, generally poor
11q23 rearrangements	MLL	Poor prognosis
t(9;22)(q34;q11)	BCR/ABL	Poor

Coexistent Chronic Eosinophilic Leukemia and T-Lymphoblastic Lymphoma (8p11-12 Stem Cell Syndrome)

- Reactive hypereosinophilia is common in T-cell malignancies.

- Hypereosinophilia associated with the *FGFR1* (fibroblast growth factor receptor-1) gene at 8p11-12 is a distinct entity that presents as coexistent myeloid and lymphoid neoplasms. The latter most often take the form of a T-ALL.

- This disorder has been called the 8p11-12 stem cell syndrome and is a rare but aggressive neoplasm. The diagnosis requires demonstration of the same translocation breakpoint at 8p11-12 in both myeloid and lymphoid cells.

Plasma Cell Neoplasms

Molecular Findings and Prognosis in Multiple Myeloma

- Several indices have long been recognized in relation to prognosis
  - The overall prognosis is relatively poor, with a mean survival of about 3 to 5 years.
  - Higher serum β2 microglobulin levels correlate with poorer prognosis.
  - A high plasma cell labeling index, which reflects the number of plasma cells in S-phase, correlates with poor prognosis.
  - Stage correlates with prognosis.

- More recently, chromosomal findings have emerged as important prognostic parameters.
  - Because it is difficult to perform cytogenetic cultures on plasma cells, FISH is typically used to detect these anomalies. Conventional cytogenetics detects only about 30% of chromosomal abnormalities in myeloma compared with interphase FISH, particularly when combined with cell-purification techniques (eg, with CD138-coated microbeads).
  - More than 80% of cases are found to have 4 or more chromosomal anomalies, the most common of which affect 13q14, 19p, 14q32, and 17p13.1.
  - Chromosome 14q32 translocations (IgH translocations) appear to be common early events and are found in more than 70% of myeloma cases and 50% of cases of monoclonal gammopathy of unknown significance (MGUS). The t(11;14)(q13;q32) translocation is the most common translocation, present in about 20% of myelomas, and affects the cyclin D1 locus. The breakpoint differs from that seen in MCL.
  - Based on FISH results, patients can be stratified into 3 distinct prognostic groups:
    - shortest survival median of about 24 months—t(4;14), t(14;16), or 17p13.1 deletion
    - intermediate survival median of 42 months—13q14 deletions alone
    - longest survival median of over 50 months—no anomalies or only the t(11;14)

263

Minimal Residual Disease

- Complete remission in multiple myeloma has been defined as the disappearance of paraprotein from serum and urine (confirmed with immunofixation electrophorosis) and fewer than 5% plasma cells in the marrow.

- The status of the marrow has traditionally been assessed with morphologic examination alone. This practice is somewhat complicated by the sometimes anomalous cytologic appearance of neoplastic plasma cells and the common presence of nonneoplastic plasma cells in the marrow. Furthermore, complete remission based on these criteria is associated with almost universal recurrence of disease.

- Several additional modalities have been explored in regard to MRD testing for myeloma, the most sensitive of which appear to be immunohistochemistry or flow cytometry.

  □ Immunohistochemistry for CD138 (syndecan-1), when used in the appropriate context, is a specific marker for plasma cells (while expressed in a wide range of tissues and neoplasms, CD138 is not expressed by other hematopoietic cells). In 1 study, CD138 immunostaining combined with immunostains for κ and λ light chains provided the highest rate of MRD detection. However, the technique has certain limitations: not all biopsy specimens are big enough to provide a useful immunohistochemical study, light chain immunohistochemistry is sometimes of poor technical quality, and plasma cell quantitation is somewhat unreliable (the denominator is at most several hundred cells).

  □ Flow cytometry, using CD38 (bright) versus CD45 (dim-absent) expression gating, can be used to detect and quantify small populations of clonal plasma cells. Assessment of CD19, CD56, and cytoplasmic κ/λ expression can confirm the neoplastic nature of the gated plasma cells (benign reactive plasma cells are CD19-positive/CD56-negative/light chain unrestricted, while neoplastic plasma cells are usually CD19-negative/CD56-positive/light chain restricted.

  □ FISH can be applied to posttreatment marrow, especially if a specific pretreatment anomaly is known. However, it appears to be less sensitive than immunohistochemistry and/or flow cytometry.

  □ PCR, for detection of IgH gene rearrangement, performs poorly in postgerminal center B cells (eg, follicular lymphomas, myelomas) because of somatic IgH hypermutation. A way around this is patient or clone-specific primers, but this is expensive and requires pretreatment PCR analysis.

T-Cell Neoplasms

The T-Cell Receptor (TCR)

- The TCR is in many ways similar to immunoglobulin (Ig), composed of 2 polypeptides instead of 4. The TCR is a heterodimer made from either (1) an α chain linked by disulfide bonds to a β chain (αβ TCR), or (2) a γ chain linked by disulfide bonds to a δ chain (γδ TCR). The αβ TCR outnumbers the γδ TCR in a ratio of about 20:1 (γδ TCR-bearing T cells are most common in skin and spleen). Each TCR is noncovalently associated with a molecule of CD3.

- The TCR genes are located on chromosomes 7 (TCRβ and TCRγ) and 14 (TCRα and TCRδ). Final TCRα and TCRδ genes are formed from somatic recombination of V, J, and C sequences. Final TCRβ and TCRγ genes are formed from recombination of V, D, J, and C sequences.

- In T-cell maturation, TCRγ rearrangement takes place first, followed by TCRδ rearrangement. If this is nonproductive, which it most often is, rearrangement of TCRα and TCRβ follows.

- Clonality assessment is commonly based on analysis of the TCRγ gene. The status of the TCRγ gene can be used to affirm clonality not only in γδ TCR-bearing neoplasms but also in αβ TCR-bearing neoplasms. This is because TCRγ rearrangement precedes TCRα and TCRβ rearrangement (TCRδ cannot be used in this way, because TCRδ is deleted in the rearrangement of the TCRβ gene). The TCRγ gene is an attractive target because it has a relatively small number of V and C sequences (the TCRα and TCRβ genes have many more), thus requiring a smaller number of consensus primers.

- Either PCR or SBA may be used to detect clonal TCR rearrangements. PCR offers many advantages, including greater yield from formalin-fixed paraffin-embedded tissue. The major drawback of PCR is the false negative rate thought to result from improperly annealing primers. The modification known as nested

15: Neoplastic Hematology

T-Cell Neoplasms>The T-Cell Receptor; Peripheral T-Cell Lymphoma; Adult T-Cell Leukemia/Lymphoma; Angioimmunoblastic T-Cell Lymphoma

PCR, which offers greater sensitivity, is presently unacceptable for clinical use because of a high rate of contamination.

- Molecular detection of a clonal TCR gene rearrangement supports the clonal and therefore the neoplastic nature of a proliferation. It is important to remember, however, that this finding cannot form the sole basis for a diagnosis of lymphoma, because clonal rearrangements can be found in several benign proliferations. Furthermore, failure to detect a clonal TCR rearrangement does not exclude lymphoma, because (1) several technical issues can lead to a false negative study, and (2) even a technically adequate study can fail to detect a small clone (particularly in cases such as angioimmunoblastic lymphadenopathy–like T-cell lymphoma in which a dense population of nonneoplastic cells may molecularly obscure the clone).

Peripheral T-Cell Lymphoma (PTCL)

- PTCL is the most common type of T-cell lymphoma in the Western world.

- Immunophenotyping is frequently used to confirm T lineage and to suggest clonality based on immunophenotypic aberrancy; however, at this time it has a limited capacity to confirm clonality. PTCL is CD4-positive and CD8-negative. There is commonly loss of 1 or several pan-T cell markers: CD2, CD3, CD5, or CD7. CD25 is negative.

- Unlike adult T-cell leukemia/lymphoma, PTCL is *not* associated with human T-cell lymphotropic virus 1 (HTLV-1).

- PTCL consistently demonstrates clonal TCR rearrangement by PCR or SBA. There is no consistent structural chromosomal abnormality, but trisomy 3 is frequent in Lennert-like variants.

Adult T-Cell Leukemia/Lymphoma (ATCL)

- ATCL is a T-cell neoplasm caused by HTLV-1, which is endemic to Southwest Japan, Southeast United States, and the Caribbean. The HTLV-1 genome encodes a protein called *Tax* that stimulates uncontrolled proliferation of infected T cells. It does this by exerting control over the expression of several cell cycle–regulatory genes while simultaneously repressing the expression of DNA repair genes. Despite these effects, it takes many years for HTLV-1 infection to produce ATCL, and it does so in only a

small minority of infected patients. It appears that an environmental (perhaps infectious) second hit is required for carcinogenesis, because the geographic incidence of ATCL does not directly parallel the incidence of HTLV-1. Furthermore, ATCL is most likely in those who acquire the infection transplacentally or in infancy.

- There are various clinical forms of ATCL: acute, lymphomatous, chronic, and smoldering. The chronic and smoldering forms are relatively indolent and do not require treatment, whereas the acute form is rapidly progressive, with a median survival of 6 months. The classic manifestations of ATCL include lymphadenopathy, splenomegaly, marked leukocytosis, hypercalcemia, and skin rash. Only lymphadenopathy is consistently present. Some patients manifest lytic bone lesions.

- The neoplastic cells have pronounced nuclear irregularity, producing cloverleaf forms, and express CD4. The most distinctive immunophenotypic finding is expression of CD25.

- Serologic screening for HTLV-1 can be performed with an enzyme-linked immunosorbent assay. Serologic confirmation requires either Western blot or another method capable of detecting multiple antibodies simultaneously; however, PCR can also be used to confirm HTLV-1 infection.

Angioimmunoblastic T-Cell Lymphoma (AITCL)

- In the past, the uncommon entities known as angioimmunoblastic lymphadenopathy (AIL) and immunoblastic lymphadenopathy (IBL) were felt to predate the development of T-cell neoplasms which became known as AIL-like and IBL-like T-cell lymphomas. It is now thought that both AIL and IBL are clonal disorders from the start, with characteristic clinicopathologic features.

- AITCL affects older adults who present abruptly with symptoms including fever, night sweats, weight loss, and generalized lymphadenopathy. Often there is a Coombs-positive autoimmune hemolytic anemia and polyclonal hypergammaglobulinemia.

- The affected lymph nodes manifest diffuse effacement with a characteristic prominence of arborizing postcapillary venules, deposition of PAS-positive extracellular material, and absence of follicles/ germinal centers. This lack of germinal centers

265

is key to distinguishing neoplasms from reactive lymphadenopathies. The cytologic findings include a mixed population of immunoblasts, lymphocytes, plasma cells, and eosinophils. An increase in the numbers of CD21-positive follicular dendritic cells is characteristic.

- The immunophenotype is CD4-positive with loss of 1 or several pan-T cell markers, such as CD2, CD3, CD5, CD7.

- AITCL is a challenging diagnosis to make based on morphologic findings alone, and molecular diagnosis is often required. PCR for TCR gene rearrangements shows a monoclonal T-cell population in nearly 100% of cases. Furthermore, conventional cytogenetic studies can detect structural chromosomal abnormalities in approximately 70% to 80% of cases. The most common findings are trisomy 3, trisomy 5 and an extra X chromosome.

Anaplastic Large Cell Lymphoma (ALCL)

- ALCL is a lymphoma of children and adults. It represents nearly half of childhood high-grade lymphomas and about 5% of adult high-grade lymphomas.

- Most ALCLs have 4 things in common: nodal involvement, anaplastic cytology, expression of CD30, and expression of the protein Alk. There are many variations on this theme, however, including Alk-negative cases, leukemic presentations, and small cell variants.

- Most commonly, ALCL presents with lymphadenopathy, histologically displaying diffuse infiltration by large and small cells, many having pleomorphic nuclei containing 1 or more nucleoli, and a variable number of anaplastic cells (multinucleated forms, horseshoe-shaped, and Reed-Sternberg–like cells).

- Cases that are Alk-positive and arise in children have the best prognosis overall (as long as there is not a leukemic component).

- Alk-negative ALCL is more aggressive than Alk-positive ALCL and occurs in older individuals.

- In the leukemic cases, small cell cytology tends to predominate. The vast majority occur in children, express Alk, and have a poor prognosis. In the small cell variant, the neoplastic cells are somewhat more uniform and the process may be mistaken for a PTCL.

- ALCL is usually positive for CD30 (membranous and Golgi staining), Alk (nucleus, cytoplasm, or both), clusterin (golgi), EMA, CD45, at least 1 T-cell antigen. The Golgi pattern of staining for clusterin appears to be highly specific for ALCL. The cells are negative for B-cell antigens, CD15, and EBV antigens.

- Alk expression correlates with t(2;5) rearrangement.

- Cases without demonstrable T antigens are called null cell type ALCL and have not been demonstrated to have any clinical differences with T-cell type ALCL. Note that anaplastic lymphomas that are CD30-positive with B-cell antigen expression are classified as DLBCL.

- Whether expressing T-cell antigens or not, PCR demonstrates a clonal TCR in over 90% of cases.

- The t(2;5)(p23;q35) rearrangement is present in more than 90% of cases. The t(2;5) results in relocation of the *ALK* (anaplastic lymphoma kinase) gene on 2p23 to the *NPM* (nucleophosmin) gene on 5q35. Since the *ALK-NPM* rearrangement occurs regularly in the same intron, PCR has no difficulty detecting the fusion gene. Less common ALK rearrangements include t(1;2), t(2;3), and inv(2).

- ALK rearrangement is not identified in most Alk-negative cases. Instead, FISH identifies trisomy 2 in most Alk-negative ALCLs (and primary cutaneous ALCL). None of the Alk-positive cases studied thus far have shown trisomy 2.

- Alk positivity is the most important prognostic factor (favorable prognosis).

Large Granular Lymphocytic (LGL) Leukemia

- The large granular lymphocytes that, in healthy adults, circulate in low numbers are a mixture of T-cytotoxic and natural killer (NK) cells. This population expands in response to viral infection, rheumatoid arthritis, other autoimmune disorders, and splenectomy. LGL leukemia is a condition in which there is an unexplained sustained (>6 month) increase (>2 × 10⁶/L) in LGLs, usually in association with neutropenia. This has previously been called large granular lymphocytosis, T-CLL, T-γ lymphoproliferative disorder.

- A small portion of cases are aggressive, a behavior linked to blastlike morphology.

15: Neoplastic Hematology

T-Cell Neoplasms>Large Granular Lymphocytic Leukemia; Hepatosplenic T-Cell Lymphoma; Blastic NK-Cell Lymphoma; Extranodal NK/T-Cell Lymphoma I Classical Hodgkin Lymphoma (CHL)

- There are 2 distinctive immunophenotypes
  - □ CD2-positive, CD3-positive, CD8-positive, CD16-positive, CD56-negative, CD7-negative, CD57-positive/negative (Tc phenotype). The distribution of CD5 is characteristically bimodal.
  - □ CD2-positive, CD3-negative, CD8-negative/positive, CD16-positive/negative, CD56-positive/negative, CD57-positive/negative (NK phenotype)
- CD3-positive (Tc) LGL has clonally rearranged TCR, whereas CD3-negative (NK) LGL has germline (unrearranged) TCR.

Hepatosplenic T-Cell Lymphoma

- Hepatosplenic γδ T-cell lymphomas is a well-recognized and distinct entity. It occurs in young males who present with constitutional ('B') symptoms, hepatosplenomegaly, cytopenias, and without lymphadenopathy. Lymphomatous infiltrates are seen in the splenic red pulp and are composed of CD8-positive cytotoxic T cells that express an γδ TCR.
- The neoplastic cells demonstrate a clonal *TCRγ* gene and/or *TCRδ* gene rearrangement. The cells often display i(7q).
- Hepatosplenic αβ T-cell lymphomas have been reported rarely.

Blastic NK-Cell Lymphoma

- This is a neoplasm involving mainly the skin, with some cases also involving lymph nodes, peripheral blood, and bone marrow.
- A lymphoblastic-appearing lymphoma with an NK immunophenotype expressing CD45, CD4, CD43, CD56, and the relatively unique antigen CD123 (shared only with so-called plasmacytoid dendritic cells).
- The tumor is nearly always negative for CD2, CD3, CD5, CD7, CD8, CD30, CD138, B-cell antigens, and myelomonocytic antigens.
- TCR and Ig genes are usually germline. About two thirds have cytogenetic anomalies, usually complex.

Extranodal (Nasal-Type) NK/T-Cell Lymphoma

- Previously known as angiocentric T-cell lymphoma or polymorphic reticulosis, this entity is 1 of the causes of the syndrome of lethal midline granuloma. This tumor tends to affect the nasal cavity, but it is also found in the skin, gastrointestinal, testis, and kidney. It is rare in the United States and other Western countries, found more commonly in Asia.
- It is an EBV-associated vasculitislike proliferation of neoplastic NK (surface CD3-, CD56+) or T (surface CD3+, CD56-) cells.
- Clonally rearranged TCR genes have been detected in some cases. Cytogenetic findings are common and include del(6)(q16-q27) and del(13)(q14-q34) most commonly.

Classical Hodgkin Lymphoma (CHL)

- There are 4 types of CHL, distinguished by clinical and morphologic features
  - □ Nodular sclerosis (NS) presents as a lymph node effaced by a nodular proliferation with intervening bands of sclerosis. Classic Reed-Sternberg and Hodgkin cells are present, but the characteristic and defining cell is the lacunar cell, a large cell with a round to convoluted vesicular nucleus and variably sized nucleoli. A cellular phase precedes the emergence of sclerosis, and it is identifiable as NS if these lacunar cells are noted. The lacune in which the cell is found is an artifact of formalin fixation not seen with other fixatives such as B5. Mummified cells are an additional characteristic finding. The large cells are scattered in a background of small mature lymphocytes, plasma cells, and eosinophils. Histiocytes, including well-formed epithelioid granulomas, are often present. NS is the most common type of Hodgkin lymphoma in the Western world, commonly affecting young females. It has a tendency to involve the mediastinum more than other types of CHL. In fact, mediastinal CHL is nearly always of the NS type, whereas intraabdominal CHL is more frequently of mixed cellularity.
  - □ Mixed cellularity (MC) causes diffuse effacement of lymph nodes by a mixture of mature lymphocytes, eosinophils, histiocytes, and plasma cells. Admixed are varying numbers of classic

Reed-Sternberg cells and mononuclear Hodgkin cells. MC is more common in underdeveloped parts of the world and in HIV-associated CHL.

- The lymphocyte rich (LR) type is morphologically similar to NLPHL but displays the typical immunophenotype of CHL.

- The lymphocyte depleted (LD) type has a predominance of classic Reed-Sternberg cells and variants, usually numbering more than 15/hpf. The number of nonneoplastic background cells are markedly decreased compared with the mixed cellularity type. LD is more common in elderly patients and presents at a higher stage.

- Immunophenotypically, the neoplastic (Reed-Sternberg) cells express CD15, CD30, fascin, and EBV. They are negative for CD45, CD20, and EMA. The background lymphocytes are predominantly T cells.

- Clinically, CHL demonstrates a bimodal peak in incidence. The first peak occurs between the ages of 15 and 35 years and is predominated by the nodular sclerosis type of CHL and NLPHL. The second peak occurs after age 50 years and contains more cases of lymphocyte depleted CHL. CHL presents with localized lymphadenopathy in the vast majority of patients. Disseminated disease is uncommon but may be seen in the LD, MC, or HIV-associated CHL. The cervical lymph nodes are most often affected. So-called "B" symptoms are present in some patients and include fever, night sweats, weight loss, and fatigue. The bone marrow is not frequently involved in CHL. The incidence of bone marrow involvement is highest in lymphocyte-depleted (50%) and HIV-associated CHL (60%), lowest in lymphocyte predominant (<1%), and about 10% overall. Marrow involvement usually takes the form of focal collections of lymphocytes, histiocytes, plasma cells, and Reed-Sternberg cells, usually with a degree of fibrosis. Finding a Reed-Sternberg cell is mandatory for the diagnosis of bone marrow involvement. In the uninvolved marrows of patients with CHL, hypercellularity, lymphoid aggregates and epithelioid granulomas are not uncommon. CHL is known for its habit of spreading via contiguous lymphatic sites. However, a tendency for noncontiguous spread is often manifested by lymphocyte-depleted CHL.

Myelodysplastic Syndrome (MDS)

- MDS is a group of diseases that have in common: cytopenias, dyspoiesis, and a tendency to progress into acute leukemia. Each MDS results from a clonal disorder of hematopoietic stem cells. The clinical presentation is reflective of progressive cytopenias, manifesting as fatigue, infection, bleeding. Splenomegaly is usually absent.

- Most cases arise de novo (primary MDS). Secondary MDS follows such things as chemotherapy (usually with alkylating agents), radiation exposure, benzene exposure, or Fanconi's anemia.

- The distinctive features in the marrow are hypercellularity and dyspoietic morphology. Blasts may be increased but by definition comprise less than 20% of cells. Dyspoiesis is recognized in the granulocytic series as aberrant granulation and abnormal nuclear segmentation. Dyspoiesis in the erythroid series is manifested as basophilic stippling, circulating nRBCs, macrocytosis, megaloblastoid changes (nuclear/cytoplasmic maturation dyssynchrony), nuclear lobulation, internuclear bridging, multinuclearity, and karyorrhexis. Additional features may include ringed sideroblasts, cytoplasmic periodic acid–Schiff positivity, and cytoplasmic vacuolization. Dyspoietic megakaryocytes show hypogranulation, micromegakaryocytes, "pawn ball"(multinucleated) nuclei, and hypolobated nuclei.

- Cytogenetic abnormalities are present in about 50% of cases overall, 30% to 40% of low-grade cases (refractory anemia, refractory anemia with ringed sideroblasts), and 70% to 80% of higher grade cases.

  - The incidence of chromosomal abnormalities is highest in secondary MDS (>80%). Overall, chromosomal losses are more common in secondary MDS, with gains being slightly more common in primary MDS, such that hypoploidy is more frequent in secondary MDS.

  - The most common (25%) karyotype, in both primary and secondary MDS, is one with complex abnormalities (2 or more clonal abnormalities), and this is associated with a poor prognosis. Recurring components of complex karyotypes in MDS, roughly in order of decreasing frequency, include 5q-, 20q-, +8 (trisomy 8), 7q-, 12p-, 11q-, and 17p-. 17p deletion may be associated with p53 mutation and rapid progression.

15: Neoplastic Hematology

Myelodysplastic Syndrome (MDS) | Myelodysplastic/Myeloproliferative Disorders(MD/MPD)>Chronic Myelomonocytic
Leukemia; Atypical Chronic Myelogenous Leukemia; Juvenile Chronic Myelomonocytic Leukemia

□ The second most common finding (15%) is isolated monosomy 7 or 7q-. Deletion of 7 is strongly associated with secondary MDS and is a frequent feature of childhood MDS. It is associated with resistance to treatment, a poor prognosis, and susceptibility to infections. The *RAS* and *NF1* genes are thought to be important in the pathogenesis of MDS with -7. Although nonspecific, monosomy 7 is the most common cytogenetic abnormality in childhood MDS.

□ Third (10%) is isolated 5q-, which is associated with a good prognosis. Del(5q) is an interstitial deletion having variable breakpoints spanning 5q11 to 5q35, all of which appear to result in deletion of 5q31. The most common form of 5q- is del(5)(q13.3q33.1). When 5q- is the sole finding, it is associated with macrocytic anemia, a normal or elevated platelet count, and hypolobated micromegakaryocytes in the marrow. This *5q- syndrome* is often identified in elderly women. Note, however, that 5q- admixed with other anomalies is common in nonspecific MDS.

■ Immunophenotyping has recently shown promise in evaluating the marrow for dysplasia. Certain reproducible patterns of abnormal antigenic maturation are demonstrable in these marrows. Among experienced observers, the sensitivity and specificity of this modality may be more than 90%, greatly exceeding that of morphology or cytogenetics alone.

■ Prognosis depends on 4 main variables: type of MDS, percentage of blasts, cytogenetics, and the number of depressed cell lines. With regard to type, refractory anemia and refractory anemia with ringed sideroblasts are the most stable. Favorable cytogenetics include loss of Y, del(5q), and del(20q). Otherwise the overall rate of progression to acute leukemia is approximately 10% for refractory anemia and refractory anemia and ringed sideroblasts, 45% for refractory anemia with excess blasts **T15.4**.

Myelodysplastic/Myeloproliferative Disorders (MD/MPD)

The MD/MPD category includes disparate entities united by the coexistence, at presentation, of dyspoiesis and increased production of some mature cells. Hence, these disorders have features of both MDS and MPD.

Chronic Myelomonocytic Leukemia (CMML)

■ CMML presents as persistent absolute monocytosis ($>1 \times 10^6$/mL) in peripheral blood, with marrow dysplasia, fewer than 20% blasts, and absence of a Philadelphia chromosome. The sum of blasts and promonocytes comprise less than 20% of the marrow.

■ There may be hepatosplenomegaly, and there is often anemia and thrombocytopenia. Despite the requisite monocytosis, about half of all CMML cases present with a normal or low white count because of offsetting neutropenia. The monocyte morphology is not overtly abnormal.

■ When the spleen is enlarged, a leukemic infiltrate of monocytes is found. When (rarely) lymph nodes are enlarged, they are found to have an infiltrate of so-called plasmacytoid monocytes having an unusual immunophenotype (CD14-positive, CD68-positive, CD56-positive, CD4-positive, CD2-positive, and CD5-positive).

■ Some cases are associated with clonal cytogenetic anomalies, but none are specific for this entity. CMML with eosinophilia ($>1.5 \times 10^9$/L) represents a distinct subset in which abnormalities of the TEL gene on chromosome 5 are common, often in the form of t(5;12).

Atypical Chronic Myelogenous Leukemia (aCML)

■ Neutrophilia composed of a spectrum of forms (mature neutrophils, metamyelocytes, myelocytes, and promyelocytes), marrow dysplasia, fewer than 20% blasts, and absence of a Philadelphia chromosome.

■ Most have clonal cytogenetic anomalies, but none are specific.

Juvenile Chronic Myelomonocytic Leukemia (JMML)

■ This is a disorder that usually affects children and presents with monocytosis and/or granulocytosis, hepatosplenomegaly, and constitutional symptoms. There is often anemia and thrombocytopenia, increased hgb F, and clonal chromosomal abnormalities (especially monosomy 7).

■ In vitro spontaneous formation of granulocyte-macrophage colonies that are hypersensitive to granulocyte-macrophage colony-stimulating factor is confirmatory.

Classical Hodgkin Lymphoma (CHL)>Juvenile Chronic Myelomonocytic Leukemia
Myeloproliferative Disorders (MPD)>Chronic Myelogenous Leukemia

T15.4
Myelodysplastic Syndromes (MDS)

Type	Peripheral blood	Bone marrow
Refractory anemia (RA)	Anemia No blasts	Dysplastic erythroids <5% blasts <15% ringed sideroblasts
Refractory anemia with ringed sideroblasts (RARS)	Anemia Dimorphic red cell population Pappenheimer bodies No blasts	Dysplastic erythroids <5% blasts >15% ringed sideroblasts
Refractory cytopenia with multilineage dysplasia (RCMLD)	Bi- or pancytopenia <1% blasts No Auer rods	<5% blasts No Auer rods Dysplasia in >10% of >1 cell line <15% ringed sideroblasts
Refractory cytopenia with multilineage dysplasia with ringed sideroblasts (RCMLD-RS)	Bi- or pancytopenia <1% blasts No Auer rods	<5% blasts No Auer rods Dysplasia in >10% of >1 cell line >15% ringed sideroblasts
Refractory anemia with excess blasts (RAEB)	Bi- or pancytopenia <5% blasts, no Auer rods - RAEB-1 5-19% blasts or Auer rods - RAEB-2	5%-9% blasts, no Auer rods—RAEB-1 10%-19% blasts or Auer rods—RAEB-2 Dysplasia
MDS with del(5q) / 5q- syndrome	Anemia, normal to increased platelets <5% blasts No Auer rods	Hypolobated megakaryocytes <5% blasts No Auer rods Isolated 5q- karyotype
MDS, unclassified	Cytopenia <1% blasts No Auer rods	Dysplasia in 1 cell line <5% blasts No Auer rods

- Nearly 10% of patients have neurofibromatosis type 1 (NF-1).
- There must be fewer than 20% blasts and no Philadelphia chromosome.

Myeloproliferative Disorders (MPD)

The distinctive features of all MPDs are the nondysplastic proliferation of marrow elements (erythrocytic, granulocytic, and/or megakaryocytic), resulting in increased production of mature cells. MPD is nearly always associated with splenomegaly at presentation. All have a tendency to progress to eventual marrow failure and/or acute leukemia.

Chronic Myelogenous Leukemia (CML)

- Without treatment, the condition of most patients with CML will progress. Within 5 years of diagnosis, patients usually proceed through an accelerated phase to an eventual blast phase. The rate of progression to acute leukemia (95%) is the highest among all MPDs (all others have rates around 10%).

- The initial chronic phase is caused by a constitutively activated tyrosine kinase, the chimeric bcr-abl, which produces marked expansion of the myeloid line. It presents with leukocytosis resulting from increased neutrophils in all stages of maturation, a myelocyte "bulge," basophilia, eosinophilia, and thrombocytosis. Blasts are rare (<1%) at this stage, and there is the distinctively low leukocyte alkaline phosphatase (LAP) score. The marrow is hypercellular with an

Myeloproliferative Disorders (MPD)>Chronic Myelogenous Leukemia

increased myeloid-to-erythroid ratio, a myelocyte "bulge," and increased megakaryocytes. One does not find a significant degree of dyspoiesis at presentation; however, dysgranulopoiesis commonly evolves in CML with chromosome 17p abnormalities and may herald an accelerated phase.

- The accelerated and blast phases result from additional chromosomal abnormalities that impair the maturation of the markedly proliferative myeloid elements. These progression-associated changes include duplication of the Philadelphia chromosome, +8, +19, or i(17q). The accelerated phase is marked by the emergence of 1 or more of the following: progressive basophilia (>20%), progressive thrombocytopenia ($<100 \times 10^9/L$), thrombocytosis ($>1000 \times 10^9/L$), progressive leukocytosis, clonal cytogenetic progression, or increasing blasts more than 10% (but less than 20%). The LAP score tends to rise. The blast phase is marked by 1 of the following: more than 20% blasts in blood or marrow, a tissue infiltrate of blasts (chloroma), or a prominent focal accumulation of blasts in the marrow biopsy. In the blast phase, 70% are of the acute myeloid leukemia (AML) type, and 30% are ALL (usually precursor B) type.

- The Philadelphia chromosome involves a reciprocal translocation of chromosomes 9 and 22, t(9;22)(q34;q11), in which the *ABL* gene at the 9q34 is translocated to *BCR* at 22q11, producing a chimeric *BCR-ABL* gene whose product has enhanced tyrosine kinase activity. This is the defining feature of CML. In about 5% of cases, the *BCR-ABL* fusion gene is present in the absence of a cytogenetically visible Philadelphia chromosome. BCR-ABL is essentially unique to CML, having been found only in some cases of ALL and extremely rare examples of MDS and AML. The absence of a Philadelphia chromosome (or better yet the absence of *BCR-ABL*) is required before making the diagnosis of another MPD **T15.5**. The recently identified *JAK-2* anomaly that is present in non-CML MPDs is not identified in CML.

- The *ABL* breakpoint may occur over a wide area of 200 kb usually within the *ABL* exon 2, whereas the *BCL* breakpoint nearly always occurs within a 5.8 kb region, which spans exons 12 to 16, called the major breakpoint cluster region (M-bcr). This breakpoint results in a 210 kD bcr-abl protein (p210). Other breakpoints, such as m-bcr and μ-bcr, are rare relative to M-bcr. The minor breakpoint cluster region (m-bcr) is located upstream from M-bcr and results in a 190-kD protein (p190). Lastly, the μ-bcr

T15.5
Molecular Anomalies in Myeloproliferative Disease

Syndrome	Finding
Chronic myelogneous leukemia (CML)	*BCR-ABL* in 100%
Polycythemia vera (PV)	*JAK2(V617F)* in 95% *JAK2 exon 12 mutation* in 5%
Essential thrombocytosis (ET)	*JAK2(V617F)* in 50%
Myeloid metaplasia with myelofibrosis (MMM/AMM/CIMF)	*JAK2(V617F)* in 50%
Chronic eosinophilic leukemia (CEL)	*FIP1L1-PDGFRA* in 100%
Mast cell disease	*C-KIT*
Chronic neutrophilic leukemia (CNL)	*JAK2(V617F)* in 20%

is located downstream from M-bcr and results in a 230-kD protein (p230); μ-bcr is associated with cases resembling chronic neutrophilic leukemia (CNL).

- Imatinib (Gleevec, Glivec, STI571, Novartis Pharmaceuticals Corp, East Hanover, NJ) functions through competitive inhibition of the ATP–binding site of bcr-abl. It is active against not only bcr-abl, but also against platelet-derived growth factor receptor and c-kit.

- Imatinib resistance is present initially in some cases (about 5%) and emerges during treatment in others.

  □ Resistance is often the result of distinct mutations in the *BCR-ABL* gene, especially the tyrosine kinase domain and the so-called P loop. In the tyrosine kinase domain, the substitution of isoleucine for threonine at position 315 (T315I) has been frequently associated with resistance.

  □ A variety of mechanisms is available for detection of BCR-ABL resistance-associated mutations. These include direct sequence analysis (limited to the kinase domain), denaturing high-pressure liquid chromatography, allele-specific oligonucleotides, and others.

  □ Additional mechanisms of imatinib resistance include P-glycoprotein (MDR-1) overexpression, amplification of *BCR-ABL* leading to increased bcr-able kinase, acquisition of additional non–BCR-ABL genetic anomalies (clonal evolution).

  □ It appears that early treatment with imatinib lessens the incidence of acquired resistance, as patients who begin therapy more than 2 years after diagnosis have a significantly higher incidence than those who begin treatment before 2 years; furthermore, those initially treated while in the accelerated or blast phase have a much higher incidence of imatinib resistance.

- The definition of minimal residual disease (MRD) has been shifting over the years, as newer technologies have emerged. Broadly speaking, it refers to a level of leukemic cells too low to produce clinical manifestations or to be visible microscopically. Several concepts are worth noting:

  □ It is estimated that, at presentation, patients with CML have around 10^{12} leukemic cells; when clinical remission is reached, there are around 10^9 to 10^{10} leukemic cells (about a 2- to 3-log reduction). Thus, MRD generally refers to a number of leukemic cells less than 10^9 to 10^{10}.

  □ There are several modalities for detecting MRD in CML, including conventional cytogenetics, FISH, PCR, and flow cytometry. Each has its unique lower limit of detection.

  □ A complete cytogenetic response (undetectable Philadelphia chromosome by conventional cytogenetics) generally is achieved when the number of leukemic cells is below 10^9 (a 3-log reduction).

  □ A true 3-log reduction at 12 months, as confirmed by quantitative PCR for the BCR-ABL transcript, predicts a nearly 0% likelihood of disease progression over the ensuing 2 years. There is a roughly 5% likelihood of progression when the reduction is less than 3 logs.

- In summary, the potential value of various molecular modalities in CML is as follows:

  □ Conventional cytogenetics can be used to (1) initially detect CML, by identifying a Philadelphia chromosome, and any additional anomalies, if any, and (2) to follow CML, by looking for cytogenetic progression. Cytogenetic remission (the lack of cytogenetically detectable Philadelphia chromosomes) is too insensitive an index of remission for clinical utility. While PCR is significantly more sensitive for detecting the *BCR-ABL* fusion gene, the major advantage of cytogenetics is its ability to find additional chromosomal abnormalities (indicative of progressive disease). *Because PCR is also of value both initially to characterize the BCR-ABL fusion gene and later to detect molecular remission*

(the lack of a molecularly detectable BCR-ABL fusion gene), it is reasonable to perform both studies whenever bone marrow tissue is obtained in patients with known or suspected CML.

  □ FISH, using a fusion probe for *BCR* and *ABL*, can detect the Philadelphia chromosome. For example, if red and green probes were used, normal cells would be expected to show 2 red and 2 green nuclear signals. In CML, cells are present with 3 signals, 1 red, 1 green, and 1 yellow (the fusion signal). FISH is more sensitive for the Philadelphia chromosome than cytogenetics, but it cannot detect additional chromosomal aberrations. Furthermore, while FISH has a level of sensitivity that is generally considered sufficient for detecting MRD, a high rate of false positive and false negative results preclude its routine use. *Thus, FISH has a limited role overall in CML diagnosis and management.*

  □ Quantitative PCR (reverse transcriptase real-time polymerase chain reaction) is considered the method of choice for MRD detection in patients who have achieved a complete cytogenetic remission. RT-PCR monitoring can be performed with equivalent efficacy on either peripheral blood or bone marrow.

  □ Nested RT-PCR is the amplification of an initial amplicon (by performing an amplification in the initial amplicon using consecutive primer sets). While capable of higher sensitivity (1 in 10^6 compared with 1 in 10^4-10^5 cells) than routine PCR, it is unclear that this degree of sensitivity offers any advantage, and nested PCR is prone to contamination. At this time it is not recommended.

Polycythemia Vera (PV)

- PV is diagnosed at a mean age of 60 years, most commonly as a result of hypertension, thrombosis, pruritus, erythromelalgia, or headache—manifestations of polycythemia. PV must be distinguished from relative polycythemia, secondary polycythemia, and CML. Relative polycythemia is seen in the setting of stress or dehydration and has been called Gaisbach's syndrome. Secondary polycythemia is associated with low arterial oxygen (Pao$_2$) states (such as smoking and living at high altitudes), abnormal hemoglobin variants, and certain neoplasms (renal cell carcinoma, cerebellar hemangioblastoma) in which there is elevated erythropoietin.

Myeloproliferative Disorders (MPD)>Polycythemia Vera; Essential Thrombocythemia; Myelofibrosis with Myeloid Metaplasia/Agnogenic Myeloid Metaplasia/Chronic Idiopathic Myelofibrosis

- The initial proliferative phase is marked by marrow hypercellularity, panmyelosis, and usually a low myeloid-to-erythroid ratio. Megakaryocyte hyperplasia and nuclear atypia is often quite prominent and may distract from the erythroid hyperplasia. The spent phase (postpolycythemic myelofibrosis with myeloid metaplasia) is heralded by a myelophthisic peripheral blood pattern, marrow reticulin fibrosis, and extramedullary hematopoiesis.

- The cause of death is most commonly thrombosis (31%), followed by acute leukemia (19%). MPDs, particularly PV, are the most common cause of the Budd-Chiari syndrome, with PV alone accounting for 10% to 40% of cases. Endogenous erythroid colony formation, a defining feature of PV, may be seen in more than 80% of patients thought to have idiopathic Budd-Chiari syndrome.

- *JAK-2* (Janus kinase 2) mutation

  □ A mutation in the *JAK-2* gene is present in 90% to 100% of PV cases and more than 50% of essential thrombocythemia (ET) and idiopathic myelofibrosis (IMF). The jak-2 protein is a tyrosine kinase involved in the pathway by which growth factor receptors alter intracellular activity once they bind ligand (growth factors such as thrombopoietin and erythropoietin). This pathway stimulates so-called signal transducers and activators of transcription (STAT) proteins, and it is called the STAT pathway.

  □ Jak-2 is a member of the Janus kinase family. These are tyrosine kinases that are activated by cell-surface growth factor receptors and, when activated, phosphorylate other proteins in the pathway (the STATs). Phosphorylated STATs enter the nucleus where they act as transcription factors for a number of genes.

  □ The common *JAK-2* mutation is a valine to phenylalanine (genotypic guanine to thymine at nucleotide 1849) substitution at codon 617 (Val617Phe or V617F). The mutation affects the protein's JH2 domain, a normally inhibitory domain. Alteration in JH2 has a net gain-of-function effect that leads to constitutive jak-2 activation, leading to cytokine-independent growth.

  □ The *JAK-2* mutation appears to be necessary for the initiation of many, perhaps all, cases of PV. It seems also to play a major role in the development of ET and IMF. Possibly other acquired mutations determine the ultimate phenotype in these cases.

  □ The major practical question at this time is in regard to the best diagnostic assay for detection of the *JAK-2* mutation. The physicochemical significance of a G to T mutation (with a 3 to 2 hydrogen bond change) has been evaluated; indeed, there appears to be somewhere between a 6°C and 10°C difference in the melting points of the wild-type and mutant alleles, as well as differences in denaturing gradient gel electrophoretic velocity and single-strand conformation. Sequence-based testing, such as allele-specific oligonucleotide (ASO) PCR and quantitative real-time PCR, remain the most sensitive assays. Direct sequence analysis is limited by dilution of cells with mutant alleles in a background of wild-type cells.

Essential Thrombocythemia (ET)

- The incidence of ET is bimodal, with a peak at age 30 years and again at age 60 years, and has a female preponderance. Overall, ET has the longest survival of the MPDs, with the lowest likelihood (5%) of transformation to acute leukemia.

- ET presents most commonly as an isolated thrombocytosis, but some patients present with thrombosis or mucosal hemorrhages. Aside from variable size, the platelets are not morphologically noteworthy, red cell indices are usually normal, and white cell indices are normal.

- The bone marrow shows an increase in mature-appearing, large, hyperlobated megakaryocytes which are clustered, paratrabecular, and display marked emperipolesis. ET must be distinguished from reactive thrombocytopenia that occurs in iron deficiency, chronic inflammation, asplenia, and other hematolymphoid malignancies (such as CML).

- The diagnosis of ET may be supported by the finding of a *JAK-2* mutation. WHO criteria specifically require the *absence* of a Philadelphia chromosome, a BCR/ABL fusion, del5q, t(3;3), and inv(3).

Myelofibrosis with Myeloid Metaplasia (MMM)/Agnogenic Myeloid Metaplasia (AMM)/Chronic Idiopathic Myelofibrosis (CIMF)

- IMF is seen in older adults, usually between the ages of 60 and 70 years. About 30% to 40% present with unexplained splenomegaly or hepatosplenomegaly.

- The cellular (prefibrotic) phase is somewhat difficult to correctly classify. It presents with anemia, mild leukocytosis, and mild thrombocytosis. There may be occasional dacrocytes and nRBCs. The marrow at this stage shows predominantly hypercellularity with an increase in megakaryocytes that are both morphologically abnormal—aberrantly lobulated with clumped, hyperchromatic, and inky chromatin—and abnormally situated—in clusters found adjacent to sinuses and trabecula.

- In the fibrotic phase, where most patients present, the peripheral smear has a leukoerythroblastic pattern, with dacrocytosis and anisocytosis. The bone marrow is often inaspirable. Characteristic bone marrow findings include reticulin and/or collagen fibrosis, intrasinusoidal hematopoiesis, and increased numbers of abnormal and clustered megakaryocytes.

Chronic Eosinophilic Leukemia (CEL)/ Hypereosinophilic Syndrome (HES)

- CEL and HES are characterized by peripheral eosinophilia ($>1.5 \times 10^9$/L), often with evidence of tissue infiltration, when no cause of secondary eosinophilia can be established. In addition to excluding secondary (reactive) eosinophilia, neoplastic eosinophilia as part of another MPD must be excluded, such as that which occurs in AML with inversion of chromosome 16 (FAB: AML-M4Eo) and CML.

- When these are excluded and evidence of clonality can be found, such as a cytogenetic abnormality or increased blasts (but not >20%), CEL is diagnosed. Traditionally, when evidence of clonality is lacking and secondary eosinophilia can be excluded, the diagnosis of HES was rendered.

- CEL/HES is predominantly a disease of men (male-female ratio, 9:1). It usually presents in males between the ages of 25 and 45 years.

- The neoplastic eosinophils may be hypogranular, in which case histochemical staining for cyanide-resistant myeloperoxidase (eosinophils are positive) can be helpful.

- Unlike most fusion genes that result from a balanced translocation, the one responsible for CEL results from a deletion of genetic material between genes. An interstitial deletion in the long arm of chromosome 4, del(4)(q12;q12), results in the *FIP1L1-PDGFRA* (Fip1-like 1 and platelet-derived growth factor

receptor-α) fusion gene. The deletion cannot be seen in routine cytogenetic studies (cryptic interstitial deletion).

- The Fip1L1-pdgfr fusion protein is a tyrosine kinase that can often be inactivated by imatinib. The dose required for inhibition is much lower than that needed for bcr-abl inhibition.

Chronic Neutrophilic Leukemia (CNL)

- CNL is characterized by splenomegaly, an elevated LAP score, and marked neutrophilia ($>25 \times 10^9$/L) which, in contrast to usual-type CML, is composed almost entirely of mature neutrophils and bands. The diagnosis rests on exclusion of CML and reactive neutrophilia.

- For the exclusion of CML, an absence of the Philadelphia chromosome is required. There are cases morphologically indistinguishable from CNL that have a μ-Bcr variant of the Philadelphia chromosome productive of a variant bcr/abl protein, p230; such cases should be classified as CML.

- For exclusion of reactive neutrophilia, clinicopathologic features are generally sufficient (ie, splenomegaly with the absence of identifiable causes of secondary neutrophilia). In research settings, the human androgen receptor gene assay (HUMARA) has been used to confirm clonality in female patients. This assay is based on the principal that in polyclonal populations, the X chromosome is randomly inactivated; thus the length of polymorphisms inherent in the human androgen receptor gene on the X chromosome can be exploited to assess clonality. In polyclonal populations, roughly half of the cells will show expression of the maternally derived allele and half express the paternally derived allele. In clonal populations, only 1 is expressed.

Mast Cell Neoplasms

- This term encompasses a group of disorders ranging from the solitary cutaneous mastocytoma to mast cell leukemia. Cutaneous mastocytosis is the most common subtype seen in routine practice. It is usually seen in children and follows a benign clinical course. The possibility of systemic mastocytosis (SM), however, must be considered in every case. SM may or may not have cutaneous involvement, can present at any age, and is characterized by multifocal mast cell infiltrates. The biologic behavior is difficult to predict, and both indolent and aggressive subtypes have been seen.

15: Neoplastic Hematology

Myeloproliferative Disorders (MPD)>Mast Cell Neoplasms | Acute Myeloid Leukemia (AML)>General Features; AML with t(8;21)(q22;q22); AML with inv(16)(p13q22) or t(16;16)(p13;q22)

At the present time, the WHO recognizes 4 major types of SM: indolent systemic mastocytosis (ISM), systemic mastocytosis with an associated clonal hematologic non–mast cell disease (SM-AHNMD), aggressive systemic mastocytosis (ASM), and mast cell leukemia.

- The bone marrow is consistently involved in SM, so bone marrow biopsy is a very important component of the evaluation. In the bone marrow, mastocytosis appears as spindled or round cell infiltrates, usually with fibrosis and a smattering of eosinophils. Both benign and neoplastic mast cell infiltrates are positive tryptase, toluidine blue, Leder stains, leukocyte common antigen, CD11c, CD33, CD43, CD117, and FcεRI. Only very immature mast cells express CD34. Neoplastic mast cell infiltrates express CD2 and CD25 (though CD2 reactivity has been difficult to reproduce). Expression of CD25 correlates with the presence of c-kit mutations and is indicative of malignancy.

Acute Myeloid Leukemia (AML)

General Features

- The diagnosis of AML is principally established on the basis of a blast percentage more than 20%. In some cases, the diagnosis can be made below this threshold, especially when certain cytogenetic abnormalities are detected, such as t(8;21)(q22;q22), inv(16)(p13q22), t(16;16)(p13;q22), or t(15;17)(q22;q12). In addition, in acute promyelocytic leukemia (APML) and acute monocytic leukemia, promyelocytes and promonocytes respectively are counted as blast-equivalents.

- Blasts in AML usually express CD13, CD117, CD33, HLA-DR (with the exception of APML), and CD45. CD34 is present frequently, but this depends on the degree of maturation. CD14 is expressed in cases with monocytic differentiation, and CD15 is expressed in cases with granulocytic differentiation. CD61 is a marker of megakaryoblastic differentiation, and CD235 (glycophorin) is a marker of erythrocytic differentiation. The blasts are usually negative for lymphoid markers, but up to 20% are positive for CD7.

- AML is segregated (WHO classification) into 4 main groups: AML with recurrent genetic abnormalities; AML with multilineage dysplasia; AML, therapy related; and AML, not otherwise categorized. The first group is considered separately in recognition of the tendency of certain genetic abnormalities to relate directly to clinical behavior. For example AML with t(8;21), inv(16), or t(16;16) tend to affect younger adults and to respond well to chemotherapy. This group represents about 30% of AML overall. The next 2 groups are marked by affinity for older adults and chemoresistance. The last group represents a miscellany of de novo AMLs that loosely recapitulate the French-American-British (FAB) classification.

AML with t(8;21)(q22;q22)

- About 10% of AMLs will be found to contain this translocation, which results in the fusion of the *AML1* and *ETO* genes. The *AML1* gene encodes the alpha chain of core binding factor (CBFα). Interestingly, the *CBFβ* gene is involved in AML with inv(16) or t(16;16).

- The blasts are characterized by pronounced azurophilic granularity, sometimes having large (pseudo Chediak-Higashi) granules, and Auer rods. Such blasts would otherwise be characterized as M2 (AML with maturation) and express CD34, CD13, CD33, HLA-DR, CD19, and usually CD15. Because CD34 is a marker of immaturity, and CD15 is acquired late in development, their coexpression is anomalous and suggestive of t(8;21) AML. CD19 expression by AML is also suggestive of this translocation. CD56 is also often expressed, indicating a worse prognosis.

- AML with *AML-ETO* fusion tends to affect younger adults and to be relatively chemosensitive.

AML with inv(16)(p13q22) or t(16;16) (p13;q22)

- These structural abnormalities result in the apposition of the *MYH11* (smooth muscle myosin heavy chain) and *CBFβ* genes. Conventional cytogenetics, FISH, or reverse transcriptase-polymerase chain reaction (RT-PCR) can commonly detect this abnormality.

- The associated leukemia shows myelomonocytic differentiation with a prominent component of morphologically abnormal eosinophils. The eosinophils have granules that are abnormally large, some of them basophilic, and alpha naphthyl acetate esterase positive (normal eosinophil granules are negative). This increase in eosinophils is something noted in the marrow, but it is not common in the peripheral blood.

Acute Myeloid Leukemia (AML)>AML with inv(16)(p13q22) or t(16;16)(p13;q22); AML with t(15;17)(q22;q21); AML with Anomalies of 11q23; AML with Multilineage Dysplasia; AML and MDS, Therapy-Related

- Immunohistochemical staining for CBFb-SMMHC protein reveals nuclear expression in this type of AML.

- The designation M4Eo (AMML Eo) was given to this morphologic appearance in the FAB classification. The blasts express CD13, CD33, CD14, CD64, CD11b, HLA-DR, lysozyme, and often express CD2.

- This type of AML tends to affect younger adults and to be relatively chemosensitive.

AML with t(15;17)(q22;q21)

- This is the FAB subtype AML M3 (APML) that is important to recognize because of its tendency to present in disseminated intravascular coagulation and its responsiveness to all trans-retinoic acid (ATRA).

- The leukemic cells are abnormal promyelocytes that have kidney-shaped or bilobed nuclei, with cytoplasm varying from intensely granulated and replete with Auer rods to hypogranulated (microgranular variant). The microgranular variant may resemble acute monocytic leukemia. The myeloperoxidase reaction is quite strong in both variants, being weak or negative in monoblasts. On flow cytometry, the neoplastic cells express CD33 strongly, express CD13 in a range of strength, and express CD15 weakly. They are negative for HLA-DR and CD34.

- The chromosomal abnormality results in juxtaposition of the retinoic acid receptor (*RARα*) gene and the *PML* gene. Several variant translocations involving *RARα* have been documented, usually resulting in morphologic APML that is relatively not as sensitive to ATRA. These include t(11;17) and t(5;17). The t(11;17)(q23;q22) translocation fuses the *RARα* gene with the *PLZF* gene. The t(5;17)(q35;q21) fuses *RARα* with *NPM* (nucelophosmin). In addition, there are 3 major breakpoints—bcr1 (located within intron 6), bcr2 (exon 6), and bcr3 (intron 3)—that lead to the production of 3 different transcripts, long, variable, and short. This last transcript (short, bcr3) more commonly have the features of variant M3 (M3v), with shorter survival and relative insensitivity to ATRA.

AML with Anomalies of 11q23 (MLL)

- This subtype is common in children and young adults, particularly those who have undergone therapy with topoisomerase II inhibitors.

- The leukemic cells usually show monoblastic (M4-M5) differentiation, with expression of CD4, CD14, CD64, CD11b, and lysozyme. CD34 is usually negative.

- Structural abnormalities of 11q23, which contains the *MLL* gene, is a finding in about 5% of ALLs and a similar percentage of AMLs. However, not all anomalies of 11q23 involve the *MLL* gene. Cytogenetics has limited sensitivity for 11q23 rearrangements; furthermore, cytogenetics cannot distinguish 11q23 rearrangements with *MLL* abnormalities from those without. FISH is significantly more sensitive and is capable of making the *MLL* distinction. The most common rearrangements are t(9;11)(p21;q23), producing an *MLL/AF9* gene fusion, and t(4;11), producing the *MLL/AF4* gene fusion and common in infants.

AML with Multilineage Dysplasia

- Affects mainly the elderly, often follows a period of MDS, but may arise de novo. By definition, there are more than 20% blasts, and dysplasia in more than 50% of the cells in at least 2 cell lines.

- Their cytogenetics are typically quite complex **T15.6**, reflecting an evolving myelodysplastic substrate. Their prognosis is relatively poor.

AML and MDS, Therapy-Related

- In addition to the aforementioned topoisomerase II–related AML with *MLL* anomalies, alkylating agent–related AML and MDS are also recognized.

T15.6
Cytogenetic Findings in Acute Myeloid Leukemia

Favorable Findings	Intermediate Risk	Unfavorable Findings
t(15;17)	Normal karyotype	Complex karyotype
t(8;21)	+8	del(7)
inv(16)	11q23	abn(3q)
	+21	del(5q)
	+22	del(5)
	del(7q)	
	del(9q)	

15: Neoplastic Hematology

Acute Myeloid Leukemia (AML)>AML and MDS, Therapy-Related; AML, Not Otherwise Categorized
Leukemia in Down Syndrome (Trisomy 21)>Transient Myeloproliferative Disorder

They have an average latency of 5 years following treatment, and the incidence is dose dependent. A period of MDS usually precedes the development of AML. The response to treatment is poor.

AML, Not Otherwise Categorized

- This group of tumors has, by definition, no highly reproducible molecular anomalies.

- Cytogenetic abnormalities are detected in up to 75% of cases, excluding the aforementioned disease-specific isolated abnormalities. In about 10% of cases, there are multiple (≥3) chromosomal rearrangements. Such cases tend to have a worse prognosis.

- Additional cytogenetic features that imply a poor prognosis include abnormalities of chromosomes 5, 7, or 8, t(6;9) and the presence of a t(9;22) Philadelphia chromosome.

- Another important molecular finding is the *FLT3* tyrosine kinase gene internal tandem duplication (FLT3 ITD). This finding can be identified in 20% to 30% of patients with AML. FLT3 ITD has been shown to be an important adverse prognostic factor in AML, independent of other chromosomal anomalies.

- The NPM1 mutation, on the other hand, implies a favorable prognosis.

Leukemia in Down Syndrome (Trisomy 21)

Acute leukemia in children with Down syndrome is somewhat evenly divided between ALL and acute myeloblastic leukemia. There is a manyfold increased risk of both. ALL in Down syndrome is in most ways similar to ALL in normal children, except for a reported increased sensitivity to methotrexate and overall favorable prognosis.

The immunophenotypic and morphologic features of AML in Down syndrome are usually those of M7 (megakaryoblastic) AML. This subtype is exceedingly rare in children who do not have Down syndrome. AML associated with Down syndrome is highly sensitive to chemotherapy. It typically arises in young children (1-5 years of age), whereas transient myeloproliferative disorder in Down syndrome arises in the first week or 2 of life.

Transient Myeloproliferative Disorder (Transient Leukemia)

- About 10% of neonates with Down syndrome (or trisomy 21 mosaicism) may manifest a transient myeloproliferative disorder (TMD). This nearly always arises in the first week of life (ranging from 30 weeks gestation to 6 months of age) with a very high white blood cell count and hepatosplenomegaly.

- It is somewhat difficult to distinguish from congenital acute leukemia, but when the infant has the obvious stigmata of Down syndrome, it is best to err on the side of TMD and withhold treatment.

- However, in many cases the child is either a trisomy 21 mosaic or, in some cases, the trisomy 21 anomaly is confined to the clone itself. Thus, in children with apparent congenital acute leukemia, a crucial first step in the evaluation, regardless of the child's morphologic features, is cytogenetics.

- The white cell count is initially quite high, and the blasts are of the megakaryoblastic or mixed megakaryoblasts-erythroblasts types. The blasts are characteristically negative for CD11b and CD13, in contrast to AML in Down syndrome, which expresses CD11b and CD13. Some develop hepatic fibrosis, attributed to megakaryoblast infiltration of the liver. In others, complete clinicopathologic resolution, without therapy, is the rule. Nonetheless, about 30% go on to develop true AML, mostly of the M7 type.

- It has recently been reported that somatic (acquired, not germline) mutations in the *GATA-1* gene are present in the blasts of both TMD and Down syndrome–associated AML.

- Congenital acute leukemia, in contrast to other childhood acute leukemias, is most commonly (about 65%) an AML. About 25% of congenital acute leukemia is ALL, and most of the remaining are mixed. It is arbitrarily defined as an acute leukemia presenting before the age of 4 weeks and must be distinguished from a leukemoid reaction (sepsis, hemolytic disease of the newborn) and TMD. While the vast majority of congenital AML falls into the M4/M5 category, TMD usually has an M7 phenotype and, of course, trisomy 21. A significant minority (about 10%) of congenital acute leukemias have abnormalities of 11q23 (MLL).

Leukemia in Down Syndrome (Trisomy 21)>Transient Myeloproliferative Disorder

T15.7
Selected Hematologic Disease-Associated Chromosomal Rearrangements

Disease	Rearrangement	Notes
Acute myelogenous leukemia (AML)	t(8;21)(q22;q22)	*ETO / AML1* M2 morphology Good prognosis
	inv(16)/t(16;16)	*CBFB / MYHII* M4 morphology Good prognosis CNS infiltration
	t(15;17)(q22;q21)	*PML / RARα* APML Good response to ATRA DIC common
	t(11;17)(q23.1;q21)	*PLZF / RARα* Variant APML Poor response to ATRA
	11q23	*MLL.* Poor prognosis. CNS involvement. Post-topoisomerase II therapy
	t(1;22)(p13;q13)	*OTT/MAL* Infantile AML-M7
Chronic myelogenous leukemia (CML)	t(9;22)(q34;q11.2)	*BCR/ABL*
	t(9;22) + Ph, +8, +19,i(17q), del(9q)	Indicates progression (clonal evolution)
Chronic eosinophilic leukemia (CEL)	t(5;12)(q33,p13)	*PDGFRβ / TEL*
B-precursor acute lymphoblastic leukemia/lymphoma (precursor-B-ALL)	Hyperdiploidy >54 chromosomes	Good prognosis
	t(12;21)	*TEL/AMLIL* Good prognosis
	t(4;11)(q21;q23)	*MLL* Neonates and infants, poor prognosis
	t(1;19)	Poor prognosis
	t(9;22)(q34;q11.2)	*BCR/ABL* Poor prognosis
Burkitt lymphoma	t(8;14), t(8;22), t(2;8)	*cMyc / IgH; cMyc / Igλ; cMyc / Igκ*
Chronic lymphocytic leukemia (CLL/SLL)	del(13q), del(11q), +12, del(17p)	20% have a normal chromosomes
Follicular lymphoma (FL)	t(14;18)(q32;q21)	*BCL2 / IgH*
Mantle cell lymphoma (MCL)	t(11;14)(q13;q32)	*BCL1 / IgH*
MALT lymphoma	t(11;18)(q21;q21)	*MLT / API2*
Lymphoplasmacytic lymphoma (LPL)	t(9;14)(p13;q32)	*PAX-5 / IgH*

T15.7 *(continued)*
Selected Hematologic Disease-Associated Chromosomal Rearrangements

Disease	Rearrangement	Notes
Myeloma	Hyperdiploidy	Good prognosis
	t(11;14)(q13;q32	*CCNDI / IgH*
	Del(13), t(4;14), t(14;16)	Poor prognosis
	t(8;14)	*cMyc/IgH*
Diffuse large B-cell lymphoma (DLBCL)	t(3;14)(q27;q32)	*Bcl-6/IgH*
Anaplastic large cell lymphoma (ALCL)	t(2;5)(p23;q35)	*ALK/NPM* Good prognosis

References

Adeyinka A, Dewald GW. Cytogenetics of chronic myeloproliferative disorders and related myelodysplastic syndromes. *Hematol Oncol Clin North Am* 2003; 17: 1129-1149.

Akasaka T, Ueda C, Kurata M, et al. Nonimmunoglobulin (non-Ig)/BCL6 gene fusion in diffuse large B-cell lymphoma results in worse prognosis than Ig/BCL6. *Blood* 2000; 96: 2907-2909.

Albinger-Hegyi A, Hochreutener B, Abdou M-T, et al. High frequency of t(14;18)-translocation breakpoints outside of major breakpoint and minor cluster regions in follicular lymphomas: improved polymerase chain reaction protocols for their detection. *Am J Pathol* 2002; 160: 823-832.

Alessandrino EP, Amadori S, Cazzola M, et al. Myelodysplastic syndromes: recent advances. *Haematologica* 2001; 86: 1124-1157.

Arber DA. Molecular diagnostic approach to non-Hodgkin's lymphoma. *J Mol Diagn* 2000; 2: 178-190.

Arber DA, Braziel RM, Bagg A, et al. Evaluation of T cell receptor testing in lymphoid neoplasms: results of a multicenter study of 29 extracted DNA and paraffin-embedded samples. *J Mol Diag* 2001; 3: 133-140.

Baens M, Maes B, Steyls A, et al. The product of the t(11;18), an API2-MLT fusion, marks nearly half of gastric MALT type lymphomas without large cell proliferation. *Am J Pathol* 2000; 156: 1433-1439.

Bain BJ. Cytogenetic and molecular genetic aspects of eosinophilic leukaemias. *Br J Haematol* 2003; 122: 173-179.

Bajwa RP, Skinner R, Windebank KP, et al. Demographic study of leukaemia presenting within the first 3 months of life in the northern health region of England. *J Clin Pathol* 2004; 57: 186-188.

Baxter EJ, Scott LM, Campbell PJ, et al. Acquired mutation of the tyrosine kinase JAK2 in human myeloproliferative disorders. *Lancet* 2005; 365: 1054-1061.

Bea S, Zettl A, Wright G, et al. Diffuse large B-cell lymphoma subgroups have distinct genetic profiles that influence tumor biology and improve gene-expression-based survival prediction. *Blood* 2005; 106: 3183-3190.

Belaud-Rotureau M, Parrens M, Dubus P, et al. A comparative analysis of FISH, RT-PCR, PCR, and immunohistochemistry for the diagnosis of mantle cell lymphomas. *Mod Pathol* 2002; 15: 517-525.

Bene MC, Castoldi G, Knapp W. Proposals for the immunological classification of acute leukemias. *Leukemia* 1995; 9: 1783-1786.

References

Bijwaard KE, Aguilera N, Monczak Y, et al. Quantitative real-time reverse transcription-PCR assay for cyclin D1 expression: utility in the diagnosis of mantle cell lymphoma. *Clin Chem* 2001; 47: 195-201.

Blum KA, Lozanski G, Byrd JC. Adult Burkitt leukemia and lymphoma. *Blood* 2004; 104: 3009-3020.

Böhm J, Kock S, Schaefer HE, Fisch P. Evidence of clonality in chronic neutrophilic leukaemia. *J Clin Pathol* 2003; 56: 292-295.

Boultwood J, Lewis S, Wainscoat JS. The 5q- syndrome. *Blood* 1994; 84: 3253-3260.

Bresters D, Reus AC, Veerman AJ, et al. Congenital leukaemia: the Dutch experience and review of the literature. *Br J Haematol* 2002; 117: 513-524.

Campo E. Genetic and molecular genetic studies in the diagnosis of B-cell lymphomas I: mantle cell lymphoma, follicular lymphoma, and Burkitt's lymphoma. *Hum Pathol* 2003; 34: 330-335.

Caraway NP, Stewart J. Primary effusion lymphoma. *Pathol Case Rev* 2006; 11: 78-84.

Cataldo KA, Jalal SM, Law ME, et al. Detection of t(2;5) in anaplastic large cell lymphoma: Comparison of immunohistochemical studies, FISH, and RT-PCR in paraffin-embedded tissue. *Am J Surg Pathol* 1999; 23: 1386-1392.

Cawley JC. The pathophysiology of the hairy cell leukemia. *Hematol Oncol Clin North Am* 2006; 20: 1011-1021.

Chadburn A, Hyjek E, Mathew S, et al. KSHV-positive solid lymphomas represent an extra-cavitary variant of primary effusion lymphoma. *Am J Surg Pathol* 2004; 28: 1401-1416.

Chan WC, Hans CP, Kadin ME. Genetic and molecular genetic studies in the diagnosis of T-cell malignancies. *Hum Pathol* 2003; 34: 314-321.

Chen Z, Issa B, Huang S, et al. A practical approach to the detection of prognostically significant genomic aberrations in multiple myeloma. *J Mol Diagn* 2005; 7: 560-565.

Cook JR, Shekhter-Levin S, Swerdlow SH. Utility of routine classical cytogenetic studies in the evaluation of suspected lymphomas: results of 279 consecutive lymph node/extranodal tissue biopsies. *Am J Clin Pathol* 2004; 121: 826-835.

Cools J, DeAngelo DJ, Gotlib J, et al. A tyrosine kinase created by fusion of the PDGFRA and FIP1L1 genes as a therapeutic target of imatinib in idiopathic hypereosinophilic syndrome. *N Engl J Med* 2003; 348: 1201-1214.

Corradini P, Cavo M, Lokhorst H, et al. Molecular remission after myeloablative allogeneic stem cell transplantation predicts a better relapse-free survival in patients with multiple myeloma. *Blood* 2003; 102: 1927-1929.

Cox MC, Panetta P, Lo-Coco F, et al. Chromosomal aberration of the 11q23 locus in acute leukemia and frequency of MLL gene translocation results in 378 adult patients. *Am J Clin Pathol* 2004; 122: 298-306.

Crespo M, Bosch F, Villamor N, et al. ZAP-70 Expression as a surrogate for immunoglobulin-variable-region mutations in chronic lymphocytic leukemia. *N Engl J Med* 2003; 348: 1764-1775.

Crossman LC, O'Brien SG. Imatinib therapy in chronic myeloid leukemia. *Hematol Oncol Clin North Am* 2004; 18: 605-617.

Cushing T, Clericuzio CL, Wilson CS, et al. Risk for leukemia in infants without down syndrome who have transient myeloproliferative disorder. *J Pediatr* 2006; 148: 687-689.

Damle RN, Wasil T, Fais F, et al. Ig V Gene mutation status and CD38 expression as novel prognostic indicators in chronic lymphocytic leukemia. *Blood* 1999; 94: 1840-1847.

Dewald GW, Ketterling RP. Conventional cytogenetics and molecular cytogenetics in hematologic malignancies. In: *Hematology: Basic Principles and Practice*. 4th Ed. Philadelphia, Pa: Elsevier, 2005.

Dohner H, Stilgenbauer S, Benner A, et al. Genomic aberrations and survival in chronic lymphocytic leukemia. *N Engl J Med* 2000; 343: 1910-1916.

Druker BJ, Sawyers CL, Kantarjian H, et al. Activity of a specific inhibitor of the bcr-abl tyrosine kinase in the blast crisis of chronic myeloid leukemia and acute lymphoblastic leukemia with the Philadelphia chromosome. *N Engl J Med* 2001; 344: 1038-1042.

References

Druker BJ, Talpaz M, Resta DJ, et al. Efficacy and safety of a specific inhibitor of the bcr-abl tyrosine kinase in chronic myeloid leukemia. *N Engl J Med* 2001; 344: 1031-1037.

Einerson RR, Kurtin PJ, Dayharsh GA, et al. FISH is superior to PCR in detecting t(14;18)(q32;q21)-IgH/bcl-2 in follicular lymphoma using paraffin-embedded tissue samples. *Am J Clin Pathol* 2005; 124: 421-429.

Facon T, Avet-Loiseau H, Guillerm G, et al. Intergroupe Francophone du Myélome. Chromosome 13 abnormalities identified by FISH analysis and serum beta2-microglobulin produce a powerful myeloma staging system for patients receiving high-dose therapy. *Blood* 2001; 97: 1566-1571.

Faderl S, Hochhaus A, Hughes T. Monitoring of minimal residual disease in chronic myeloid leukemia. *Hematol Oncol Clin North Am* 2004; 18: 657-670.

Fais F, Ghiotto F, Hashimoto S, et al. CLL B-cells express restricted sets of mutated and unmutated antigen receptors. *J Clin Invest* 1998; 102: 1515-1525.

Gascoyne RD, Aoun P, Wu D, et al. Prognostic significance of anaplastic lymphoma kinase (ALK) protein expression in adults with analplastic large cell lymphoma. *Blood* 1999; 93: 3913-3921.

Gotlib J, Cools J, Malone JM III, et al. The FIP1L1-PDGFR fusion tyrosine kinase in hypereosinophilic syndrome and chronic eosinophilic leukemia: implications for diagnosis, classification, and management. *Blood* 2004; 103: 2879-2891.

Gottschalk S, Rooney CM, Heslop HE. Post-transplant lymphoproliferative disorders. *Annu Rev Med* 2005; 56: 29-44.

Greiner TC. Diagnostic Assays for the JAK2 V617F mutation in chronic myeloproliferative disorders. *Am J Clin Pathol* 2006; 125: 651-653.

Hagland U, Juliusson G, Stellan B, et al. Hairy cell leukemia is characterized by clonal chromosome abnormalities clustered to specific regions. *Blood* 1994; 83: 2637-2645.

Hamblin TJ, Davis Z, Gardiner A, et al. Unmutated Ig VH genes are associated with a more aggressive form of chronic lymphocytic leukemia. *Blood* 1999; 94: 1848-1854.

Hochhaus A, Hughes T. Clinical resistance to imatinib: mechanisms and implications. *Hematol Oncol Clin North Am* 2004; 18: 641-656.

Hodges E, Krishna MT, Pickard C, et al. Diagnostic role of tests for T cell receptor (TCR) genes. *J Clin Pathol* 2003; 56: 1-11.

Huang L, Abruzzo LV, Valbuena JR, et al. Acute myeloid leukemia associated with variant t(8;21) detected by conventional cytogenetic and molecular studies: a report of four cases and review of the literature. *Am J Clin Pathol* 2006; 125: 267-272.

Hughes TP, Kaeda J, Branford S, et al. Frequency of major molecular responses to imatinib or interferon alfa plus cytarabine in newly diagnosed chronic myeloid leukemia. *N Engl J Med* 2003; 349: 1423-1432.

Ibrahim S, Keating M, Do K, et al. CD38 expression as an important prognostic factor in B-cell chronic lymphocytic leukemia. *Blood* 2001; 98: 181-186.

Iqbal J, Sanger WG, Horsman DE, et al. BCL2 translocation defines a unique tumor subset within the germinal center B-cell-like diffuse large b-cell lymphoma. *Am J Pathol* 2004; 165: 159-166.

Jaffe, Harris, Stein, Vardiman Eds., *Tumours of Haematopoietic and Lymphoid Tissues.* Lyon, France: International Agency for Research on Cancer, 2001.

Kadin ME. Genetic and molecular genetic studies in the diagnosis of T-cell malignancies. *Hum Pathol* 2003; 34: 322-329.

Kansal R, Sait S, Block A, Ward PM, et al. Extra copies of chromosome 2 are a recurring aberration in ALK-negative lymphomas with anaplastic morphology. *Mod Pathol* 2005; 18: 235-243.

Kobayashi Y, Nakata M, Maekawa M, et al. Detection of t(11;18) in MALT-type lymphoma with dual-color fluorescence In situ hybridization and reverse transcriptase-polymerase chain reaction analysis. *Diagn Mol Pathol* 2001; 10: 207-213.

Kralovics R, Passamonti F, Buser AS, et al. Gain-of-function mutation of *JAK2* in myeloproliferative disorders. *N Engl J Med* 2005; 352: 1779-1790.

References

Krober A, Seiler T, Benner A, et al. VH mutation status, CD38 expression level, genomic aberrations, and survival in chronic lymphocytic leukemia. *Blood* 2002; 100: 1410-1416.

Kussick SJ, Fromm JR, Rossini A, et al. Four-color flow cytometry shows strong concordance with bone marrow morphology and cytogenetics in the evaluation for myelodysplasia. *Am J Clin Pathol* 2005; 124: 170-181.

Kussick SJ, Wood BL. Four-color flow cytometry identifies virtually all cytogenetically abnormal bone marrow samples in the workup of non-CML myeloproliferative disorders. *Am J Clin Pathol* 2003; 120: 854-865.

Kyle RA, Gertz MA, Witzig TE, et al. Review of 1027 patients with newly diagnosed multiple myeloma. *Mayo Clin Proc* 2003; 78: 21-33.

Lange B. The management of neoplastic disorders of haemopoiesis in children with Down's syndrome. *Br J Haematol* 2000; 110: 512-524.

Levine RL, Loriaux M, Huntly BJ, et al. The JAK2V617F activating mutation occurs in chronic myelomonocytic leukemia and acute myeloid leukemia, but not in acute lymphoblastic leukemia or chronic lymphocytic leukemia. *Blood* 2005; 106: 3377-3379.

Lin P, Hao S, Medeiros LJ, et al. Expression of CD2 in acute promyelocytic leukemia correlates with short form of PML-RARα transcripts and poorer prognosis. *Am J Clin Pathol* 2004; 121: 1-9.

Lindvall C, Nordenskjold M, Porwit A, et al. Molecular cytogenetic characterization of acute myeloid leukemia and myelodysplastic syndromes with multiple chromosome rearrangements. *Haematologica* 2001; 86: 1158-1164.

Litzow MR. Imatinib resistance: obstacles and opportunities. *Arch Pathol Lab Med* 2006; 130: 669-679.

Liu H, Ye H, Ruskone-Fourmestraux A, et al. t(11;18) is a marker for all stage gastric MALT lymphomas that will not respond to *H. pylori* eradication. *Gastroenterology* 2002; 122: 1286-1294.

Look AT. Molecular pathogenesis of MDS. *Hematology Am Soc Hematol Educ Program* 2005: 156-160.

Lossos IS, Czerwinski DK, Alizadeh AA, et al. Prediction of survival in diffuse large-B-cell lymphoma based on the expression of six genes. *N Engl J Med* 2004; 350: 1828-1837.

Macdonald D, Reiter A, Cross NC. The 8p11 myeloproliferative syndrome: a distinct clinical entity caused by constitutive activation of FGFR1. *Acta Haematol* 2002; 107: 101-107.

MacDonald D, Sheerin SM, Cross NC, et al. An atypical myeloproliferative disorder with t(8;13)(p11;q12): a third case. *Br J Haematol* 1994; 86: 879-880.

Macon WR, Levy NB, Kurtin PJ, et al. Hepatosplenic αβ T-cell lymphomas: a report of 14 cases and comparison with hepatosplenic γδ T-cell lymphomas. *Am J Surg Pathol* 2001; 25: 285-296.

Marasca R, Maffei R, Morselli M, et al. Immunoglobulin mutational status detected through single-round amplification of partial vh region represents a good prognostic marker for clinical outcome in chronic lymphocytic leukemia. *J Mol Diagn* 2005; 7: 566-574.

Merchant SH, Amin MB, Viswanatha DS. Morphologic and immunophenotypic analysis of angioimmunoblastic T-cell lymphoma. *Am J Clin Pathol* 2006; 125: 1-10.

Merzianu M, Medeiros LJ, Cortes J, et al. Inv(16)(p13q22) in chronic myelogenous leukemia in blast phase: a clinicopathologic, cytogenetic, and molecular study of five cases. *Am J Clin Pathol* 2005; 124: 807-814.

Miranda RN, Briggs RC, Kinney MC, et al. Immunohistochemical detection of cyclin D1 using optimized conditions is highly specific for mantle cell lymphoma and hairy cell leukemia. *Mod Pathol* 2000; 13: 1308-1314.

Murugesan G, Aboudola S, Szpurka H, et al. Identification of the JAK2 V617F mutation in chronic myeloproliferative disorders using FRET probes and melting curve analysis. *Am J Clin Pathol* 2006; 125: 625-633.

Natkunam Y, Rouse RV. Utility of paraffin section immunohistochemistry for C-kit (CD117) in the differential diagnosis of systemic mast cell disease involving the bone marrow. *Am J Surg Pathol* 2000; 24: 81-91.

References

Ng A, Taylor GM, Wynn RF, et al. Effects of topoisomerase 2 inhibitors on the MLL gene in children receiving chemotherapy: a prospective study. *Leukemia* 2005; 19: 253-259.

Ng SB, Lai KW, Murugaya S, et al. Nasal-type extranodal natural killer/T-cell lymphomas: a clinicopathologic and genotypic study of 42 cases in Singapore. *Mod Pathol* 2004; 17: 1097-1107.

Nikiforova MN, Hsi ED, Braziel RM, et al. Detection of clonal IGH gene rearrangements: summary of molecular oncology surveys of the College of American Pathologists. *Arch Pathol Lab Med* 2007; 131: 185-189.

Nishino HT, Chang C. Myelodysplastic syndromes: clinicopathologic features, pathobiology, and molecular pathogenesis. *Arch Pathol Lab Med* 2005;129: 1299-310.

Onciu M, Behm FG, Raimondi SC, et al. Alk-positive anaplastic large cell lymphoma with leukemic peripheral blood involvement is a clinicopathologic entity with an unfavorable prognosis: Report of three cases and review of the literature. *Am J Clin Pathol* 2003; 120: 617-625.

Onciu M, Schlette E, Medeiros LJ, et al. Cytogenetic findings in mantle cell lymphoma: cases with a high level of peripheral blood involvement have a distinct pattern of abnormalities. *Am J Clin Pathol* 2001; 116: 886-892.

Orchard JA, Ibbotson RE, Davis Z, et al. ZAP-70 expression and prognosis in CLL. *Lancet* 2004; 363: 105-111.

Pagliuca A, Mufti GJ, Janossa-Tahernia M, et al. In vitro colony culture and chromosomal studies in hepatic and portal vein thrombosis: possible evidence of an occult myeloproliferative state. *Q J Med* 1990; 76(281): 981-989.

Pedersen B, Jensen IM. Clinical and prognostic implications of chromosome 5q deletions: 96 high resolution studied patients. *Leukemia* 1991; 5: 566-573.

Petrella T, Bagot M, Willemze R, et al. Blastic NK-cell lymphomas (agranular CD4+, CD56+ hematodermic neoplasms). *Am J Clin Pathol* 2005; 123: 662-675.

Rai KR, Chiorazzi N. Determining the clinical course and outcome in chronic lymphocytic leukemia. *N Engl J Med* 2003; 348(18): 1797-1799.

Raimondi SC, Chang MN, Ravindranath Y, et al. Chromosomal abnormalities in 478 children with acute myeloid leukemia: clinical characteristics and treatment outcome in a cooperative Pediatric Oncology Group study-POG 8821. *Blood* 1999; 94: 3707-3716.

Rainis L, Bercovich D, Strehl S, et al. Mutations in exon 2 Of GATA-1 are early events in megakaryocytic malignancies associated with trisomy 21. *Blood* 2003; 102: 981-986.

Rassenti LZ, Huynh L, Toy TL, et al. ZAP-70 compared with immunoglobulin heavy-chain gene mutation status as a predictor of disease progression in chronic lymphocytic leukemia. *N Engl J Med* 2004; 351: 893-901.

Remstein ED, Dogan A, Einerson RR, et al. The incidence and anatomic site specificity of chromosomal translocations in primary extranodal marginal zone B-cell lymphoma of mucosa-associated lymphoid tissue (MALT lymphoma) in North America. *Am J Surg Pathol* 2006; 30: 1546-1553.

Renne C, Martın-Subero I, Hansmann M, et al. Molecular cytogenetic analyses of immunoglobulin loci in nodular lymphocyte predominant Hodgkin's lymphoma reveal a recurrent IGH-BCL6 juxtaposition. *J Mol Diagn* 2005; 7: 352-356.

Ross JS, Ginsburg GS. The integration of molecular diagnostics with therapeutics. *Am J Clin Pathol* 2003; 119: 26-36.

Schafer AI. Molecular basis of the diagnosis and treatment of polycythemia vera and essential thrombocythemia. *Blood* 2006; 107: 4214-4222.

Schlette E, Rassidakis GZ, Canoz O, et al. Expression of bcl-3 in chronic lymphocytic leukemia correlates with trisomy 12 and abnormalities of chromosome 19. *Am J Clin Pathol* 2005; 123: 465-471.

Sen F, Lai R, Albitar M. Chronic lymphocytic leukemia with t(14;18) and trisomy 12: report of 2 cases and review of the literature. *Arch Pathol Lab Med* 2002; 126: 1543-1546.

Shanafelt TD, Geyer SM, Kay NE. Prognosis at diagnosis: integrating molecular biologic insights into clinical practice for patients with CLL. *Blood* 2004; 103: 1202-1210.

References

Slack GW, Wizniak J, Dabbagh L, et al. Flow cytometric detection of ZAP-70 in chronic lymphocytic leukemia: correlation with immunocytochemistry and Western blot analysis. *Arch Pathol Lab Med* 2007; 131: 50-56.

Staudt LM. Molecular diagnosis of the hematologic cancers. *N Engl J Med* 2003; 348: 1777-1785.

Stilgenbauer S, Dohner H. Molecular genetics and its clinical relevance. *Hematol Oncol Clin North Am* 2004; 18: 827-848.

Still IH, Chernova O, Hurd D, et al. Molecular characterization of the t(8;13)(p11;q12) translocation associated with an atypical myeloproliferative disorder: evidence for three discrete loci involved in myeloid leukemias on 8p11. *Blood* 1997; 90: 3136-3141.

Tan AY, Westerman DA, Dobrovic A. A simple, rapid, and sensitive method for the detection of the JAK2 V617F mutation. *Am J Clin Pathol* 2007; 127: 977-981.

Tischkowitz M, Dokal I. Fanconi anemia and leukemia: clinical and molecular aspects. *Br J Haematol* 2004; 126: 176-191.

Valent P, Akin C, Sperr WR, et al. Mast cell proliferative disorders: current view on variants recognized by the World Health Organization. *Hematol Oncol Clin North Am* 2003; 17: 1227-1241.

Valla D, Casadevall N, Lacombe C, et al. Primary myeloproliferative disorder and hepatic vein thrombosis: a prospective study of erythroid colony formation in vitro in 20 patients with Budd-Chiari syndrome. *Ann Intern Med* 1985; 103: 329-334.

Verdonck K, González E, Van Dooren S, et al. Human T-lymphotropic virus 1: recent knowledge about an ancient infection. *Lancet Infect Dis* 2007; 7: 266-281.

Vyasa P, Crispino JD. Molecular insights into Down syndrome-associated leukemia. *Curr Opin Pediatr* 2007; 19: 9-14.

Xu Y, Dolan MM, Nguyen PL. Diagnostic significance of detecting dysgranulopoiesis in chronic myeloid leukemia. *Am J Clin Pathol* 2003; 120: 778-784.

Yin CC, Glassman AB, Lin P, et al. Morphologic, cytogenetic, and molecular abnormalities in therapy-related acute promyelocytic leukemia. *Am J Clin Pathol* 2005; 123: 840-848.

Zhao W, Claxton DF, Medeiros LJ, et al. Immunohistochemical ANALYSIS of CBFb-SMMHC protein reveals a unique nuclear localization in acute myeloid leukemia with inv(16)(p13q22). *Am J Surg Pathol* 2006; 30: 1436-1444.

Zhao X, Huang Q, Slovak M, Weiss L. Comparison of ancillary studies in the detection of residual disease in plasma cell myeloma in bone marrow. *Am J Clin Pathol* 2006; 125: 895-904.

Chapter 16

Pharmacogenetics and Pharmacogenomics

Introduction

Pharmacogenetics is a term that refers to the study of individual genes, especially ones that encode drug-metabolizing enzymes, as they related to drug effects. *Pharmacogenomics* refers to the study of multiple genetic factors as they simultaneously relate to drug effects. Essentially, pharmacogenetic is to pharmacogenomic as gene is to genome; nonetheless, the terms are often used loosely and interchangeably.

With regard to pharmacogenomics, it is useful to recall the concept of polymorphism. Polymorphisms are variations in genes (sequences other than the wild type) that exist stably in the population (present in >1% of the population) and have no adverse effects (ie, are not disease-causing). Single nucleotide polymorphisms (SNPs) are the most common type of polymorphism. In specific circumstances, however, a polymorphism may be pathologic (eg, many of the genetic variations considered in this chapter are polymorphisms that have no clinical effects unless the patient is exposed to a toxin or drug **T16.1**); alternatively, they may be beneficial in comparison with the wild type (eg, some red cell polmorphisms have no clinical effects but are protective against malaria). For example, it has long been recognized that certain individuals become ill on ingestion of fava beans. This phenomenon, favism, is an example of a genetic polymorphism that highlights another recurring feature in pharmacogenomics: the frequency of a particular polymorphism varies significantly from 1 population group to another.

Cytochrome P-450 Enzymes

A large group of enzymes (and genes) is associated with the cytochrome P-450 system, whose purpose is the oxidative metabolism of toxins (including medications). The cytochrome P-450 genes are expressed mainly in the liver. 1 gene, *CYP2D6* is also highly expressed in brain. Genetic anomalies in P-450 genes may lead to enhanced, reduced, or absent activity.

CYP2D6 (Cytochrome P-450 2D6, Debrisoquine Hydroxylase)

- Several *CYP2D6* polymorphisms result in reduced activity and a *poor- (slow-) metabolizer* phenotype. This phenotype is found in around 5% of Caucasians. Alternatively, other *CYP2D6* polymorphisms cause a *rapid-metabolizer* phenotype, and in some cases an *ultrarapid-metabolizer* phenotype (the latter often on the basis of gene duplication). Thus, the clinical effect

of a polymorphism on drug action can range from enhanced toxicity to reduced efficacy.

- The *CYP2D6* gene is located on chromosome 22q13.1. At this time, there are over 40 different known polymorphic CYP2D6 alleles. The most common allele in the Asian population, with a frequency of around 50%, is CYP2D6*10. The CYP2D6*10 allele encodes an enzyme with markedly diminished activity. In American Blacks, the most common polymorphism is CYP2D6*17, which encodes an enzyme with mildly reduced activity. The overall incidence of poor metabolizers in the American Caucasian population is about 10%, and the incidence of ultrarapid metabolizers among American Caucasians is about 2%. The ultrarapid metabolizers represent anywhere from 1% to 30% (the highest rate found among Ethiopians), depending on the population studied.

- It is estimated that the metabolism of around 25% of all commonly administered drugs is dependent on CYP2D6. Major drug classes affected include the antidepressants, neuroleptics (antipsychotics), antiarrhythmics, chemotherapeutic agents, and β-blockers. Patients receiving tamoxifen therapy may display variable responses based on CYP2D6 polymorphisms. The present data are in favor of CYP2D6 genotypes as a predictor of response to tamoxifen, but additional studies are necessary to recommend testing to all breast cancer patients contemplating tamoxifen. Patients with variant forms of the gene CYP2D6 may not receive the full benefits of tamoxifen.

CYP2C9 (Cytochrome P-450 2C9)

- CYP2C9 is responsible for the metabolism of warfarin (coumadin) and phenytoin (dilantin). There are several polymorphisms, most of which result in decreased warfarin metabolism.

- Warfarin acts through the inhibition of VKORC1 (vitamin K epoxide reductase). VKORC1 is involved in maintaining high levels of vitamin K, which is necessary for γ–carboxylation of vitamin K–dependent coagulation factors.

- Several *CYP2C9* polymorphisms have been associated with reduced CYP2C9 activity. 2 of these are fairly common, CYP2C9*2 (R144C mutation) and CYP2C9*3 (I359L mutation), each present in around 10% of the Caucasian population. Their incidence is considerably lower in African American, Latin American, and Asian groups.

T16.1
Selected Pharmacologically Significant Genetic Polymorphisms

Gene	Drug	Comment
Catechol-O-methyltransferase (COMT)	Levodopa	Polymorphism with decreased function present in 25% of population, leading to enhanced drug toxicity
CYP2D6 (cytochrome P-450 2D6)	Codeine Nortryptyline Sparteine	Polymorphism with decreased function leads to enhanced drug effect
CYP2C9 (cytochrome P-450 2C9)	Warfarin (coumadin) Phenytoin (dilantin)	Polymorphism with decreased function leads to enhanced drug effect
CYP2C19 (cytochrome P-450 2C19)	Omeprazole	Polymorphism with decreased function leads to enhanced drug toxicity. Present in 20% of Japanese and 15% of Chinese.
Dihydropyrimidine dehydrogenase (DPD)	Pyrimidines (5-FU)	Polymorphism with decreased function leads to enhanced drug effect
N-acetyltransferase (NAT)	Isoniazid Hydralazine Procainamide	Polymorphism causing decreased enzyme function present in nearly half of Caucasians, leading to enhanced drug toxicity
Thiopurine methyltransferase (TPMT)	6-mercaptopurine 6-thioguanine	Polymorphism causing decreased enzyme function present in <1% of Caucasians and leads to enhanced drug toxicity
Angiotensin converting enzyme (ACE)	ACE inhibitors	
Glycoprotein IIIa	Aspirin GBIIb/IIIa inhibitors	
Antitrypsin	Heparin	Inability to achieve therapeutic heparinization
UGT1A1	Irinotecan	Polymorphism causes inefficient metabolism and buildup of toxic byproduct (SN38) resulting in severe neutropenia and diarrhea.
ERCC	Cisplatinum	Polymorphism causes increased expression of the ERCC1 enzyme, which recognizes the tumor cells affected by platinum-based chemotherapy. ERCC1 expression impairs the DNA repair mechanism and allows the tumor cells to proliferate unaffected.

- Warfarin response is also modulated by the *VKORC1* gene polymorphisms. There are several variant alleles, referred to as H1, H2, etc. H1 and H2 haplotypes have been associated with enhanced sensitivity to warfarin (thus requiring lower doses). H7, H8, and H9 have been associated with relative warfarin resistance (thus requiring higher doses).

CYP2C19 (Cytochrome P-450 2C19)

- CYP2C19 is responsible for metabolism of omeprazole, as well as several other agents, including diazepam and phenytoin (dilantin).

- Several polymorphisms have been identified— CYP2C19*2 through CYP2C19*8—that are associated with slow metabolism of these agents. This may result in enhanced activity of omeprazole but enhanced toxicity of phenytoin. This example illustrates 1 of the features of pharmacogenetic polymorphism; that is, the effect has to do with the width of the therapeutic window. In agents with a narrow window (phenytoin), the effect may be profound toxicity with normal doses, whereas in agents with wide windows (omeprazole), the effect may be merely enhanced activity with lower doses.

Other Drug-Metabolizing Enzymes

N-Acetyltransferase (NAT)

- NAT types 1 and 2 catalyze the transfer of an acetyl group from acetyl CoA to several nitrogen-containing agents. Polymorphisms in the *NAT* gene may result in enhanced or reduced activity.

- 1 of the major drugs metabolized in this way is isoniazid, used in tuberculosis treatment (recall that the NAT enzyme is present in some antimicrobial resistant strains of *Mycobacterium tuberculosis*).

16: Pharmacogenetics and Pharmacogenomics

Other Drug-Metabolizing Enzymes>Thiopurine Methyltransferase; 5,10-methylenetetrahydrofolate Reductase; Uridine Diphosphoglucuronisyl Transferase 1A1; Excision Repair Cross Complementation, Group 1

Thiopurine Methyltransferase (TPMT)

- The efficacy of thiopurine drugs (6-mercaptopurine, azathioprine, and 6-thioguanine) depends on metabolic activation, a process dependent on the enzyme hypoxanthine guanine phosphoribosyl transferase (HGPRT). Thiopurine inactivation is mediated by TPMT and xanthine oxidase (XO), administered as anti-cancer chemotherapy.

- Polymorphisms have been identified in the *TPMT* gene that result in increased activity (reduced therapeutic effect) or decreased activity (increased toxicity). Reduced activity alleles—TPMT*2, TPMT*3A, and TPMT*3C—have been identified in about 5% of the population.

5,10-methylenetetrahydrofolate Reductase (MTHFR)

- Methotrexate is an inhibitor of dihydrofolate reductase and other folate-related enzymes, including MTHFR.

- The substitution C677T is a very common *MTHFR* gene polymorphism, present in about 30% of Caucasians, and is associated with reduced MTHFR activity.

- An increased incidence of toxicity is seen in those with reduced MTHFR activity as a result of the C677T polymorphism.

Uridine Diphosphoglucuronisyl Transferase 1A1 (UGT1A1)

- Irinotecan (Camptosar, Pfizer) is a treatment option for colorectal cancer. It is derived from a class of therapeutic agents, camptothecins, that interact specifically with the enzyme topoisomerase I.

- It is known that at least 10% of the North American population has a genetic polymorphism which causes reduced production of the enzyme uridine diphospho-glucuronisyl transferase 1A1 (UGT1A1). This enzyme is essential for the metabolism and excretion of the active metabolite of irinotecan, SN-38.

- Inefficient metabolism of the drug leads to serious and potentially life-threatening side-effects in patients who are already in a compromised state of health.

Excision Repair Cross Complementation, Group 1 (ERCC1)

- ERCC1 is a protein involved in the DNA repair mechanism. It plays a major role in the resistance of some tumors to platinum-based chemotherapy.

- As many as 44% of patients with non–small cell lung cancer (NSCLC) express ERCC1. Increased expression of the ERCC1 enzyme, which recognizes the tumor cells affected by platinum-based chemotherapy, impairs the DNA repair mechanism and allows the tumor cells to proliferate unaffected.

- Platinum-based chemotherapy is currently considered 1 of the treatment options for patients with locally advanced NSCLC. Individuals who have an ERCC1 polymorphism or gene alteration may not respond favorably to platinum-based chemotherapy. Because platinum-based chemotherapy is associated with serious side effects and only provides a modest improvement in overall survival, identification of these polymorphisms could be used as predictive factors for tumor response to platinum-based chemotherapy.

References

References

Abraham BK, Adithan C. Genetic polymorphism of CYP2D6. *Indian J Pharmacol* 2001; 33: 147-169.

Adcock DM, Koftan C, Crisan D, et al. Effect of polymorphisms in the cytochrome P450 CYP2C9 gene on warfarin anticoagulation. *Arch Pathol Lab Med* 2004; 128: 1360-1363.

Chou W, Yan F, Robbins-Weilert DK, et al. Comparison of two CYP2D6 genotyping methods and assessment of genotype-phenotype relationships. *Clin Chem* 2003; 49: 542-551.

David SP. Pharmacogenetics. *Prim Care Clin Office Pract* 2004; 31: 543-559.

Evans WE, McLeod HL. Pharmacogenomics: drug disposition, drug targets, and side effects. *N Engl J Med* 2003; 348: 538-549.

Gage BF. Pharmacogenetics-based coumarin therapy. *Hematology Am Soc Hematol Educ Program* 2006: 467-473.

Gasche Y, Daali Y, Fathi M, et al. Codeine intoxication associated with ultrarapid CYP2D6 metabolism. *N Engl J Med* 2004; 351: 2827-2831.

Gonzalez FJ, Fernandez-Salguero P. Diagnostic analysis, clinical importance and molecular basis of dihydropyrimidine dehydrogenase deficiency. *Trends Pharmacol Sci* 1995; 16: 325-327.

Hawkins GA, Weiss ST, Bleecker ER. Asthma Pharmacogenomics. *Immunol Allergy Clin North Am* 2005; 25: 723-742.

Hines RN, McCarver G. Pharmacogenomics and the future of drug therapy. *Pediatr Clin North Am* 2006; 53: 591-619.

Ingelman-Sundberg M. Genetic polymorphisms of cytchrome P450 2D6 (CYP2D6): clinical consquences, evolutionary aspects and functional diversity. *Pharmacogenomics J* 2005; 5: 6-13.

Ito RK, Demers LM. Pharmacogenomics and pharmacogenetics: future role of molecular diagnostics in the clinical diagnostic laboratory. *Clin Chem* 2004; 50: 1526-1527.

McMurrough J, McLeod HL. Analysis of the dihydropyrimidine dehydrogenase polymorphism in a British population. *Br J Clin Pharmacol* 1996; 41: 425-427.

Marsh S, McLeod HL. Pharmacogenomics: from bedside to clinical practice. *Hum Mol Genet* 2006; 15(review issue No. 1): R89-R93.

Olaussen KA, Dunant A, Fouret P, et al. DNA Repair by ERCC1 in Non–small-cell lung cancer and cisplatin-based adjuvant chemotherapy. *N Engl J Med* 2006; 355: 983-991.

Rieder MJ, Reiner AP, Gage BF, et al. Effect of VKORC1 haplotypes on transcriptional regulation and warfarin dose. *N Engl J Med* 2005; 352: 2285-2293.

Sconce EA, Khan TI, Wynne HA, et al. The impact of CYP2C9 and VKORC1 genetic polymorphism and patient characteristics upon warfarin dose requirements: proposal for a new dosing regimen. *Blood* 2005; 106: 2329-2333.

Shikata E, Ieiri I, Ishiguro S, et al. Association of pharmacokinetic (CYP2C9) and pharmacodynamic (factors II, VII, IX, and X; proteins S and C; and γ-glutamyl carboxylase) gene variants with warfarin sensitivity. *Blood* 2004; 103: 2630-2635.

Siddiqui A, Kerb R, Weale ME, et al. Association of multi-drug resistance in epilepsy with a polymorphism in the drug-transporter gene ABCB1. *N Engl J Med* 2003; 348: 1442-1448.

Ulrich CM, Yasui Y, Storb R, et al. Pharmacogenetics of methotrexate: toxicity among marrow transplantation patients varies with the methylenetetrahydrofolate reductase C677T polymorphism. *Blood* 2001; 98: 231-234.

Van Kuilenburg AB, Vreken P, Beex LV, et al. Severe 5-fluorouracil toxicity caused by reduced dihydropyrimidine dehydrogenase activity due to heterozygosity for a G→A point mutation. *J Inherit Metab Dis* 1998; 21: 280-284.

Weinshilboum R. Genomic medicine: inheritance and Drug Response. *N Engl J Med* 2003; 348: 529-537.

Yuan HY, Chen JJ, Lee MT, et al. A novel functional VKORC1 promoter polymorphism is associated with inter-individual and inter-ethnic differences in warfarin sensitivity. *Hum Mol Genet* 2005; 14: 1745-1751.

Index